Calming Your Anxious Child

Calming Your Anxious Child

Words to Say and Things to Do

Kathleen Trainor, PsyD

JOHNS HOPKINS UNIVERSITY PRESS | Baltimore

Note to the reader: This book is not meant to substitute for medical care of children with anxiety, and treatment should not be based solely on its contents. Instead, treatment must be developed in a dialogue between the individual and his or her physician. This book has been written to help with that dialogue.

Drug dosage: The author and publisher have made reasonable efforts to determine that the selection of drugs discussed in this text conform to the practices of the general medical community. The medications described do not necessarily have specific approval by the U.S. Food and Drug Administration for use in the diseases for which they are recommended. In view of ongoing research, changes in governmental regulation, and the constant flow of information relating to drug therapy and drug reactions, the reader is urged to check the package insert of each drug for any change in indications and dosage and for warnings and precautions. This is particularly important when the recommended agent is a new and/or infrequently used drug.

© 2016 Kathleen Trainor
All rights reserved. Published 2016
Printed in the United States of America on acid-free paper
9 8 7 6 5 4 3 2 1

Johns Hopkins University Press
2715 North Charles Street
Baltimore, Maryland 21218-4363
www.press.jhu.edu

Library of Congress Cataloging-in-Publication Data

Trainor, Kathleen, 1955– author.
  Calming your anxious child : words to say and things to do / Kathleen Trainor.
Description: Baltimore : Johns Hopkins University Press, 2016. | Includes
  bibliographical references and index.
Identifiers: LCCN 2015034014| ISBN 9781421420097 (hardcover : alk. paper) |
  ISBN 9781421420103 (pbk. : alk. paper) | ISBN 9781421420110 (electronic) |
  ISBN 1421420090 (hardcover : alk. paper) | ISBN 1421420104 (pbk. : alk.
  paper) | ISBN 1421420112 (electronic)
Subjects: LCSH: Anxiety in children--Popular works. | Anxiety
  disorders--Treatment--Popular works. | Parent and child--Popular works.
Classification: LCC RJ506.A58 T73 2016 | DDC 618.92/8522--dc23 LC record available at
http://lccn.loc.gov/2015034014

Special discounts are available for bulk purchases of this book. For more information,
please contact Special Sales at 410-516-6936 or specialsales@press.jhu.edu.

Johns Hopkins University Press uses environmentally friendly book materials, including recycled text paper that is composed of at least 30 percent post-consumer waste, whenever possible.

To all my patients, past and present,
who have been my greatest teachers.

To my children, Dagan, Brian,
and Kara, and my daughters-in-
law, Lori and Liza, and my beautiful
grandchildren, Dallan, Nevan,
and Braden.

My family has provided my inspiration
through their endless love and support.

Contents

Calming Your Anxious Child

Anxious about Anxiety

Responding to a Call for Help

Anxiety among children and adolescents is now considered an epidemic, and its prevalence continues to increase dramatically. After thirty-plus years of treating thousands of patients as a social worker and a child psychologist, I am amazed by the current pervasiveness of anxiety-related disorders such as obsessive compulsive disorder, separation anxiety, post-traumatic stress disorder, phobias, and selective mutism.

Why are anxiety disorders so prevalent?

There's no definitive answer, but I believe it's a combination of nature and nurture influences. Looking at environmental factors, our society has changed dramatically, becoming much faster paced and more complex. And family life is now more hectic and challenging than ever. As a key dynamic today, technology has had positive effects in reducing stress in some ways, but it has raised it in many other ways.

Our world is an increasingly anxious place. We have experienced 9/11, subsequent terrorist attacks, a financial crash, unthinkable school violence, devastating natural disasters, accelerated drug abuse, school bullying, more academically high-pressured kids, dramatic racial divides, and much more general tribulation. In short, familial, social, technological, economic, natural, and political forces have all stressed us out to the max—but these have also informed us about how to raise our kids and manage stress.

Certainly, we have advanced in diagnosing and treating anxiety, although most anxious kids receive no—or inadequate—treatment. Many families have been frustrated because various forms of therapy, however well meaning, and medication have not worked.

Family functioning is deeply affected when a child experiences anxiety. Parents are usually not prepared to help their anxious child, and dealing with an anxious child can be confusing. Parents may feel desperate as they search for effective guidance and support.

An Answer

The good news is that cognitive behavioral therapy (CBT) is an extremely useful approach for identifying and managing anxious thoughts and feelings. Through a family approach based on CBT (explored in depth in the book's first chapter), parents and their children can learn strategies together, creating teamwork and strengthening family bonds.

This book describes a proven approach—cognitive behavioral therapy— to help anxious kids while actively engaging parents in the process. Other books effectively address some important issues, but none presents a behaviorally grounded how-to strategy to confront these problems. Accordingly, with so many families crying out for help, I felt compelled to construct the CBT-based 7-Step TRAINOR Method as a simple and pragmatic way to find solutions.

This book puts the TRAINOR Method to work. It is written primarily for parents, to help them learn more about anxiety disorders and symptoms of child anxiety. It also gives a voice to these anxious children, who are often misunderstood. Families and mental health and related professionals all will find this approach beneficial.

The children and teenagers I have treated differ in many respects, but children with anxiety can all benefit from many common strategies and lessons learned from the step-by-step TRAINOR approach. These strategies are mapped out in the book through case studies based on my interactions with real patients and parents, though in some instances I provide a composite view of the sessions in an attempt to be more comprehensive and informative for readers. In most chapters I outline my meetings with parents and then with the kids; sometimes I see them separately and sometimes as a group, starting with a younger child's experience and continuing with an adolescent's case study. I describe the initial challenges, the strategy, and the results.

At the end of chapters 3–8 the reader will find the *DSM-5* criteria that are used in diagnosing a child with the anxiety disorder described in that chapter. The *Diagnostic and Statistical Manual of Mental Disorders* (DSM) is the standard catalog of mental disorders that mental health professionals in the United States refer to in making diagnoses; it includes a list of diagnostic criteria for every psychiatric disorder recognized by the U.S. healthcare system. (The *DSM-5*, which is the fifth edition of the manual, was published by the American Psychiatric Association in 2015.) Many anxious children do not meet the full criteria of a formal diagnosis but can benefit from the strategies outlined in this book. The *DSM* criteria are included for readers' information only. There is no expectation or even wish for parents to learn to diagnose or to practice diagnosing; diagnoses must be done by professional mental health providers who have expert training in diagnosis and treatment.

I focus on the most common anxiety problems and provide a fair amount of detail, since understanding the nuances is critical to success. I also provide information on additional resources, with the understanding that this therapy isn't a quick fix; although we expect positive results, the process of overcoming anxiety requires a commitment to work together as a team.

Those who share their experiences in this book represent the voices of my greatest teachers—the many children and parents I've worked with through the years. Each parent and child described in this book illuminates the experiences of wonderful children and loving families dealing with anxiety. The parents all have one thing in common: anxious children and a desire to help them.

I hope this book offers parents and professionals an understanding of anxiety in children and how to help anxious children overcome their problems.

Chapter 1

Fighting Anxiety

Applying CBT with a Step-by-Step Approach

As a therapist, I see many parents of anxious children who feel exhausted and isolated because their child seems happy in so many ways yet causes unbelievable chaos, confusion, and frustration at home—stressful reactions mostly hidden from the outside world. How can we best understand what it means when a child is anxious? Is there anything particular a parent can do when raising a child who has anxiety problems?

This chapter begins to explore these questions, providing an overview about anxiety and how children and parents can work together to treat it. I also discuss what to consider in using medication as part of the treatment. Finally, I address cognitive behavioral therapy (CBT) and introduce the 7-Step TRAINOR Method as a framework for successful outcomes. (The specifics of this step-by-step approach are illustrated in greater detail in chapter 2.)

I begin with a discussion of the biological bases of anxiety. Although understanding the scientific explanations of anxiety is not required in order to benefit from treatment, children and families are encouraged to be active partners on their therapy team, and healthcare providers should at least review this information with families.

Anxiety Overview and Biological Underpinnings

Anxiety is the most common psychiatric disorder among children and adolescents, with statistics suggesting epidemic levels: an estimated 12.3 percent of children have met the criteria for an anxiety disorder by the time they're in middle childhood, and up to 30 percent of all children and adolescents have been diagnosed with an anxiety disorder at some point.[1] Those numbers are astounding, considering that many anxious children may not meet the full criteria for a "disorder" but are still negatively affected by their irrational fears.

Anxiety doesn't go away with time; kids don't "outgrow" it. If anything, it tends to worsen over time. Anxiety can be normal at certain developmental stages, but when it persists, it can become problematic. Left untreated, it's likely to affect emotional, social, academic, and occupational functioning. Most people underestimate the impact of anxiety, not only in childhood but throughout life. Childhood anxiety has been shown to precede adult anxiety, alcohol and drug addiction, and poor physical health in young adulthood. For example, research shows that 35 to 45 percent of people struggling with alcohol and drug addictions also have an anxiety disorder. They may be "self-medicating" their anxiety with substance abuse.[2]

Anxiety is caused by biological vulnerabilities, chronic stress, traumatic life events, or some combination of these. And it runs in families. Anxious parents have a greater chance of having anxious children.[3] The nature versus nurture debate is ongoing, but the source of anxiety seems most often to be a combination of both. The cause of childhood anxiety is a complicated interplay of genetics, brain function, environmental stressors, and parenting styles.[4] The biological underpinnings of anxiety; the cognitive aspects, or the distorted thinking that comes with anxiety; and the dysfunctional reaction parents may have to their child's anxiety; all are important to understand.

Later in this chapter, I review the critical role that parents play in the development and treatment of anxiety as well as in its prevention. But overall, what is most important is that when parents learn how to raise a child who is anxious, they can make a huge difference in reducing the child's anxiety symptoms and in fostering healthy growth and development.[5]

Several parts of the brain constitute the "fear circuitry," which controls emotional regulation and the processing of fear. These include the amygdala, the ventromedial prefrontal cortex, and the anterior cingulate cortex, which I describe below. It's believed that anxious children may have structural as well as functional differences in these areas of the brain. Parents often feel their anxious child is simply "wired differently." Recent research on the anxious brain is proving parents to be right in some respects.[6]

The *amygdala* is almond shaped and located deep within the temporal lobe of the brain. The temporal lobe is involved in processing sensory input into meanings for the retention of visual memories, language comprehension, and emotion association. The amygdala is the part of the brain that controls the fear response. It processes and consolidates memories associated with emotional events. The amygdala imprints in the brain the reaction of synapses that elicit fear (synapses transmit and receive impulses from nerves). The amygdala can trigger release of stress hormones, which create the physical response of anxiety, including rapid heartbeat, sweating, stomach discomfort, shaking, and other panic symptoms. Increased activation in the amygdala along with possible structural differences have been identified in anxious children relative to children who don't suffer from anxiety.

When a child has an anxious reaction to an experience, the amygdala retains that memory of fear. This intense memory causes the child's extreme response to be maintained. Activation of the amygdala influences the strength of anxious, emotional memories and promotes fear conditioning.[7] This can explain what parents observe in their anxious child's automatic, intense, and irrational reaction when anxious. Parents will often say, "When she gets anxious, she can go from 0 to 100 in seconds." They are witnessing their child's automatic, poorly modulated fear response.

The *ventrolateral prefrontal cortex* modulates the activity of the amygdala and has also been shown to have increased activation in anxious children. This part of the brain attempts to provide emotional regulation and to process fear. It processes past emotional associations with events. When this function isn't working effectively, emotions may become confused, and the experience of fear can feel overwhelming. This explains why a child who becomes flooded with anxiety acts in a way that appears to her parents to be irrational and agitated.

The *anterior cingulate cortex* (ACC) processes cognitive and emotional information and the functional integration of both. It regulates blood pressure and heart rate and influences rational cognitive functions and modulation of emotional response to stimuli. MRIs (magnetic resonance images) have shown increased activation in this part of the brain too in

anxious children.[8] When these three parts of the brain are not func
well together, anxiety takes over. Parents often recognize their anxious child
as having a "panic attack," with a rapid heartbeat and obvious physical
symptoms of intense fear.

As we learn more about brain development, it appears that the brains
of children with anxiety function differently from the brains of children
without anxiety. Children with anxiety more easily become activated by
fear, and their thinking quickly becomes irrational. They have trouble controlling their anxious feelings, and their bodies seem to experience stronger
reactions to fear. This is all because of how their brains are "wired."[9]

It's important to consider this brain connection and remember that
anxious children don't choose to be afraid; rather, they are likely experiencing intense anxiety because their brains are overactive in the areas
that process fear. This brain processing likely has a genetic component,
which is why some kids and parents are more anxious than others.

Overall, the brain is a powerful controlling organ that we know too
little about, but we're learning more and more. We do know that, due to
the brain's "wiring," anxious children have a distortion in their ability
to perceive their surroundings and to process information. They tend to
react to ambiguous stimuli as negative and interpret benign information
as a threat. They see danger when there is no danger. They tend to be
hypervigilant and automatically imagine that if something bad has even a
remote chance of happening, it will happen. When anxious, their thinking
becomes impulsive and distorted, causing them to feel fear when there is
nothing to be afraid of. Their strong emotional reactions limit their ability
to access and apply coping strategies.

When flooded with anxiety, anxious children feel the fear in their bodies
because their overactive brains release stress hormones. This reaction is
confusing for the children and causes more fear and distorted thinking,
which in turn causes anxiety to spiral. This is also known as the "worry
loop." It's real, and kids can get stuck in it, escalating their arousal and
fear, quickly leading to a panic response, with rapid breathing, dizziness,
stomach pain, nausea, shakiness, and often yelling and tears.

Different kids may respond differently when anxious. Some kids shut
down and appear very frightened. They "implode" and may look frozen,

with a "deer in the headlight" look. Other kids become emotionally dys-regulated when they're anxious, and they "explode." That's another way of saying they have angry tantrums. There's evidence that the neural mecha-nisms of emotional regulation are different in anxious kids. This can easily fool parents and others who expect a frightened child to be withdrawn and helpless looking, not kicking and screaming.

Understanding these tantrums as a child's version of a panic attack can change the response to them. Rather than responding with anger, it's more effective to try to help calm the child. When a child's brain is overactive in this manner, attempts to be rational or to discipline only escalate the anxiety.

Medication: When Is It Appropriate?

Medications are being prescribed for anxious children and adolescents now more than ever.[10] This is big business, with psychiatric medications bringing in billions of dollars for pharmaceutical companies. We are all influenced by this business, because pharmaceutical ads are everywhere. Unfortunately, too many kids are prescribed medication as a first line of treatment, without any therapy involved. In addition to the pharmaceutical companies, insurance companies also benefit from this practice because it's cheaper to medicate a child than it is to cover the cost of therapy. Parents are often reluctant to medicate their children, but when a medication is recommended by a professional, it can be hard to resist.

Research is incomplete on the long-term effect of these medications on children's developing minds and bodies. We do know, however, that children who take medications often experience side effects. And, perhaps most important, children treated with medication for anxiety may not be learning the strategies and skills that will help them manage their anxious feelings. The message is: a pill will take care of it.

Anxiety can be mild, moderate, or severe. In some cases of severe anxiety, medication can help a child function and access therapy. When a child is flooded with severe anxiety, learning and applying strategies can feel impossible. With medication, the anxiety can be reduced to facilitate learning.

So the caveat with medication is to proceed with caution and use medication as part of the treatment plan only when necessary and always in addition to therapy.

Cognitive Behavioral Therapy and the TRAINOR Method

Cognitive behavioral therapy (CBT) is an evidence-based treatment for child anxiety.[11] *Evidence based* means there's strong research proving its effectiveness in helping children significantly reduce their anxiety symptoms. In short, it's treatment that's been proved to work, even with very young children.[12] In addition, it has demonstrated long-term effectiveness, with the positive treatment effects maintained many years after the CBT treatment.[13] The cognitive part of the therapy involves changing the way a child thinks about irrational fears; the behavioral part engages the child in changing avoidant behavior.

The TRAINOR Method illustrated in this book applies CBT in a family-based approach that is individualized and engages both child and parents in the change process. Involving parents—not just through brief parent training, but through active engagement in working with their child—has been shown to be an effective treatment approach for anxious children. In addition to reducing children's anxiety, a CBT approach that involves parents improves family functioning.[14]

The TRAINOR Method simplifies and structures CBT in a manner that parents can use to help their anxious child. This therapy doesn't happen only in the therapist's office; it happens every day, with parents and teachers helping the anxious child apply and practice strategies and achieve goals to reduce anxiety. Applying CBT strategies has been shown to actually change the brain. We are learning more and more about brain *plasticity,* meaning the brain changes for the better with environmental influences such as CBT, and for the worse with exposure to trauma or chronic stress. Many clinical studies have shown that CBT changes the wiring of the brain. It changes dysfunctions in the nervous system. Through the technologies of positron emission tomography (PET) and functional magnetic resonance imaging (fMRI), by which we take pre- and post-CBT-treatment brain scans, dramatic brain changes have been proved to happen as a result of CBT. Feelings and behaviors involve specific brain circuits, and changes in thinking and behavior are associated with cerebral alterations.[15] This is exciting research that integrates neurobiology, psychopathology, neuropsychology, and psychotherapy.

Families are deeply affected by an anxious child and often seek treatment, desperate for guidance, because family functioning seems to have been turned upside down by the anxious child's symptoms. Working together, parents and children can learn strategies that increase understanding and promote change.

Parenting an Anxious Child: A Closer Look

Effective methods for parenting an anxious child may seem counterintuitive. The natural parenting response to a child who's exploding with anxiety is to want to take control and set limits. An anxious child is a child who needs to learn how to calm down and gain greater control of his thoughts and emotions. This is something the child has to learn through CBT, and parents can't do it for him. Reacting with anger only increases the child's arousal and explosive behavior. Attempting to talk to a child in this anxious state is also ineffective because the aroused brain interferes with the child's ability to be rational. When in fear mode, the anxious child's ability to solve problems and use coping strategies becomes impossible.

To avoid these explosive outbursts, parents often find themselves giving in or accommodating the anxiety. Parents "walk on eggshells," wanting to avoid major disruptions that can affect the whole family. This doesn't feel right for parents but often is necessary. When this happens, parents may feel angry and frustrated with their child and lose confidence in their ability to parent. In this situation, both parents and child are held hostage by anxiety.

When the child is imploding, rather than exploding, with anxiety, the child provokes a different response from parents. This child looks shut down, frozen, pale, and often sick. The instinctual response is to protect your child from pain. Yet this parenting style promotes avoidance behavior and accommodates the anxiety. Parental accommodation has been shown to cause more severe anxiety symptoms and longer term negative consequences for the child.[16]

When not confronted with anxiety-producing challenges, anxious children look very relaxed. This is what makes accommodation so tempting. For example, letting a scared child sleep with parents is disruptive but easier. The child goes to sleep peacefully, and everyone sleeps well. Not letting the child in the bed feels far more disruptive, with the child screaming in fear in the middle of the night, waking everyone up. Though everyone knows having a big kid in the parental bed isn't helpful in the long run because the child's fears aren't confronted, the drive to avoid the fear reactions and keep the peace so that everyone sleeps is very understandable. But again, the short-term gains usually lead to longer term, more severe problems with anxiety.[17]

Anxious parents are often described as overprotective in the literature, and this is interpreted as a causal factor in the development of a child's anxiety. An anxious parent, like an anxious child, has the tendency to see danger when there is none and to imagine all kinds of catastrophes happening. Helping an anxious child to change means that anxious parents have to change as well. Parents may be transmitting verbal and behavioral messages to their child that promote anxiety. This is the "nurture" aspect of the development of childhood anxiety. This parenting style, added to genetic tendencies passed down from parent to child, creates a combination that almost guarantees the development of severe childhood anxiety.[18]

Overprotective parenting and accommodating anxiety may not be a cause of anxiety so much as a reaction when parenting an anxious child. When how the child is wired is the primary cause of anxiety, accommodating feels like an automatic reaction. This is made most clear when parents of multiple children notice how differently they parent when challenged by their child who is anxious than they do when challenged by their child who is easygoing. Without an understanding of the biological underpinnings of anxiety, it's easy to blame parents. All children are not born equal when it comes to the genetic predisposition for anxiety. Terrific parents who are praised for their "calm child" are the same parents who can be harshly judged by others when their anxious child is acting out. Parents are often blamed, and feel blamed, when others witness their anxious child at her worst.

Fortunately, as noted before, CBT has been shown to be very effective in treating children with anxiety disorders. It focuses on changing the cognitive distortions of anxiety and the behavioral reactions children have to anxious feelings. Research consistently demonstrates that parents play critical roles in the development and transmission of anxiety in their children. Whether we lean toward nature or nurture, parents need to be very involved in treatment. They need to learn how to recognize when anxiety is playing a role in their child's thinking and behavior, and they need to learn to recognize their dysfunctional parental responses.

How Cognitive Behavioral Training and the TRAINOR Method Work

The TRAINOR Method helps parents feel more comfortable changing their parenting approach to promote exposure, instead of protection and avoidance. Parents are very engaged in the TRAINOR Method because they are the most important change agents for their anxious child. Anxiety for children is a daily, minute-to-minute, hour-to-hour experience. Parents live with their children and are in the unique position to promote their child's work toward making cognitive and behavioral changes every day. Anxious children need to apply specific CBT strategies daily to make a difference. It's this practice that changes the brain. For an anxious child, talking or playing with a therapist once a week is well meaning but not enough.

Anxiety is brain and behavior driven, and to change a child's thinking and behavior demands a more intensive approach. For children, this means parents must be actively involved with an approach that is reinforced and involves accountability. The TRAINOR Method guides parents and children to work together in this process of learning how to manage anxiety.

Involving parents also educates them about anxiety and the most effective parenting approaches for their child. Parents of anxious children are desperate to learn strategies that work. Even the smartest, most relaxed parents, when confronted with a very anxious child, often feel totally incompetent. Everything they think should work often doesn't. These parents are eager to learn how to help their anxious child calm down.

As noted before, CBT works by changing the way a child thinks (the cognitive part) and by changing how a child behaves in response to anxious feelings (the behavioral part). The two parts go hand in hand. If children think they're in danger, the smart thing is to avoid it. If a car is coming, and a child is in the middle of the street, he better get out of the way. When there's an anxiety disorder, kids feel like they're in danger when they're not. They want to run and avoid these feelings. But pushing through the experience, absorbing the anxious feelings, and experiencing that nothing bad happens help challenge these anxious thoughts. And changing anxious thinking and behaviors will change the brain and reduce the anxiety.

Denial and avoidance, which I address further in the next chapter, are the major defenses against anxiety. Kids have to learn to stop avoiding and to take on challenges step by step, knowing that with experience and practice, the anxious feelings will go away and will be replaced with positive feelings of mastery. This is the behavioral part of the therapy, and in many ways, the behavioral part of CBT is the most important. If a child understands there's nothing to be afraid of but continues to avoid anyway, change won't happen. Changing behavior reinforces that there's nothing to fear.

It's like the kid who can swim, standing at the edge of the diving board, afraid to jump. Understanding there's nothing to be afraid of, and talking about it over and over again, is fine but not enough. Taking that jump into the water and coming up, experiencing pride in overcoming fear, is what makes the difference. That behavioral change also makes a difference in the child's brain. Experiences change the brain, far more than thinking or talking about change does. Doing it, experiencing the challenge to anxiety, is far more powerful than talking about it. The CBT-based TRAINOR Method is effective because of the concrete behavioral goals that are agreed on and practiced by the child, with the support of her parents.

The anxious child has to do the work to get better, and parents have to learn how to set behavioral goals for their anxious children that are challenging but not overwhelming. Again, parents have to learn not to accommodate anxiety, even though accommodating feels like the best and sometimes only course of action. A child who never challenges her anxious feelings will continue to be afraid, and that fear will increase. As parents of anxious children, the message can't be "If it makes you uncomfortable, you don't have to do it." With the TRAINOR Method, the message is "If it makes you uncomfortable, we will break it down into steps, because there's nothing to be afraid of; you can do it, and it's very important that you do it."

The TRAINOR Method depends on parents acting as coaches with the "You can do it" attitude and the expectation that their child will push through the anxious feelings to function at a higher level.[19] Establishing cognitive and behavioral goals begins the change process. The TRAINOR Method stresses the importance of reasonable goals that are not forced on children but that both parents and child agree on. This promotes a collaborative approach to overcoming anxiety. Parents providing positive daily reinforcement strengthens the effectiveness of CBT treatment for the child.

To be sure, anxious children are scared children who feel a strong need to be in control, which makes them seem stubborn. Getting them to agree on goals that push them out of their comfort zone involves the use of incentives and rewards. They are being asked to do things that will initially make them feel anxious. This will feel uncomfortable. They are also being asked to gain self-control and not become so dysregulated. Learning how to calm down can be very hard work. Without incentives, this is a hard sell, and parents can't do this work for their child. Incentives motivate, and as the child begins to feel successful and less anxious, success builds on success, and the incentives often become less important for motivation.

The 7-Step TRAINOR Method recognizes that anxiety is not a child's problem alone; it affects the whole family. It's not a cookie cutter approach because every child and family is different, and anxiety comes in many forms and may be mild, moderate, or severe. Accordingly, this approach is individually tailored for each child and family. It engages parents in the treatment process with great respect for the role of parents in helping their child. Parents, as leaders of the family, become leaders in helping their anxious child become free of fear. This empowers parents to empower their children to live more full and productive lives, not burdened by the destructive, lifelong effects of untreated anxiety.

I invite you to learn more!

Chapter 2

Stepping Up to the Challenge
How the 7-Step TRAINOR Method Works

The 7-Step TRAINOR Method will guide you toward finding your way out of the grips of anxiety and regaining some peace of mind for your entire family.

TRAINOR is an acronym that aids you in remembering each of the seven steps:

Target
Rate
Agree
Identify
Note
Offer
Reinforce

In the first chapter, I provided general notes about cognitive behavioral therapy and how it is connected to the TRAINOR Method. In this chapter, I examine each of the seven steps and illustrate how they are applied to help anxious kids.

Denial

The TRAINOR Method starts by confronting the number-one defense against anxiety: denial. Both children and parents experience denial—an unconscious defense mechanism that often limits acknowledging the painful realities, thoughts, or feelings of dealing with anxiety or raising an anxious child. Parents adapt, or give in, to not rock the boat. As one parent described it: "We walk on eggshells, doing things—some that seem crazy—because we don't want to set her off. If we don't give in to her, she has a meltdown lasting an hour or more. We do these bizarre things—that we know other parents of kids her age don't do—to avoid a struggle."

You and your child will learn to work together to confront the denial. You will change how you think and respond to the anxiety invading your home.

This chapter details the seven steps of the TRAINOR Method to get you started.

TRAINOR Method Step 1: Target Anxious Thoughts and Behaviors

Target: To direct an action at something.

Begin by zooming in on your child's trouble areas, which will help you identify the stressors. Do this by noticing what precedes the reactive behaviors and considering two questions:

- What are the anxious thoughts?
- What are the anxious behaviors?

Moving from a place of denial to one of perspective, with the ability to back away and observe the problem, is a vital first step. This may not seem easy at first, and you may think, "But I am too frazzled at the moment to think about the anxious thoughts and behaviors." This is true: in the moment may not be the right time, but taking the time later to sort through the anxieties that create difficult behaviors will bring you one step closer to improvement. Until we face the fact that anxiety problems are not fixable by denial, wishful thinking, or hoping for different circumstances next time, the problems will likely persist.

The following is an example of how this worked for one family.

Ally and Steven came to talk about their 10-year-old daughter, Missy. Ally explained: "Missy is a great girl—loving, caring. She has lots of friends. We get compliments about her all the time. But she worries way too much about one thing: vomiting. The weird thing is she's probably thrown up twice in her life, yet this is her big fear. No matter what we tell her, it doesn't help."

Nobody enjoys the thought of vomiting, but for Missy, this fear immediately induced panic. Fear of vomiting is one of the most common phobias children and teens have. But Missy's fear of vomiting was so extreme, it literally made her sick, interfered with her life, and drove her family crazy.

Steven went on to explain how Missy expressed this fear. "She asks a zillion questions about getting sick," he said. "Every morning, it's 'Daddy, am I going to get sick at school today?' Every night, the same thing: 'Promise me I won't get sick.' If I don't promise her, she flips out. I feel like an idiot, but sometimes ten or fifteen times a day I find myself saying, 'You are not going to get sick; I promise you, you will not get sick.' It's senseless to us how worried she is about this."

Ally explained that instead of getting better, the problem was getting worse. "She goes to the nurse at school several times a day, worried about her stomach," Ally said. "If she eats a little too much at dinner and feels full, she panics. If she learns that anyone at school has been sick, she avoids them. The questions come all day long, at school and at home. She even has me come into the bathroom to check her bowel movements and make sure I don't see any signs of the stomach bug." Ally paused and looked away a second. "That's actually the first time I said this out loud," she continued. "I can't believe how ridiculous it sounds. She's 10 years old, and I check her poops; I think I may be losing it." Ally and Steven were finally facing the reality that these abnormal actions had become their "new normal." Anxiety had taken control not only of their daughter, but also of them.

In order to guide Missy, Ally and Steven first needed to consider their thoughts and behaviors in reaction to their daughter's behaviors. They had become sucked into this unsettling world ruled by anxiety. They hated it and found it frustrating. ("We argue about it; nothing we try works.") At times it made them feel angry. ("Stop with the questions. Go to bed. I've had enough!") They both experienced guilty feelings. ("She can't control herself, and she's so miserable over this. We should have more patience. We must be bad parents if we can't manage a 10-year-old.") They also felt terribly confused. ("We just don't know what to do anymore.")

We had to target their thoughts and behaviors—as well as Missy's—for change to occur. In fact, the whole family needed to learn how to help Missy manage her anxiety. Once they understood this, it would help them break through their denial and recognize the huge role they play in either helping her fight her anxiety or continuing to reinforce it.

Of course, Missy experienced denial, too. She believed strongly that her anxious thoughts were based on reality. She needed to challenge these thoughts, accept that she had to change, and most important, believe she was strong enough to control her worries about getting sick and vomiting, which induced panic.

What were Missy's anxious thoughts and behaviors? She avoided anything that might make her uncomfortable—a common reaction to anxious feelings. She sought reassurance from her parents for these anxious feelings every morning before school, every night before bed, and throughout the day at random times; at school, she frequently went to the nurse, and the nurse would call her parents. At first, her mother came to take her home, thinking she was sick. Soon, it became clear that her worries *made* her sick. Missy felt so anxious that she caused her stomach to hurt, which made her more worried about vomiting. Her mother stopped taking her home, but the nurse kept calling her to try to calm Missy down over the phone. Sometimes Missy felt okay after speaking to her mom, and she returned to class; other times, after talking to her mother, she cried more. The nurse would take her temperature, let her lie down, and eventually Missy would return to class. She would usually be back soon, however, and it would start all over again. She became a "frequent flier" to the nurse.

The more Missy asked about vomiting, the more she was stuck on it. She felt she needed reassurance to feel better, and this reassurance held a special power. Thoughts like these kept her reliant on frequent reassurance from others: "If Daddy doesn't promise, then I'll get sick." "I have to go to the nurse or I might vomit."

Another anxious behavior was worrying about food. She restricted her eating, afraid some foods would make her sick. And she stopped having breakfast. She said her stomach hurt every morning, and because she felt so scared she would vomit, she couldn't eat. Another behavior, which everyone dismissed as no big deal, was keeping a bucket next to her bed "just in case." If she needed to vomit in the night, she felt prepared. When I mentioned that this was not normal, her parents looked puzzled. They were so used to it that they never questioned it. It was a potent example of the family's denial.

Avoidance

The second major defense against recognizing and beginning to treat anxiety is avoidance. The parents' avoidance behaviors included all the abnormal things they did for her. They would do anything to avoid her meltdowns and to keep the peace—from checking her poops, to saying things over and over again "just the right way," to even being afraid to discipline her at all, for fear of setting her off. They hoped all this would just pass, even though it was getting worse. They found themselves focusing on how happy she could seem, laughing with her friends, playing soccer, and fooling around with her sister. She was even acting in a play. How could there be something wrong with her? They tried not to talk about it, except when the issues flared. Missy's worries about vomiting caused them to say, "We need help," but they continued to avoid doing anything about it, until they came for treatment.

Missy had many avoidance behaviors of her own. She stayed far away from anyone she thought might have been sick and even someone whose brother or sister was sick. She avoided hearing the word "vomit," freaking out and holding her hands over her ears if someone said the word. She also washed her hands too much to avoid getting germs on her hands. Missy's long list of avoidances included avoiding breakfast, spicy foods, and feeling full after eating—because then she would worry more.

Missy and her parents discussed openly her worries and her behaviors in reaction to her worries. They also described all the behaviors they were doing to reassure Missy when she was worried. It became clear how much Missy's anxiety was not only controlling her, but also controlling her parents. This is initially difficult to talk about, and reminding them that many, many families experience anxiety helped them feel less ashamed. After facing their denial and avoidance defenses, and analyzing the anxious thoughts and behaviors, Missy and her family were ready for Step 2.

TRAINOR Method **Step 2:** Rate the Anxious Behavior

Rate: Measure the value of something.

How do you begin to change all this? Where do you start? Once you have targeted the behaviors, it is important to have a rating system to chart progress.

One method for change that doesn't work is threats and punishments, as Ally, Missy's mom, experienced. "We tried getting her to stop all her talk and worries about sickness. We even threatened to punish her if she didn't stop," Ally began. "She just looked at us and started crying. She can't stop focusing on her fear of throwing up. We have no idea how to help her stop."

So together, we made a list of her anxious behaviors, and Missy then rated them, based on level of difficulty. She guided us to know where to start. She rated how hard it would be, on a scale of 0 (meaning it is easy) and 10 (meaning it is impossible), to

- Not ask Mom about getting sick 9
- Not ask Dad about getting sick 6
- Not ask Mom to check my poops 3
- Not sleep with a bucket 7
- Not avoid kids who have been sick 4
- Go on play dates 6
- Say the word vomit without holding my hands on my ears 5
- Watch a show where somebody vomits 7
- Let myself eat enough to feel full 6
- Go on sleepovers 9
- Not go to the nurse 9

Missy was clear about her hierarchy of difficulty. As her parents listened to her make and rate her list, they learned a lot and looked surprised by some of her responses. For instance, they had no idea the school nurse was so important to her. They had noticed Missy refusing play dates and sleepovers, but they'd had no idea it all came back to her fear of vomiting. Feeling afraid she would get sick at a friend's house, she stayed home. Ally was glad to learn that not asking her to check her poops was pretty easy for Missy, because her mother felt so ridiculous doing it. We all gained a good sense of the hardest and the easiest things for Missy and developed a much better understanding of her anxiety.

As you can see, the process of rating helps the child and parents understand the level of anxiety around particular anxious behaviors; it is a key tool for getting started. To think about goals for Missy to work on, we needed to understand which things were easier for her to work on and which were, at that time, too difficult.

TRAINOR Method Step 3: Agree on Challenges to Work On

Agree: Have the same opinion about something; concur.

Anxious children often do not want to work on changing the anxious behaviors they have rated: it feels too difficult. Easing them into it with gentle empowerment and excitement makes it easy.

In Missy's case, she felt afraid. She looked around her, anticipating that all the grownups in the room, including this *doctor*, would now force her to do things she felt way too scared to do. Like a kid at the edge of the diving board for the first time, scared to jump, she did not want to be pushed.

I started by saying, "We'll fight this step by step. You'll be the leader of the fight, and we're all part of your team."

Missy broke into a smile, looked at her parents, and felt a bit of power. She had never been the leader before with her parents. Then I mentioned that she would earn prizes doing this hard work, and her smile grew. She started to get excited, imagining what those prizes could be.

We looked at her working list together. The easiest thing was not asking Mom to check her poops. She had been asking her mom to do this at least four or five times a week. Every day she did not ask, she earned 1 point, and when she went seven days in a row without asking anyone to check her poops, she earned a bonus 5 points.

Not avoiding someone who had been sick was also not too difficult. Talking to a child who was back at school after being sick, or even touching them or their things, gained her another 5 points.

Not going to the nurse was a big one, rated very high. Her parents felt urgency about this one, because Missy missed a lot of class time. We usually start with the lower numbers and work our way up gradually to the harder things, but Missy's mom took a chance and asked if she was ready to work on staying in class and not going to the nurse. The mood in the room changed immediately. Missy hesitated. Tears welled up in her eyes. She looked at her parents with a mixture of fear and anger. A meltdown fast approached. The thought that we would say she could never go to the nurse overwhelmed her. She needed to know we would not force her to do something she was not ready to do. She felt she needed those visits to the nurse.

The more you push an anxious child too far, the more they push back with great force. Remember the kid at the edge of the diving board? Try to push him, and he will push back, turn around, and walk off the board angry, without jumping. Too many parents of anxious children know this battle too well, a battle you will never win.

I quickly chimed in and told Missy we would not take away her visits to the nurse. She was the leader of this team; we were there to help and support her. I also reminded her that the harder the work, the bigger the prize. She calmed down a bit. Prizes can be a great mood shifter. We discussed how often she went to the nurse. She told us she went at least once a day, sometimes four or five times a day. Her parents looked surprised and concerned. No wonder her grades had slipped so quickly. Not going to the nurse at all, at this point, would be too hard. By establishing this baseline, however, we figured out how to choose a challenging goal that would not overwhelm her. We broke it down: 10 points for not going to the nurse at all in a day, 5 points for going once, 2 points for going twice, and 0 points for going three or four times. Missy agreed. We couldn't set the goals too high, or she would fail; too low, and she would earn points without challenging her anxiety—making no progress.

We reviewed our plan all together so it was clear. She would work on not asking for her poops to be checked, cutting back on her visits to the nurse, and not avoiding anyone who had been sick. I asked her if she also wanted to work on anything else. Her look of fright said it all. We all agreed that this was enough to start. Working intensely on a few goals is better than trying to work on too many at once. If a child is overwhelmed by the goals in the beginning, effort is diminished. The child feels defeated before the work has even started.

TRAINOR Method Step 4: Identify and Teach Strategies to Practice

Identify: Establish or indicate who or what.

Now Missy and her parents knew what she would work on, but that was not enough. They needed to know how to do this—easier said than done. I explained to Missy that lots of kids get worries and have to learn to fight them and get rid of them. I explained to her that there are two kinds of worries: real worries and silly worries. Real worries are like when she is in the middle of a street and a car is coming. That is a real worry. She needs to get out of the street. If she has trouble at school and can't get help, that is a real worry. She needs to talk to someone and ask for help. These are problems that can be solved.

Silly worries are worries that lots of kids get when there is no danger. Some kids worry about aliens or monsters. Her silly worry is about throwing up. She is not silly; her worries are silly. She needed to reframe them by changing the way she thought about her worries.

Missy needed to remember that her worry about vomiting was a "silly worry." When she started thinking about it, she needed to refocus her attention on something else—to let it go and not be stuck on it. I suggested that her thoughts not be, "Don't think those scary thoughts about vomiting." Instead, I suggested she think, "Those thoughts are silly, not important. I want to think about other things." She began learning how to "talk back" to the anxiety.

We made a list of what she could focus on when she started to get the silly worries—how she could "change the channel in her head" off the worry channel. When home, she could listen to music, and she loved singing. She could make her own special calm-down playlist of songs and sing along. It's difficult to be worried and singing at the same time. We made a list of all the relaxing activities she could choose from when she began worrying about vomiting. She loved to read, draw, make up stories, ride her bike, and make special snacks. When she started to get the silly worry about vomiting and used this list to change her channel, she earned another 5 points.

What about at school? Missy needed to remember the vomiting worry as a silly worry and focus on what was going on around her: listening to the teacher, participating in class, talking to her friends at lunch, or keeping her attention on what is important at school, not on the silly worries.

We discussed how everybody's behavior would change to fight the anxiety and not be ruled by it. For Missy to get better, she had to first feel uncomfortable and experience a manageable level of distress. Her parents had to learn to do things that are counterintuitive for parents. As parents, from the time our newborn is placed in our arms, we have an instinct to protect and shelter our child from pain. Parenting anxious children demands the opposite response: we must support our children to push through their discomfort to get to the other side. We help our children learn to push themselves, even when it feels difficult, knowing that those anxious feelings will go away.

Protecting and sheltering your anxious child fuels the anxiety and makes it worse. An anxious child who is too comfortable is limited by the anxiety—her world will become smaller and smaller over time.

We discussed how Mom and Dad could help. They could remind Missy that she could meet her goals, praise her for her accomplishments in fighting the silly worries, and, of course, provide the rewards.

Not talking to her about the worries is important. We agreed, specifically, not to talk about her poops. If Missy forgot and asked, her mother could say "silly worry" as her reminder. If Missy felt worried, she could pick from her list of options to "change the channel" in her head. Her mother would avoid the repetitive conversation about how her poops are fine, that she is not going to vomit, and so on. Talking about her worries with Missy would only model that they were something she needed to talk about, something important. This would give Missy's worries too much attention and bring Missy and her parents back into the worry loop of "But Mom, what if . . . I need you to . . . It could be true . . . How do you know?" Such conversation rapidly escalates until Mom is once again staring down into a toilet bowl looking at perfectly normal poops, assuring her child she is not sick. Anxiety wins again, and everyone feels defeated. Instead, Missy and her parents had to learn, "No talking about it—silly worry—move on." Every time Missy did this, she would earn more points. Missy and her parents agreed to this plan and felt optimistic that they could now work together to help her manage her anxiety.

In addition, exposing herself to her fear is also very important to desensitize her to her fear of vomiting, which for Missy will include saying "vomit" and "throw up" and watching videos of people vomiting and rating her anxiety level until it goes down to zero. This graduated exposure would significantly help reduce her anxious response to vomiting.

TRAINOR Method Step 5: Note and Chart Progress Made

Note: To notice or pay particular attention to.

Once the wheels are set in motion, the next step is to note the desired actions and create a chart as a means of tracking results toward goals.

Missy and her parents made a chart that included what Missy was working on. She made her chart with her parents and decorated it. This was her chart, made in a way that she and her family deemed easiest to use. Some families use paper or poster board; others prefer the computer, an iPad, or a calendar. Whatever is clear, visual, simple, and easy for the family to use works best. Missy's chart, which they hung in the kitchen on the refrigerator, looked like this:

Missy Silly Worry Chart

- ☐ No checking P [code for poops in case non–family members might see the chart]
- ☐ Nurse: No? Yes? How many times?
- ☐ Not avoiding kids who have been sick
- ☐ Changing the channel in my head by picking from my activity list

Next we created another chart using a calendar format, because Missy needed to work on reducing her anxiety every day. Missy found a calendar on the computer and copied her list of worries onto every day on the calendar. Then she printed the calendar out. Every day that she did something from her list, she checked it off. Under the check, she gave it a number, 0 to 10, to show how hard it was. The more she practiced, the lower the numbers went, measuring how her anxiety decreased. Next, she recorded how many points she had earned for that worry on that day.

She and her parents chose a time each day to go over her points earned and add them all up. This kept the process positive and reminded her to keep working at her goals and not slip back. The first two weeks of Missy's calendar looked like the illustration on pages 28 and 29.

This wasn't always easy, of course. Some days the process went smoothly; some days Missy needed a boost, which was usually as simple as reviewing her rewards. And on days when her parents were busy with work issues or just typical active family life, they needed to force themselves to make time to sit with Missy and review the day. Their motivation? The baby steps of progress they were beginning to observe. Missy's motivation? The points and the powerful feelings of accomplishment. She was very proud of herself.

TRAINOR Method Step 6: Offer Incentives to Motivate

Offer: To present for acceptance or rejection.

As families proceed with the steps, the reward system needs to be carried out, to be sure the message is clear that prizes will come. Of course, for the parents, the reward is the child's changing behaviors, but the behavior changes may fall apart without carrying out the actual offers made when setting up the chart.

What do all these points mean for a child or adolescent? What can they cash them in for?

The younger the child, the quicker they need the rewards. Most children need a reward within a week of working hard. Some kids are motivated to work for something large. If the reward is too far in the future, it becomes abstract and not motivating; however, they can "bank" their points for something large and, in the meantime, receive smaller things along the way.

Missy and her parents agreed on prizes, which do not have to be purchased items but can also be activities or privileges; this can help alleviate concerns about spending money on rewards. The prizes can even replace treats that in the past did not have to be earned. Now, when Missy wanted a treat, instead of just getting it, she earned it through this hard work.

Missy's Silly Worry Calendar

How hard? Rate each worry on a scale of 0 to 10, with 10 the hardest.

How many points?

Not checking P: Every day without asking = 1 point; 7 days in a row without asking = bonus 5 points.

Talking to a child who was back at school after being sick, or even touching them or their things = 5 points.

Not going to the nurse at all in a day = 10 points; going once = 5 points; going twice = 2 points; going three or four times = 0 points.

Changing the channel in her head by picking from list = 5 points.

Missy's total points for this month: ___

Sunday 1	Monday 2	Tuesday 3	Wednesday 4	Thursday 5	Friday 6	Saturday 7
☐ Not checking P How hard? ___ How many points? ___	☐ Not checking P How hard? ___ How many points? ___	☐ Not checking P How hard? ___ How many points? ___	☐ Not checking P How hard? ___ How many points? ___	☐ Not checking P How hard? ___ How many points? ___	☐ Not checking P How hard? ___ How many points? ___	☐ Not checking P How hard? ___ How many points? ___
☐ Not avoiding kids who have been sick How hard? ___ How many points? ___	☐ Nurse: No? Yes? How many times? How hard? ___ How many points? ___	☐ Nurse: No? Yes? How many times? How hard? ___ How many points? ___	☐ Nurse: No? Yes? How many times? How hard? ___ How many points? ___	☐ Nurse: No? Yes? How many times? How hard? ___ How many points? ___	☐ Nurse: No? Yes? How many times? How hard? ___ How many points? ___	☐ Not avoiding kids who have been sick How hard? ___ How many points? ___
☐ Changing the channel in my head by picking from my activity list How hard? ___ How many points? ___	☐ Not avoiding kids who have been sick How hard? ___ How many points? ___	☐ Not avoiding kids who have been sick How hard? ___ How many points? ___	☐ Not avoiding kids who have been sick How hard? ___ How many points? ___	☐ Not avoiding kids who have been sick How hard? ___ How many points? ___	☐ Not avoiding kids who have been sick How hard? ___ How many points? ___	☐ Changing the channel in my head by picking from my activity list How hard? ___ How many points? ___
Today's total points: ___	☐ Changing the channel in my head by picking from my activity list How hard? ___ How many points? ___	☐ Changing the channel in my head by picking from my activity list How hard? ___ How many points? ___	☐ Changing the channel in my head by picking from my activity list How hard? ___ How many points? ___	☐ Changing the channel in my head by picking from my activity list How hard? ___ How many points? ___	☐ Changing the channel in my head by picking from my activity list How hard? ___ How many points? ___	Today's total points: ___
	Today's total points: ___	Today's total points: ___	Today's total points: ___	Today's total points: ___	Today's total points: ___	

8	9	10	11	12	13	14
☐ Not checking P	☐ Not checking P	☐ Not checking P	☐ Not checking P	☐ Not checking P	☐ Not checking P	☐ Not checking P
How hard? __	How hard? __	How hard? __	How hard? __	How hard? __	How hard? __	How hard? __
How many points? __	How many points? __	How many points? __	How many points? __	How many points? __	How many points? __	How many points? __
	☐ Nurse: No? Yes?	☐ Nurse: No? Yes?	☐ Nurse: No? Yes?	☐ Nurse: No? Yes?	☐ Nurse: No? Yes?	
	How many times? __	How many times? __	How many times? __	How many times? __	How many times? __	
	How hard? __	How hard? __	How hard? __	How hard? __	How hard? __	
	How many points? __	How many points? __	How many points? __	How many points? __	How many points? __	
☐ Not avoiding kids who have been sick	☐ Not avoiding kids who have been sick	☐ Not avoiding kids who have been sick	☐ Not avoiding kids who have been sick	☐ Not avoiding kids who have been sick	☐ Not avoiding kids who have been sick	☐ Not avoiding kids who have been sick
How hard? __	How hard? __	How hard? __	How hard? __	How hard? __	How hard? __	How hard? __
How many points? __	How many points? __	How many points? __	How many points? __	How many points? __	How many points? __	How many points? __
☐ Changing the channel in my head by picking from my activity list	☐ Changing the channel in my head by picking from my activity list	☐ Changing the channel in my head by picking from my activity list	☐ Changing the channel in my head by picking from my activity list	☐ Changing the channel in my head by picking from my activity list	☐ Changing the channel in my head by picking from my activity list	☐ Changing the channel in my head by picking from my activity list
How hard? __	How hard? __	How hard? __	How hard? __	How hard? __	How hard? __	How hard? __
How many points? __	How many points? __	How many points? __	How many points? __	How many points? __	How many points? __	How many points? __
Today's total points: __	Today's total points: __	Today's total points: __	Today's total points: __	Today's total points: __	Today's total points: __	Today's total points: __

Note: The TRAINOR method works best when the child can see the difficulty level going down and the points going up.

Missy decided she would like to earn

- a special doll
- a sleepover with two friends
- being able to choose what the family would eat for dinner (within reason)
- having breakfast on the weekend alone with Dad
- an iTunes gift card
- an ice cream sundae

She and her parents agreed on how many points she needed for each prize. Missy's doll was worth 250 points, but every 20 points she earned got her a smaller prize. Missy was excited, and the process of working hard doing so many things that initially felt uncomfortable was actually manageable. She could do it!

TRAINOR Method Step 7:
Reinforce Progress and Increase Challenges

Reinforce: to strengthen by additional assistance, material, or support.

After a couple of weeks, Missy's calendar was all filled in. She'd earned prizes, and she felt excited to show me how many points she'd earned. We looked at her accomplishments. Not having Mom check poops was now easy, rated a 0, down from an initial rating of 3. Zero meant we could cross it off the list—she did it!

In the beginning, not going to the nurse was difficult, but after a while, she'd earned more days of maximum points for not going to the nurse at all. She rated that behavior a 2, down from an initial rating of 7; it was still a bit hard, but so much better.

Not avoiding kids who have been sick was another 0, down from a 4—she crossed that off the list. Missy was making great progress. What to work on next? We needed to increase her challenges.

She agreed to work on not asking Dad about getting sick. If she slipped and asked, she agreed Dad could say "silly worry" to remind her to let it go and move on. When it felt difficult, she would pick from her calm-down list. Every day that she did not ask Dad about getting sick, she would earn 5 points; every day that she asked but could stop and move on, she earned 3 points. And if she really needed him to give her reassurance because she felt so worried, he would, but she then would receive no points. She agreed.

Saying the word "vomit" without covering her ears still challenged her. She hated that word. Every day that she worked on saying the word "vomit" over and over, she earned 2 points. The more she did it, however, the quicker she would improve; exposure works so well with scenarios like this.

We agreed that Missy would keep working on not going to the nurse, but now she would earn her points by not going at all for five days in a row. She agreed to that challenge. She also agreed to go on play dates with her friends, a step in the direction of being able to do sleepovers again, since social isolation is often a symptom of anxiety and an important area to work on.

Missy now had a new chart, new work to be done fighting the anxiety, and more points and prizes to be earned.

Missy's parents came to meet with me privately a few times during these weeks to talk about their changing role and behaviors. They wanted to understand more about anxiety and how to help Missy. They also talked to me about her sister, who had some anxiety problems as well. When there are siblings involved, I often recommend that the siblings get a chart so that they can be working on things too. Since anxiety tends to run in families, often more than one child in a family has anxiety. If the other siblings are not anxious, there is always something they can work on, from making their bed to doing their homework without a fuss. This reinforces the message that every kid has something to work on and normalizes this process. It also discourages jealousy from the other siblings over getting prizes. As Missy's parents have demonstrated, the TRAINOR Method's seven steps provide a process for parents to leap out of their out-of-control zones and into a new and guided means of helping their child and themselves. It helped them move from feeling powerless and controlled by their child's anxiety to feeling united as a family empowering her to exercise control.

Next Steps

Missy continues to work hard and is now doing sleepovers with friends. She has an overnight school trip she wants to go on, however, and it's making her feel scared. We are discussing strategies, and this is giving her the confidence she needs to meet this goal and go with her friends. Her parents are also learning how to help her sister, Grace, with her anxiety, which is very different. Grace is relaxed in many ways but worries way too much about schoolwork. We are all working together to help both children feel free of anxiety.

Chapter 3

Daytime, Bedtime, Worry, Worry

Generalized Anxiety Disorder

All kids worry, but some kids worry to the extreme. Kids with generalized anxiety disorder (GAD) have worries that are more pervasive and persistent than others. They often think in terms of "What if . . . ?" They are highly sensitive to thinking that if something bad happens to someone, anywhere in the world, it could easily happen to them, or to their family. The natural response, to reassure them, leads to more anxiety and more "What if . . . ?"

Children with GAD have trouble keeping things in perspective. Parents intuitively know that these kids can't handle watching the news and often try to protect them from hearing anything "bad." They know it will start them worrying, which can be distressing and hard to stop. Once children with GAD get stuck on a worry, they may have trouble sleeping, and their fears can become so intense that they have crying meltdowns and are difficult to soothe. They get caught up in a "worry loop" of repeating the same "what ifs," and it can be hard to get out of this cycle.

Kids with GAD usually want to know exactly what to expect in their day-to-day life. When things become unpredictable, they seem unable to cope. Flexibility, change, and failure create extreme discomfort for them. As a result, getting them to engage in new activities can be difficult, and getting them to stick it out and not quit can seem impossible. Uncertainty can be hard for them to tolerate, and learning new things involves risk and possible failure.

These feelings can feel too overwhelming for kids with GAD to bear. They are often driven by perfectionism, and when engaged in learning, they quickly become self-critical. As we know, learning involves the opposite of perfectionism. We have to work and struggle, and we often make mistakes as we learn. When faced with challenges, kids with GAD become filled with anxious thoughts, including, "I'm not as good as everyone else. Kids will make fun of me, and I can't do it. This is too hard. I hate it. I don't want to do it." Kids never say, "I don't want to do it because it makes me feel too anxious." They say, "I don't like it. I hate doing that, and you can't make me do it." So parents are faced with a dilemma: they want their kids to participate in activities, but they don't want to force them to do things they don't like.

How can you force your child to do something he hates, especially considering that avoidance is the number-one defense against anxiety? Anxious children often avoid doing after-school activities or worse, refuse to go to school.

These kids may "hate" almost everything except staying home riveted to a screen. When that's the case, anxiety is making their choices for them. Screens and snacks become their companions and their preferred after-school activities. They are often most comfortable at home, eating the limited foods they like, and playing games or watching videos. Kids with GAD are often labeled "picky eaters," "homebodies," "gamers," "shy," or "just not into sports."

Kids with GAD often worry excessively about school performance. Their parents say they don't pressure them about grades, but the children seem to be internally driven to be perfect, which translates into getting perfect grades. This can cause them to spend way too much time on homework. They may make a simple homework assignment into a much bigger deal. When homework has to be perfect, it can take twice as long as it should. Anxiety about homework often leads to meltdowns. Some kids worry too much about tests, so the night before a test can be tense. Even when they are great students, anxious kids worry about failing. All this is usually happening in the evening, when everyone is tired—a recipe for an ugly scene. The more kids get anxious, the less they can focus on their work. Parents often dread homework time because of the stress it causes.

Kids with GAD may also have physical symptoms, most frequently headaches and stomachaches. Pediatric gastroenterologists are usually aware that a large proportion of their patients struggle more with anxiety than with any significant gastrointestinal problem. These physical symptoms often become the focus of parents' attention, with frequent visits to doctors and medical test after test coming back normal. Being physically sick also becomes a reason to avoid anxiety-producing activities.

Again, parents are in a dilemma: "How can I push her to go to school when she's sick?" Being sick may be a way for a child with GAD to defend against anxious feelings. And anxiety can actually make kids sick. The stomach and the brain are closely tied together. Kids may have stomach pain and may even vomit, but the worries are causing the pain, not an illness. Reducing the anxiety reduces the pain.

Kids may also have trouble sleeping, because at night, when all is quiet, there is more time to worry. Children with GAD need their sleep, exercise, and a healthy diet, or their symptoms can worsen. Knowing this can be frustrating for parents because getting kids with GAD to calm down and do the healthy things they need to do can be so difficult. Sleeping issues and eating problems often go hand and hand with anxiety.

Many of the above issues manifested themselves in the experiences described below.

Mike and Sarah's Story

Mike and Sarah came to me because they were very concerned about Lily, their 9-year-old daughter. Sarah spoke first. "Lily is a great little girl, but she worries all the time about everything. She's always been like this, but lately it's getting worse, and we don't know what to do to help her. I'm at my wits' end. She's a kid. She should be happy. She's a great student, but she worries every time there's a test. When she's studying the night before a test, she often ends up crying and screaming over the littlest thing. The strange thing is, she always gets fine grades. She also worries about her friends not liking her, but she has a good group of girls who always seem happy to play with her."

Sarah paused, then continued. "Her big worry, every night, is someone's going to come in our house and . . . I don't know what. Hurt her? Kidnap her? She doesn't say. She can't sleep in her bed. This has always been a problem with her, but now she's so old, and it's impossible to get her in her bed. Her room is at the top of the stairs, and she thinks this 'bad guy' will come into the house and get to her first. She seems terrified, so she sleeps with us every night. I know it sounds crazy, but within minutes, she goes right to sleep in our bed. We live in a safe neighborhood, have an alarm system, and our dog barks at everything. It doesn't matter to her. No matter how many times we tell her she's safe, she can't seem to get it through her head. It's always 'What if . . . ?' from her, no matter what we say. It can get ridiculous."

Sarah seemed exasperated. "Last night it was 'What if someone comes in, and the alarm doesn't work, and he gets the dog to be silent, and he's so quiet he doesn't wake you up, and he comes up the stairs and into my room?' It can go on and on. There's no getting through to her. Some nights she seems to almost have a panic attack if we try to make her stay in her bed, as if she's in total danger of being attacked."

Mike then jumped in. "She sleeps with you. I have to find a bed to sleep in; I usually end up in her bed or on the couch. It's ridiculous, but we all need our sleep." Sarah continued. "Another thing, I don't know if it's all related, but she has temper tantrums like a 2-year-old. She's almost 10—way too old for this behavior. She gets herself so worked up sometimes, she becomes hysterical, and there's no talking to her. We've tried punishing her, talking to her, ignoring her—nothing works. It's usually before we have to go somewhere, like her soccer games or practices, or in the morning before school. The littlest thing causes her to explode. This morning it was that she wanted to wear a short-sleeve shirt, and it's thirty degrees outside. That caused a screaming fit for almost a half hour. We barely made it to school on time.

"I can't tell you how disruptive this is for the whole family. Her little brother runs away scared when she gets like this. Then once she's out the door and goes to school or to her sports, wherever, she is this normal, happy girl for the most part. Change is hard for her to handle, and it's not summer anymore—she has to wear warm clothes."

Mike added, "She's always complaining of a stomachache and asking to go to the doctor. We have taken her to the doctor many times, and the pediatrician says there's nothing wrong with her. Lately she has been going to the school nurse and calling to get picked up. If we pick her up, as soon as she gets home, she's fine. Is she making this up, or is her anxiety really making her sick? This is so frustrating. We both work and can't keep missing work over this."

Sarah nodded, then said, "I know we're telling you all these bad things, but Lily is a terrific kid, kind, sensitive, and sweet. When you meet her, you'll see. She's adorable. No one would imagine this same girl acts so scared and out of control at home. I always get the best reports from teachers, coaches, and other parents. In fact, her teacher told me, at the last conference, she wishes all the kids were like her. I bit my tongue, but I felt like saying, come and live with us for twenty-four hours and you might change your mind!"

"I must admit, I lose my patience with her," said Mike. "Nothing I do seems to work. If I try to joke about it, she gets mad. If I try to talk seriously with her about how crazy these fears are, she starts screaming at me that I don't understand. If there's something to worry about, she will find it. Lily has had a very stable home. No big changes in her life."

Then Mike added an interesting wrinkle to the discussion: "She reminds me of my mother. When I was a kid learning to swim, my mom talked endlessly about drowning and how I needed to learn to swim, not because it was fun, but so I wouldn't drown. I would go to the playground, and she would imagine me falling off the jungle gym and cracking my skull open."

He then looked at his wife and said, "Honestly, you know, that's the way Mom is, and sometimes Lily seems like mini-Mom. Seeing this anxiety in Lily drives me crazy. I love my mother, but she's a stress machine. Lily is not my mother, I know. I just don't want her growing up to be anxious like my mom. What can we do to help her? What did we do wrong? We have a younger son, and he's just the opposite. Nothing bothers him. Why can't she be more like him? What really upset both of us was the other night, after I tried and failed once again to get her to sleep in her own bed, she had a meltdown, crying and screaming, and at one point, she said she wished she was dead. To hear my little girl say such a thing really tore me apart. We know we need help with this."

Clearly, it sounded like Mike's mother had anxiety issues, and I explained to Mike and Sarah that anxiety is often genetic. I then asked them more about family history. Sarah laughed and said, "Aha! She gets this from your side."

Mike laughed too. "Yes, it's my fault ... but let's talk about your family. Your father, for starters!"

Sarah laughed again. "Yes, he's right. My father was always a worrier and very overprotective of me and my sisters. We needed to sneak around to go out with our friends, knowing he would want us to stay home. We were all so glad to go to college and get freedom. My mother was great, but my aunt had a lot of problems. I remember she would just stay in her house and not go out. I could never understand it. She even had groceries delivered, and she never came to family functions. I think I met her once when she was sick and my mom brought some soup to her. My mom would say, 'She's just a homebody,' whatever that meant. Could that have been anxiety?"

She then smiled at Mike and said, "Okay, maybe it's not all your fault."

Mike said, "I guess the poor kid has no chance with our genes. She gets it from both sides, and we just need to know how to help her. I love my mother, but I don't want Lily growing up with my mother's anxiety. There has to be a way we can prevent that and help her."

I reassured them that there was a way. We needed to hear from Lily.

Lily's Story

Lily did seem like the sweet, engaging child her parents described, but she was obviously conflicted, and she echoed many of her parents' comments while meeting with me.

"I worry about lots of things. I can't help it. My biggest worries are at night. I'm so scared someone could come into the house and into my room. I can't sleep in my room; I keep hearing noises and think someone's coming. I can't stand it. I need to run into Mom and Dad's bed. Then I feel safe and can sleep. I know other kids my age sleep alone, and I don't want anyone to know I sleep with my parents. At night, when it's dark out, I can't even go upstairs when everyone else is downstairs. I get so scared. I feel like someone could be hiding up there. I hate when it's dark."

She shuddered a bit, then continued. "I have other worries too. I worry about school all the time. Tests are the worst. I hate tests. I worry that I could fail or forget everything, and it makes me so scared. My teacher is nice, but what if she gets mad at me? And my friends—sometimes I think they don't like me. Sometimes I think I have no friends, and I get so upset. I know I have friends, but what if they are mad at me? My mom wants me to have a birthday party, and I want to, but I'm scared no one will come, or if they come, they won't have fun. What if no one comes to my party? I told her I don't want a party."

Lily caught her breath. "Then there's sports. My mom and dad want me to play, and I like soccer and basketball, but I worry. What if I mess up and everyone sees it? Maybe they won't want me on the team any-more. Before the games and the practices, I get so upset sometimes, my stomach starts to hurt, and I just wish I could stay home. I don't know why, but before I leave the house, everything just makes me crazy, and I start screaming and crying. I just get so upset and angry. I want to stay home. My parents get so mad at me when I'm like this. I know it's bad, but I can't help it. I don't know why it happens. Once I get to soccer and start playing, it's fun, and I feel so happy. One of my coaches even said I was a great soccer player."

Lily began feeling more comfortable as she continued: "My parents tell me to never watch the news. It scares me to hear about bad things. I can't stop thinking these bad things could happen to me. When it gets cloudy out, I start to worry about things like hurricanes and tornadoes, and sometimes, I just don't want to go outside. If there are big clouds, I get too scared. I have a lot of things that make me worry.

"I know sometimes I get really angry and upset, especially at night or before tests. I always feel so sorry after. My mom understands, I think, but my dad, he can be mean. Mom always lets me in their bed and doesn't get so mad, but Dad can get angry. He says 'Lily, you have to go in your room. Don't be silly. You can do it.' When I get upset, he tells me to stop crying. I wish I could! It's not that easy. I don't want to be like this. He doesn't understand. I'm really scared. Why am I like this? Nobody understands that I can't change this; it's just the way I am. My parents brought me to another doctor, and she was nice, and we played games. They stopped taking me because they said nothing was getting better. I can't change this, and I want everyone to leave me alone. I don't want anything to change. There's not such a big problem."

It appeared that Lily wanted help but was convinced she couldn't change. This was a girl who hated failure and had no confidence she could get help. We were now ready to start working together and giving her more confidence in her ability to gain self-control and learn how to manage her worries.

Step 1: Target Anxious Thoughts and Behaviors

Not surprisingly, when Lily and her parents came together for the next session, she made it clear that she wanted no part of continued therapy. When she came into my office, she made no eye contact, sat really close to her mother, and whispered to her, "When can we go home?" She then took one of the pillows on my couch and put her head behind it. She was showing me how mad and oppositional she could be. Her father just looked down at the floor, and her mother's face started getting red. It was like both parents were saying, "Here we go again. What are we supposed to do?"

Her mother then said, "It was a huge battle to get her here." Then she turned to Lily and said in a stern voice, "Lily, don't be rude."

With that, Lily started crying. We were off to a horrible start.

Lily was like many kids with anxiety who are high functioning and, as a result, hate feeling so helpless and out of control. Lily wanted to be the girl teachers love and friends invite to parties, the girl who is a great athlete. She didn't want to be the weird girl who needed to see a therapist. She felt ashamed and hopeless about this part of herself, her anxious self. She was angry about having these problems, and her anger was directed at her parents and anyone who wanted to help her with her anxiety. Instead, she needed to learn to get angry at her worries so that she could work to be free of them. She needed help to integrate her strengths and her struggles. She needed to learn that one doesn't negate the other, and we all have both. After all, Lily was smart, athletic, popular, and, at times, struggling with painful anxiety. She needed to know that lots of great kids have these same worries and that she would learn how to free herself from them.

To normalize her experience, we talked about how many kids struggle with worries. I let her know that I see other kids from her school. She looked surprised. She had thought she was the only kid in the world, never mind in her school, who had worries.

She perked up. "Who else in my school comes here?"

I explained that I couldn't tell her because it's private. She looked both curious and relieved that no one would find out she had these problems. She was still sitting very close to her mom but was making eye contact and even smiling a little.

We started talking about what her worries were, and I explained that all the kids who see me start by making a list of what they're afraid of. I let her know that she could earn prizes for making the worries go away. She became quiet again; it was hard to talk about her fears.

Her mom jumped in. "Is it okay if I start?" Lily nodded.

Mom started with the list of things we needed to work on:

- Staying in her bed
- Going upstairs at night
- Going to sports without a fuss
- Going to school without a fuss
- Doing homework without a fuss
- Taking tests without a fuss the night before
- Not seeking reassurance, since she has the "What if's" about a lot of things (for example, she randomly said things like, "What if I touched the floor and then put my finger in my mouth—could I die?")

I reiterated to Lily that I see lots of kids who have the same problems. Realizing that she was not alone helped her feel less ashamed and more engaged in the process.

We then listed her anxious thoughts:

- For staying in her bed, she said, "I worry about a bad guy coming into my room."

- For going upstairs at night, she said, "I worry there's someone up there."
- For going to her sports, she had to think, but then said, "I worry that I will mess up, and everyone will be mad at me, and when my stomach hurts, I worry I will get sick."
- For school, she said, "I just keep thinking I hate school, and I don't want to go. I know I don't really hate school, but in the morning that's what I think. I just want to stay home and not have to go, and I get really angry about having to go to school."
- For the test anxiety, she said, "I worry I'll fail the test, and I worry the teacher will get mad at me."
- For her other random worries, she said, "I just worry I could do something that could make me sick or die."

As her parents listened, I could see they were surprised at how strong her fears were. Her father moved toward her and kissed her forehead. He understood more how hard this was for his little girl.

Then we forged ahead.

Step 2: Rate the Anxious Behavior

We went through the list again, and Lily rated how hard she thought it would be to work on these symptoms. She rated them on a scale of 0 to 10, with 0 being easy and 10 being impossible:

- Staying in her bed she immediately said was a 10. She started to cry and say, "I can't do it! I get too scared." I quickly explained to her that we would break it down so she could accomplish this in steps. The first step would be for her to try to stay in her bed. If she went into her parents' room, her dad would bring her back to her bed but stay there in her room until she fell back asleep. She looked relieved and said, "I think that would be about a 7. Okay, I guess I could do that, maybe." She didn't sound too convincing. Of course, both parents would have to be on board and ready to do this. I recommended that they think about it and perhaps start when there was a long weekend, so getting sleep was not such an issue.
- Next was going upstairs at night. Again Lily said that was a 10. We discussed breaking it down. We agreed that it would be a 6 if she went upstairs at night but one of her parents was in the room at the bottom of the stairs, and she just went up to get something and then came right down.
- Next was going to her games and practices without a struggle. She seemed

to think that was a 3, although her parents looked surprised at such a low rating. She also rated going to school and doing homework and taking tests with a similarly low rating. She was perhaps overconfident in her ability to control her anxiety. We also knew she was very ashamed of this behavior and confused by it. We discussed how sometimes, when you rate things in my office, it might be different when you actually try to do it; it could be a higher or a lower number. Lily said, "No, I think it really is a 3. I can do it."

- Having her birthday party she rated as a 4. Her parents were surprised that she was so worried about this. Her dad said, "Lily, what's the big deal about having a party?" She then looked sad and became very quiet. She said, "I just don't want a party." I reminded them that worries don't make sense, and lots of kids worry about things that they don't need to worry about. Birthday parties can create anxiety for some kids. Lily worried about her friendships, and she worried that her friends wouldn't come to the party, or if they came, maybe they wouldn't have a good time. She couldn't decide if she wanted a party or what kind of party to have. Making these decisions felt overwhelming for her. So the solution was to avoid the whole party thing altogether.

Now it was time to move on to specific goals and get to work.

Step 3: Agree on Challenges to Work On

Lily agreed to try to go upstairs at night, with at least one of her parents staying in the room at the bottom of the stairs. She also agreed to try to control her meltdowns when she was anxious about school and sports. But she didn't want to work on staying in her bed.

Her dad's immediate reaction was "This is not an option, Lily. You have to do this." He clearly was frustrated by this sleep situation.

She then started crying again and said, "I can't do it!" Her anxiety in even talking about it was all over her face. She even started shaking.

This goal seemed too hard for her right then, and if we pushed her to do something she was not ready to do, we could cause this whole plan to fail. If the goal is too high, kids often shut down, feeling they can't do it. They then can become angry and resistant. We knew this was Lily's pattern. She also needed a sense of control because her anxiety could make her feel so out of control. So we needed to respect her limits at this point, to get her to agree to do this work. Lily needed to gain more confidence in her ability to manage her anxiety, and then she would be more ready to tackle sleeping independently.

So, it was agreed. Dad had to wait until Lily was ready to work on her sleeping. Dad was not happy, but he reluctantly supported the plan.

Next was the birthday party. At first Lily insisted that she just didn't want a party. Her mom and dad felt that this was strange since she went to parties and had lots of friends. The anxiety this caused her was confusing for them. Lily didn't want to recognize that this was anxiety related but said, "Okay, if it means that much to you, I'll have the party." Her birthday was in four weeks, so that was a timely goal.

Now, we needed to move from goals to strategies.

Step 4: Initiate and Teach Strategies to Practice

Lily needed to understand how to challenge her anxious thoughts. This is the cognitive part of the therapy. We talked about how to label these thoughts and see them as something to observe, without reacting to them, and not to believe anxious thoughts are true. We discussed what to label them; she thought for a few minutes, and then said, "fake fears." Okay, we would call her worries fake fears. This was her label that she thought of. She needed to think of these thoughts as lies in her head that she would not believe.

Her biggest fear was that an intruder would come into the house. She knew that was not realistic, yet when she had these thoughts, she became very frightened.

Her dad reminded her that their dog barks at flies that come into the house, never mind a stranger. Lily laughed, which was wonderful because anxious kids need to learn to laugh at their irrational worries and not be so serious. Laughing puts the worries in perspective.

Then he added, "On our block the biggest intruder has been that skunk we've all smelled."

Now she was really laughing. Humor works beautifully to take the power out of anxious thoughts, when the anxious person is not currently flooded with fear. When Lily was not experiencing anxiety, that was the time to help her begin to change the way she thought about her worries.

Eventually, she needed to realize that these thoughts were "fake fears."

Our goal was to help her take the power out of the thoughts. She could learn to label them and practice putting her attention on what was important, in the here and now. This mindfulness would allow her to accept these thoughts as irrational and let them go. She could then focus on soothing, calm, happy thoughts or on the activities she was engaged in.

We discussed how this practice would help her at bedtime. Music or an audiobook helps a lot of kids relax at night. Even though she clearly stated that she was not ready to work on sleeping alone, the seed was planted for her to know strategies that could help her, when she was ready.

Since she agreed to work on no fussing before school, sports, or tests, we needed to discuss strategies to help her. She needed to review her anxious thoughts and have "replacement thoughts." These are thoughts that are based on reality, not her fears.

For all her worries about the "bad guy," we discussed what she could say to herself to "talk back" to the anxiety. "I am safe in my room and in my home. My parents are here, and they take care of me. These are my fake fears, and I don't need to pay any attention to them."

For her school anxious thoughts, she said, "I don't love school, but it's okay. I'm smart, and I have friends who like me. Recess is always fun."

For her fears before tests, she said, "I'm a smart girl. I studied, and I will do the best I can. If I get things wrong, no one will be mad at me. It's okay; I don't have to be perfect." I also encouraged her to write down her worries before a test. Writing down the specific worries helps kids make them concrete and more able to let them go, instead of going into the test with this vague dark cloud of nervousness over their heads.

For sports, Lily said, "I'm a good player. I am getting better, and no one's perfect. I don't have to be perfect. I always have fun when I play, and I will have fun."

As we were discussing these thoughts, her mother was writing the replacement thoughts down, so Lily could read them when she was feeling anxious. That was an excellent strategy to help Lily stay focused on what's real, and not on her irrational thoughts, when she starts to get anxious.

Lily also agreed to have a "calm-down list," which included things that she could use to calm herself down when she started to worry.

Lily's Calm-Down List:

- She agreed to make a special playlist on her iPod of her favorite happy songs to listen to.
- She likes the feeling of playing with silly putty.
- She's a good artist and enjoys drawing pictures of animals.
- She loves to write stories about mermaids.
- She always feels happy riding her bike.
- She likes to play basketball and focus on getting the ball in the hoop.
- She loves to sing and dance by herself in her room in daylight.

We discussed how she needed to use this list. When she noticed she was getting anxious and upset, she needed to try to calm herself down. If her parents noticed, they could prompt her to calm herself down. I reminded her parents that they can't calm Lily; she needed to learn to calm herself. Lily and her parents were getting the message that Lily had to take control of her emotions. Her parents could support her, but she needed to do the work.

The work continued with practice.

Step 5: Note and Chart Progress Made

Lily and her parents agreed on how to chart her progress. They decided to record the date, what she worked on, the difficulty rating, and how many points she earned. Her parents figured out how many points she could earn and what the points were worth.

Lily agreed and was excited, but she wondered what the points meant. This led us to the "perks."

Step 6: Offer Incentives to Motivate

We now discussed what she could cash in her points for—what rewards she wanted to earn. Right away, Lily said, "I want a new puppy!" This family already had a dog. A pet is often what kids want for a prize, but it's not a good reward, unless the family has already agreed on it. Mom and Dad had clearly said no more pets. So we had to move on.

Lily was deflated for a few minutes, but we quickly started coming up with other ideas. I reminded her that prizes didn't have to be things; they could be experiences.

So we made a list of rewards she could earn points for:

- Breakfast with Dad **30 points**
- Picking the restaurant the next time her family goes out to dinner **20 points**
- Extra 20 minutes on the iPad **20 points**
- Miniature golf **30 points**
- Picking a movie to watch **25 points**

- Sleepover with two friends (her parents hate sleepovers!) **75 points**
- Getting a manicure with Mom **40 points**
- Going on a hike with Dad, without brother **15 points**

She was now very excited about earning her points and receiving prizes.

Step 7: Reinforce Progress and Increase Challenges

After two weeks, we met again.

Lily was thrilled to tell me her progress. She had struggled at first with going to sports without a fuss. It was harder than she thought, but she was having success. She was proud to show me her chart and how her numbers had gone down.

She showed me her latest ratings for all the goals she'd been working on:

- Going upstairs. This was now a 0! She proudly told me she was not scared anymore as long as Mom or Dad was in the room at the bottom of the stairs when she went up. We discussed increasing that goal, with Mom or Dad able to be anywhere in the house when she went upstairs. She agreed and said that would probably start out at a 5 rating of anxiety.
- Mornings with no fuss. This had been going very well. Most of the time she did it, but on some days, she lost it and melted down, crying and screaming. We discussed what had happened on those days. Usually the meltdowns were triggered by something not going smoothly in the morning, including fighting with her brother, having a hard time picking what to wear, or not being hungry for breakfast. We discussed how to use music in the morning to help her keep calm. We also discussed again how to talk

back to her anxious feelings. She still wanted to work on this, so it stayed on her chart.

- No fussing with sports. This was something she had been mastering. She now said it was about a 3 and much easier. She'd been reading her positive thoughts before getting in the car and enjoying music in the car. Now she said she didn't have to read the positive thoughts—she remembered them— but would continue to use music. This also stayed on her chart.

- Fussing before tests. This was also much better. She had a big standardized test coming up soon, so we decided to keep this on the chart until she got through that test. We identified her anxious thoughts about the test, and she would write them down.

- Birthday party. She had planned for her birthday party and was looking forward to it. It was in less than a week. We discussed how, right before the party, she might get worried and might need to use her calm-down list to help her. She had to remember to challenge her anxious thoughts. She could now get points for working on staying calm before the party and not having a meltdown. Her parents now understood, in advance, what could trigger her anxiety and were learning to help her be prepared with strategies that would help avoid difficulties.

Overall, Lily had done a great job meeting these challenges and seemed very happy with herself. But we still had to address her hardest goal: sleeping in her bed, something she hadn't been able to do for years. She looked upset and didn't want to talk about it. We discussed breaking it down, with the first step being a parent sitting next to her bed until she falls asleep. I reassured her that they would not leave until after she was asleep. Lily said she would like to listen to a book instead of music at night. We agreed it should be a book she'd already read, so she wasn't staying up to hear what came next—distracting but not stimulating. Her mother or father would stay with her, but after they said goodnight, the lights would go out, and the book would go on.

At that point, there would be no more talking. It would be as if the parents were not in the room. I made it clear that if Lily tried to talk to her mom or dad after this point, they would ignore her. It was time to go to sleep. She agreed to start with that.

Once Lily was comfortable with this approach, which would probably take several days, her parents would then move their chair closer to the door but do the same routine. When she was comfortable with that, they would move the chair out of the room, step by step, until she could fall asleep alone in her room.

Lily was reminded that her fears at night were "fake fears," and that she needed to label them and focus on the book she was listening to. We discussed the points, and I suggested she get 10 points for the first night she does every new step, and 5 points for practicing the same step until she was comfortable. She agreed and was excited to earn so many points.

We discussed when she would start this. A long holiday weekend coming up seemed ideal, because no one had to get up early for school or work, so there would be less anxiety about getting sleep. We all agreed that she would start then, and we talked about one new prize she wanted to earn, another audiobook. Lily's dad had never looked happier. He was eager to sleep in his bed instead of on the couch.

In short, while Lily continued to make progress, getting through all the steps was a process. She was learning that she was the "boss" of her brain and that she could control her worries. That is always a breakthrough.

Next Steps

Lily continued to make progress with her worries. After a few weeks of working on sleeping in her own bed, she was sleeping independently through the night. Her parents were thrilled. They didn't realize it could be changed so quickly. They've learned how to anticipate Lily's triggers for her worries and help her in advance to use her strategies to relax and stay in control. Now, Lily continues to earn prizes, and things are much better. They don't need to meet together anymore but agreed that if things get difficult again, they will come back for a "tune-up."

Dagan and Sheila's Story

GAD affects kids of all ages. Eric is a teenage example. His parents met with me first.

His father, Dagan, started: "We are here because of our 16-year-old son. Eric's a great student, a star soccer player, who plays year round, and a terrific kid. The problem is, he worries way too much. He worries not only about getting into college, but the other night, he was worrying about never finding a good job after college, and not having enough money to live . . . For god's sake, he's 16 years old! He worries about other things too. He's always studying like crazy before a test, and then he can't sleep because he worries he won't get a good enough grade. He stays up to all hours of the night doing homework. His grades, by the way, are fine. He tells us he always has trouble sleeping, because, I guess, there's always something this kid can worry about. I don't get it. He has a great life, and what does he have to worry about, really?"

Sheila then added, "What really has us concerned is that he's a great athlete, but he worries that he doesn't have strong enough muscles. I know teenage girls worry about their bodies, but I didn't know boys did. He wants to get a six pack, and he worries that he's fat. He's not fat. He works out in the gym and plays soccer all the time, and he's in great shape. For the last couple of months, he's been worrying about food. Out of the blue, he doesn't want to eat this or that, because it has too much fat or too many calories. I don't want him to start getting some crazy eating disorder on top of everything else. He still eats his ice cream and French fries, but he has a lot of worries about it."

Sheila wondered about the differences between their children. "He has an older sister, and we never had these problems with her. Are boys different with puberty? Do you think he could have other worries about his body? He needs help to stop worrying so much and to enjoy these teenage years."

Dagan added, "He also is a bit of a hypochondriac. I mean, any little ache or pain or minor illness, he blows way out of proportion. He worries he has a tumor or some horrible disease and is going to die. We have to keep telling him he's fine. And Sheila and I are in good health, but I swear, we even sneeze and he's all over us with questions about what's wrong with us. He worries we are going to get sick and die. He's done this since he was a little kid."

When I asked about family history, both Dagan and Sheila were very open.

"I'll be honest with you," Dagan said. "My brother died of a heroin overdose. Eric doesn't know the whole story. He thinks it was a heart attack. It happened seven years ago, and Eric was so young, we didn't want him to get all worried and upset. My brother used to be a worrier, just like Eric, but then he got into drugs, and there was no helping him. God knows we tried. He was in and out of treatment centers. My poor parents, what they went through with him . . . I tell my kids, whatever you do, stay away from drugs. I think this whole legalizing marijuana is a big mistake."

Sheila interrupted. "Dagan, let's not get into that now. Tell her about your cousins."

"Oh yeah, my cousins, three of them actually, were all diagnosed with ADHD. They were a wild bunch, and one of my sisters, she told me she takes medicine for anxiety, but I thought that was just because of my brother's death. His death really shook us all up. I don't want my kids getting into any of that. It really scares me about Eric."

Sheila then talked about her family. "Well, I certainly am an anxious person. It got really bad after Eric was born. Something about having two kids and the responsibility of it all freaked me out. Then I started worrying that I was going to hurt the baby. It was terrible, and I couldn't sleep. They said it was postpartum depression, but I think it was my anxiety getting out of control. So I started taking medicine, and I still take it. It helps me not to get so worried all the time. My father was a big-time worrier too.

"Mr. Worst Case Scenario. If there was something that could go wrong, he had already worried about it. He was always convinced that the worst thing possible was going to happen. My poor dad, he was always wound tight." Her eyes filled up. "I'm sorry. He just passed away last year, and I still miss him. That was hard for Eric. He was close to his grandfather. I think his anxiety got worse after that."

Dagan agreed. "Yes, that was tough for all of us. He was a great man. Eric became more of a health nut after his death. He was constantly worrying that he might die or we could die. Remember that? He couldn't stop talking about death and dying and how scared he was."

Sheila nodded. "He's better with that now, but you're right. It took months for him to tone down all his worries about death. I guess that isn't normal."

"I have to ask this," Dagan said to me. "Could all this worrying lead Eric into drugs and alcohol? My brother's death killed my parents. They have never been the same. I still feel so haunted by it, wondering if there was something I could've done to help my brother. I couldn't bear to lose my son that way."

I explained to Dagan and Sheila that having an untreated anxiety disorder does increase the risk for substance abuse because it can become a way to self-medicate to reduce anxiety.

Dagan immediately looked worried. We discussed how alcohol and drugs can be relaxing and make the worries, for some kids, go away temporarily, but then they have more problems. On the other hand, I have treated many anxious kids who are afraid of alcohol and drugs because they can't bear to lose control. I had recently worked with a teen who had ended up in the emergency room after smoking marijuana because the feeling of being out of control had caused him to panic, and then he had thought he was dying.

I emphasized that it's important for Eric to learn how to manage his anxiety so he doesn't experience difficulties later. I also suggested that they tell Eric the real story about his uncle's death. Better he hear the facts from them than from someone else, and it might motivate him to stay away from drugs because they took the life of his uncle. With the family history of addiction, he's at higher risk and needs to be very careful about drugs and alcohol. They agreed to tell him.

Okay, Eric was up next.

Eric's Story

Eric wanted to meet alone with me to talk about his concerns.

"I worry about everything. I can't help it. I love soccer, and I really want to get a soccer scholarship. I want to play in college, so of course, in every game I worry about a zillion things. Getting goals, obviously, but then I worry about getting injured. Can you imagine? One big injury, and that's the end of my days as a soccer player. I'm one of the best players on the team, so that has me worried. I feel like, lately, I've been holding back in the field. If I mess up . . . I can't mess up. Even my coach said something about it. He said, 'Keep your head in the game, Eric. What's going on with you? Get out there and score!' Now I'm worried about the coach being upset with me. So much pressure."

He added, "I worry about tests, grades, getting into the right college, getting a job after college. I know I take longer than anyone else doing my homework. I can never feel like I've done enough. How much is enough? What does 'doing my best' mean? Most nights I'm up way past midnight working. When I'm not working on my schoolwork, I feel guilty and worried, thinking I need to work harder."

The worries go on. "I'm starting to worry more about getting fat. I should be in better shape and . . . this is embarrassing, but I worry I'm not developed enough down there, that girls won't like me or guys will laugh at me in the locker room. There's a girl I like in science class, but I'm afraid to ask her out. I keep looking in the mirror, and I don't like what I see. I think I'm fat, and I know I'm not big enough. I can't stop thinking about this.

"I get good grades, although lately it's been harder and harder to keep them up. I have lots of friends, if only I didn't worry so much. I'm tired of it. It's exhausting, and I wish I was like everybody else. Even my friend Rob said, 'Eric, loosen up. What's wrong with you?' I know this can't be normal."

Like most kids with anxiety, Eric thought he was the only one who had these feelings. I let him know that lots of kids share these worries, and we could work on freeing him from worrying so much. After I explained to Eric how cognitive behavioral therapy works, he was eager to begin.

Step 1: Target Anxious Thoughts and Behaviors

We explored Eric's anxious thoughts and behaviors. They generally fell into two categories: the first was worrying and ruminating over various issues. The second was perfectionism, which included worrying about his performance in school and sports. His perfectionism led to working too hard on homework, to the point where he often got fewer than five hours of sleep at night. Most of Eric's anxiety involved thoughts and not behaviors. It was fueled by how he put so much pressure on himself at school, in sports, and with friends, especially girls.

Eric started making his list of anxious thoughts:

- My homework is not good enough.
- I'm going to fail the next test.
- I'm going to stink in soccer.
- I'm not going to have a good life (job, family, money, etc.).
- I'm not strong enough or big enough, and I'm fat.
- I have a fatal disease.
- My parents have a fatal disease and will die.

He also listed his anxious behaviors:

- Overproducing on my homework and spending too much time making it perfect.
- Studying much more than is needed for tests.
- Becoming more restrictive in my eating, due to worries about getting fat.
- Examining myself in the mirror to make sure I'm not getting fat.
- Checking the size of my penis and researching penis size on the Internet.
- Seeking reassurance from my parents.

At this point, I needed to explore whether Eric was depressed in addition to his anxiety. Depression is a serious illness that affects many teens. When I asked him about his mood, he denied any depression. He said he can get down about the worrying, but if he didn't have all those worries, he'd be fine. Significant anxiety can be depressing, a normal reaction to anxiety, not an additional diagnosis. Eric had great friends, a supportive family, and a general optimism about his future.

A thorough assessment of depression is always important to do. After assessing Eric, I felt confident that he was not suffering from any mood disorder but was experiencing the saddening effects of his anxiety disorder. I also screened him for suicide risk, which is critical to do with every patient. Sometimes parents are afraid to bring up suicide for fear that it might give their child this idea. To the contrary, openly asking about suicidal thoughts is crucial. Eric was clear that he had no suicidal thoughts or other thoughts about wanting to hurt himself. He just wanted relief from his anxiety.

"Most of the time, I'm pretty happy," he said. "I'm just exhausted from worrying so much. I wish I could make it stop."

I told him we were on the right track.

Step 2: Rate the Anxious Behavior

We talked about how Eric had to change the way he thinks as well as some of his behaviors. We discussed how hard it would be to make these changes. Eric then rated the difficulty on a scale of 0 (easy) to 10 (impossible).

- Not worry about college and his future **8**
- Not worry about soccer **6**
- Be more aggressive in soccer and not hold back **3**
- Not worry about tests **8**
- Set limits with homework **8**
- Not worry about girls **5**
- Ask a girl out **4**
- Not worry about his body **4**
- Not examine his body in the mirror **5**
- Not seek reassurance about his body **8**

- Not be picky about his food **3**
- Not seek reassurance about the fat content of food **2**
- Not worry about having a serious illness **4**
- Not seek reassurance about a serious disease when he is not feeling well **7**
- Not worry about his parents being so sick they will die **3**
- Not seek reassurance from his parents when they are sick **4**

Step 3: Agree on Challenges to Work On

Eric looked seriously at his list for what seemed like a long time. He couldn't decide what to work on. He was demonstrating for me how he tends to overthink everything and become overwhelmed. He then seemed to get lost and unfocused on what he needed to do. He needed to be reminded that there was no perfect choice. I suggested he break it down by focusing on the easiest first. It was clear how tasks could take him a long time because he got very caught up in the details and couldn't see the whole picture. I had to remind him that this choice didn't have to be perfect; he should just pick.

Once I helped him break it down, he agreed to the following:

- Be more aggressive in soccer.
- Stop being picky about his food.
- Not examine his body in the mirror.
- Not seek reassurance about his body or food.
- Ask a girl out.

The goals felt challenging but not too overwhelming, so he was willing to start with these and then work up to the harder goals.

Step 4: Initiate and Teach Strategies to Practice

Eric identified his thoughts about soccer. He said, "When I'm playing, and even before the game, I start thinking, *What if I mess up in front of every-one? I will be letting my team down, the coach will be disappointed, and no one will think I'm such a good player anymore. I won't get a scholarship, I won't go to college, and I will have a terrible life.* Once I start thinking this way, I get more afraid to even try to score."

We then discussed what the realistic thoughts are:

- I'm a good player. I work hard at developing my skills, I want to score, and no one's a perfect soccer player.
- If I mess up, everyone will not be focusing on that, and it won't change the way they think of me.
- My coach likes me and has confidence in me.
- My team needs me to put myself in the game and play the best I can.
- If I don't get a scholarship, I can still go to college.

He then identified his anxious thoughts about food:

- If I eat this, I will get fat.
- If I get fat, girls won't like me.

Next, we worked on replacement thoughts:

- I don't have a weight problem.
- I'm a healthy eater.
- Everything is fine in moderation, and I enjoy food.

Then he listed his anxious thoughts about his body:

- I'm getting fat.
- I don't have enough muscles.
- Girls won't like my body because I don't look strong enough, and my penis is too small.

Replacement thoughts:

- I'm healthy and fit; there is nothing wrong with how I look and how strong I am.
- I'm not too small, and my penis is normal. My doctor told me everything about my body is normal.

Eric revealed that there's a girl, Lucy, in his science class that he's friendly with and wants to ask out but has been too afraid.

His anxious thoughts are:

- What if she says no? I'll be humiliated.
- I don't know how to ask her.
- I can't think of where to go with her.
- What if she really doesn't like me?

Replacement thoughts:

- She's always friendly and seems to like me.
- I could text her and ask her if she wants to go to the movies this weekend.
- If she says no, I tried, and it doesn't have to be such a big deal.

We discussed his seeking reassurance. He agreed to stop it and, when he gets the urge, to remind himself that it's just his anxiety and he doesn't need to focus on it. He then agreed to read these lists of anxious thoughts and replacement thoughts every day to help him keep focused on what is rational.

Eric seems to have a lot of free-floating anxiety. "I feel like I'm always stressed, and I can't relax."

We discussed the use of mindfulness in managing his anxiety. He agreed to work on meditation, using a meditation app on his phone, for fifteen minutes a day. I also talked with him about observing his anxious thoughts but not engaging with them—keeping a distance from them. Labeling them helps with this, as does realizing that these anxious thoughts are meaningless and not important. Keeping his focus on the here and now, what is really going on around and within him, will help him relax.

Next, we discussed other relaxing activities he could build into his life. He already exercised, which was helpful. We talked about using music, which he loves. He agreed to listen to music before bed as a way of relaxing and turning off his worries. He needed to get more sleep, but he was still very driven to work too much on homework. That was something he needed to work on, so he agreed to practice these strategies to help manage his stress and to proceed with our steps.

Step 5: Note and Chart Progress Made

Like most teenagers, Eric had his phone with him all the time, so keeping track of his work on his phone made the most sense. In the notes section of his phone, he listed his anxious thoughts and replacement thoughts. He put in a daily reminder to review them.

Before each soccer game, he would write concrete goals for himself, and after the game, he would review how well he did with them. For example, he decided to take a shot at a goal anytime the ball was near and he had a chance, instead of avoiding it.

He thought afternoons, after school, would be the ideal time for him to take fifteen minutes to meditate. He put reminders in for that.

He also made a playlist to listen to at night to help him relax before bed.

Step 6: Offer Incentives to Motivate

Eric felt that he did not need incentives, but he wanted his parents to know what he was working on. We invited them to join us toward the end of the session to learn about his goals. Eric shared that he was going to really make an effort at not seeking reassurance from them. They were very supportive and asked if they could do anything to help. Eric suggested that if he forgot and asked for reassurance, they could remind him that his anxiety was talking and not answer his anxious questions. Dagan then asked what they should say to Eric if he asks for reassurance. Eric thought for a few minutes and then said, "Just say 'Stop.'" They agreed.

Step 7: Reinforce Progress and Increase Challenges

After three weeks, Eric was happy to report his progress. He had gone to the movies with Lucy. He had been much more engaged in soccer, and his coach had recently commented on how his game had improved. He had worked on not seeking reassurance about food and his body, and his worries about both were much lessened.

Eric had been applying the music and meditation strategy, but not every day. He complained that his life was so busy, it was hard to find time. He said that even with the reminders, he would be busy doing something else, and then forget. He reported that his school worries had gotten worse, and he was still getting very little sleep. Math was particularly difficult, and his grades were falling. He was getting worried about taking the SAT, even though it was six months away. He said, "I can't stop thinking about college and getting into a good school and worrying I won't be able to. I'm getting more and more stressed. All my friends are starting to talk about college, and that's really making me crazy."

We invited his parents into the conversation. They agreed that he'd made good progress with the things he'd worked on, but they were seeing him get less sleep and worry more and more about school.

Sheila said, "He got a C on his last math test, and I thought it was going to put him over the edge. He's never gotten a C before, and he's working so hard. We don't know what to do to help him."

We discussed several options. One was to consider a medication evaluation. Another was to consider having a neuropsychological battery of tests done to see if there might be something, other than anxiety, that could be making it harder for him to reduce his time on homework. He might have organizational or attention difficulties, or an undiagnosed learning disability. Once we had more information, the skills and strategies to help him would be clearer.

Eric and his family decided to get the testing and postpone discussion of medication. He agreed to keep working at the CBT as well, since there had definitely been progress.

Next Steps

Eric got the results from his neuropsychological evaluation and it showed that, in addition to anxiety, he had attention deficit hyperactivity disorder (ADHD), which was contributing to his academic difficulties. He was a smart kid, so the ADHD had not been a problem until he encountered the increased demands of high school. In the earlier grades, he was able to do well even without paying attention. High school was different. If he got distracted, he quickly fell behind. Falling behind triggered his anxiety, which distracted him more. This had become a vicious circle for Eric and was a major reason his homework took so long.

Anxiety disorders and ADHD often go together, and each one makes the other worse. An anxious child who is distracted and unable to concentrate and know what is going on becomes more anxious. An impulsive child who blurts out answers or interrupts others becomes more anxious due to feeling so out of control. In addition, anxiety can be distracting; sitting in class and worrying about things can make it difficult to concentrate. Anxiety can also make some kids appear hyperactive. Noticing if the symptoms of inattention and hyperactivity are still present when a child is not anxious can give a clue as to whether these are symptoms of generalized anxiety or of two separate conditions. It is important to tease this out, and sometimes that's best done through a comprehensive neuropsychological evaluation, which is what helped Eric and his parents understand his challenges.

The combination of a neuropsychological evaluation and the clinical information about anxiety can be useful in sorting out the cause of a child's distraction level. Many kids have both ADHD and anxiety, and on the surface, the symptoms can look the same, but asking key questions helps figure out what is causing the distraction. A common example is parents complaining about the long showers their kids are taking. With ADHD, the long showers are caused by kids standing in the shower spaced out, relaxing, and not realizing how the time is passing. Kids with anxiety are in the shower for a long time worrying that they might not be clean enough and feeling they need to wash more and more. On the surface, the symptom is the same: forty-five-minute showers. But the cause is very different. The same dynamic is seen with a child who is distracted in school. Is the child daydreaming or busy worrying? It looks the same to the teacher, since the child is not paying attention, but the cause is either lack of attention, intense worrying, or, as in Eric's case, both.

Eric had a difficult time maintaining attention and then would panic when he realized he had missed what he needed to be doing in school. The more anxious he was, the more difficult it was for him to pay attention. His ADHD fueled his anxiety, and his anxiety fueled his ADHD. Both needed to be addressed. He is now working with a tutor to help him stay organized, and his parents have requested accommodations at school, including extra time for tests and being able to sit in the front of the class so he has fewer distractions.

Eric also had a medication evaluation and has been taking medication for his anxiety and to improve his attention. Eric and his parents report much progress, and they have a greater understanding about what has made things so difficult. His grades have improved, he's getting more sleep, and he is worrying less. He tells me that it's easier to use the strategies we discussed, and he can more easily push away the worries. His parents report the most important thing for them: Eric seems much happier.

Eric is a good example of how complicated kids can be. Because he has always had high anxiety, it was easy to assume that anxiety was his only problem. Yet his ADHD was greatly contributing to his anxiety. Understanding this helped us work on all the issues he was struggling with, not just his anxiety.

DSM-5 Guidelines

The *DSM-5* identifies the diagnostic criteria necessary for a diagnosis. The assumption is that many readers will have children who meet some but not all the criteria.

Generalized Anxiety Disorder

A. Excessive anxiety and worry (apprehensive expectation), occurring more days than not for at least 6 months, about a number of events or activities (such as work or school performance).

B. The individual finds it difficult to control the worry.

C. The anxiety and worry are associated with three (or more) of the following six symptoms (with at least some symptoms having been present for more days than not for the past 6 months):

Note: Only one item is required in children.

1. Restlessness or feeling keyed up or on edge.

2. Being easily fatigued.

3. Difficulty concentrating or mind going blank.

4. Irritability.

5. Muscle tension.

6. Sleep disturbance (difficulty falling or staying asleep, or restless, unsatisfying sleep).

D. The anxiety, worry, or physical symptoms cause clinically significant distress or impairment in social, occupational, or other important areas of functioning.

E. The disturbance is not attributable to the physiological effects of a substance (e.g., a drug of abuse, a medication) or another medical condition (e.g., hyperthyroidism).

F. The disturbance is not better explained by another mental disorder
    (e.g., anxiety or worry about having panic attacks in panic disorder,
    negative evaluation in social anxiety disorder [social phobia], contami-
    nation or other obsessions in obsessive-compulsive disorder, separation
    from attachment figures in separation anxiety disorder, reminders of
    traumatic events in post-traumatic stress disorder, gaining weight in
    anorexia nervosa, physical complaints in somatic symptom disorder,
    perceived appearance flaws in body dysmorphic disorder, having a
    serious illness in illness anxiety disorder, or the content of delusional
    beliefs in schizophrenia or delusional disorder).

American Psychiatric Association. "Generalized Anxiety Disorder." In *Diagnostic and
Statistical Manual of Mental Disorders.* 5th ed. Washington, DC: American Psychiatric Association, 2013.

Attention-Deficit/Hyperactivity Disorder

A. A persistent pattern of inattention and/or hyperactivity-impulsivity that
    interferes with functioning or development, as characterized by (1) and/
    or (2):

    1. **Inattention:** Six (or more) of the following symptoms have persisted for at
        least six months to a degree that is inconsistent with developmental level
        and that negatively impacts directly on social and academic/occupational
        activities.

        Note: The symptoms are not solely a manifestation of oppositional behavior, defi-
        ance, hostility, or failure to understand tasks or instructions. For older adolescents
        and adults (age 17 or older), at least five symptoms are required.

        a. Often fails to give close attention to details or makes careless mistakes
            in schoolwork, at work, or during other activities (e.g., overlooks or
            misses details, work is inaccurate).

        b. Often has difficulty sustaining attention in tasks or play activities (e.g.,
            has difficulty remaining focused during lectures, conversations, or
            lengthy reading).

        c. Often does not seem to listen when spoken to directly (e.g., mind seems
            elsewhere, even in the absence of any obvious distraction).

        d. Often does not follow through on instructions and fails to finish
            schoolwork, chores, or duties in the workplace (e.g., starts tasks but
            quickly loses focus and is easily sidetracked).

e. Often has difficulty organizing tasks and activities (e.g., difficulty managing sequential tasks; difficulty keeping materials and belongings in order; messy, disorganized work; has poor time management; fails to meet deadlines).

f. Often avoids, dislikes, or is reluctant to engage in tasks that require sustained mental effort (e.g., schoolwork or homework; for older adolescents and adults, preparing reports, completing forms, reviewing lengthy papers).

g. Often loses things necessary for tasks or activities (e.g., school materials, pencils, books, tools, wallets, keys, paperwork, eyeglasses, mobile telephones).

h. Is often easily distracted by extraneous stimuli (for older adolescents and adults, may include unrelated thoughts).

i. Is often forgetful in daily activities (e.g., doing chores, running errands; for older adolescents and adults, returning calls, paying bills, keeping appointments).

2. **Hyperactivity and impulsivity:** Six (or more) of the following symptoms have persisted for at least six months to a degree that is inconsistent with developmental level and that negatively impacts directly on social and academic/occupational activities:

Note: The symptoms are not solely a manifestation of oppositional behavior, defiance, hostility, or a failure to understand tasks or instructions. For older adolescents and adults (age 17 and older), at least five symptoms are required.

a. Often fidgets with or taps hands or feet or squirms in seat.

b. Often leaves seat in situations when remaining seated is expected (e.g., leaves his or her place in the classroom, in the office or other workplace, or in other situations that require remaining in place).

c. Often runs about or climbs in situations where it is inappropriate. (**Note:** In adolescents or adults, may be limited to feeling restless.)

d. Often unable to play or engage in leisure activities quietly.

e. Is often "on the go" acting as if "driven by a motor" (e.g., is unable to be or uncomfortable being still for extended time, as in restaurants, meetings; may be experienced by others as being restless or difficult to keep up with).

f. Often talks excessively.

g. Often blurts out an answer before a question has been completed (e.g., completes people's sentences; cannot wait for turn in conversation).

h. Often has difficulty waiting his or her turn (e.g., while waiting in line).

i. Often interrupts or intrudes on others (e.g., butts into conversations, games, or activities; may start using other people's things without asking or receiving permission; for adolescents and adults, may intrude into or take over what others are doing).

B. Several inattentive or hyperactive-impulsive symptoms were present prior to age 12 years.

C. Several inattentive or hyperactive-impulsive symptoms are present in two or more settings (e.g., at home, school, or work; with friends or relatives; in other activities).

D. There is clear evidence that the symptoms interfere with, or reduce the quality of social, academic, or occupational functioning.

E. The symptoms do not occur exclusively during the course of schizophrenia or another psychotic disorder and are not better explained by another mental disorder (e.g., mood disorder, anxiety disorder, dissociative disorder, personality disorder, substance intoxication or withdrawal).

American Psychiatric Association. "Attention-Deficit/Hyperactivity Disorder." In *Diagnostic and Statistical Manual of Mental Disorders*. 5th ed. Washington, DC: American Psychiatric Association, 2013.

Chapter 4

Silent Liza and Hidden Patrick

Selective Mutism and Social Anxiety

Selective mutism is an anxiety-based disorder in which the anxiety is focused on speaking. It is an extreme form of social anxiety, which is why these disorders are grouped together in this chapter.

Selective Mutism

Children with selective mutism usually speak freely and normally at home but are mute in other situations, particularly at school. The disorder is often evident when they go to preschool and do not speak at all. Their anxiety can be so severe that they are often described as having the "deer in the headlight" look of sheer terror when expected to speak. There are many myths about these children, including that they have been traumatized or that they are just stubborn, with overprotective mothers. Nothing could be further from the truth. Selectively mute children all have one thing in common: anxiety.

With a phobia about speaking, children with selective mutism often don't want any attention from others. Birthday parties with singing and a cake can feel overwhelming, and eye contact can be difficult when others are speaking to them. At the same time, most of these children, to the surprise of others, are chatty and outgoing at home with their immediate family.

Early intervention with these children is crucial. The longer this disorder goes on untreated, the harder it is to treat. Teenagers with selective mutism have already lived silent lives. They get by; schools often make accommodations for them, enabling their silence. They frequently have no friends, because it is hard to be a nonverbal friend. Silent play dates may work in preschool, but not in adolescence. They have become the child who doesn't speak, and staying in that environment makes it difficult to speak. If they are known as the child who doesn't speak, they think that to start speaking would draw attention to them. These kids hate that attention; it increases their anxiety. Ironically, selectively mute kids who are placed in a different environment, among people who don't know they don't speak, will often have an easier time speaking.

Selectively mute teens may seem odd because they have not had normal social development. Their lives are limited yet all too comfortable because of the well-meaning accommodations given to them. Motivating these older children with selective mutism becomes very difficult. At that point, parents are desperate; many have tried traditional therapy or medications, which have failed. They worry about how their child can ever become independent. These teens are not easy to treat, because they are so used to getting by without speaking.

Unfortunately, I have seen far too many of these teens, which motivates me to advocate strongly for early intervention with selectively mute kids. Many of these older kids who have been selectively mute for many years often have an additional diagnosis of being on the autism spectrum. They often speak fully at home, however, without any language difficulties.

In the following pages, you will hear one family's story about their daughter's selective mutism and how they used the TRAINOR Method to change behaviors. The TRAINOR Method focuses the cognitive behavioral therapy on training parents to apply CBT strategies to help their child speak in social and school environments, without focusing on getting the child to speak with the therapist. The idea is that spending a lot of time getting children to speak with the therapist does not easily translate to the children speaking where they really need to speak, to their friends and in school. Focusing the intervention specifically on the child's environment, with parents and teachers working together to directly apply CBT strategies, is a more effective and powerful approach to curing selective mutism.

Isabella's Story

Isabella came to me because her daughter, Liza, was in kindergarten and not speaking. At our first visit, this is how she described the situation: "Liza is 5—smart, funny, and a delight to be around. We have a 3-year-old daughter, Ariel, and our son, Patrick, is 7. Liza plays well with her brother and sister, and honestly, if you saw her running around our house screaming and laughing with her brother and sister, you would think nothing's wrong." Isabella began enthusiastically, but then she turned serious. "Obviously something is very wrong. She doesn't speak at all in school, not even to her teacher. She doesn't talk to the other children, although she plays with them, and they like her, and she gets invited to all their birthday parties. Liza talks at home when she gets ready for school, but her silence begins when I walk her to the bus stop. As soon as we get close, she becomes silent, even though her best friend is there."

Isabella sighed, then continued. "Her problem with speaking is not just in school. She doesn't speak to some of her aunts and uncles. She speaks to my mother, but not much to my father. My husband's parents live out of state, and when they come to visit, she's quiet at first but then warms up to them and talks. In restaurants, she talks freely to us but usually asks us to order her food." I was beginning to get a picture of Liza, and the family's dynamics, as Isabella went on to share more.

"Her best friend, Annie, is in her class and lives on our street. They play together almost every day. She talks to Annie when she comes to play at our house, and she is normal with her when she plays at Annie's house, but she doesn't speak to Annie's parents. And at the bus stop and school, she doesn't even speak to Annie, which must be confusing for her." I asked Isabella how long this had been going on.

"I first realized this was a problem in preschool," she said. "I spoke to her pediatrician, and he said I should 'leave it alone' and she would 'grow out of it.' Now she's in kindergarten. She's not growing out of it. If anything, it may be getting worse." Isabella took a deep breath, then slowly exhaled. "I worry because other people never get to see the real Liza—the bubbly, chatty girl we know. They see this silent girl. Liza can already read, but her teachers don't know that because she's so silent at school. She's smarter than they realize. She likes school and is happy to go," Isabella explained. "But when she comes home, she talks and talks and is really hyper and can be mean to her younger sister. I wonder if it's because she's been so silent at school all day."

At this point, I asked Isabella what Liza had told her about her silence. "When I try to talk to her about talking, she gets angry and won't discuss it. I've tried ignoring it, and I've tried getting angry about it. Nothing works. Frankly, when she doesn't answer people who talk to her, she looks rude. I usually answer for her and say something about her being shy. I feel embarrassed. I don't know what to do to help her." Then Isabella introduced information about her husband. "Her father tries, too," she said, looking away a moment, then back at me. "He jokes about it with Liza, and tells me to lighten up about it. He had anxiety as a child, so he's more tolerant than I am. I find myself getting so annoyed, feeling like those two are buddies and I'm the bad guy." Here, Isabella stopped and leaned her head in her hand. "I'm very worried about her."

The parents' story, of course, is from their perspective. When the child finally feels safe talking to someone about it, her story begins to unravel the mystery.

Liza's Story

Having worked with many hundreds of kids with selective mutism, I know Liza's story. I know it from what these children tell their parents, and I know it from what they tell me when they are cured. I am very practical in my approach to working with these children. My goal is not to get them to speak to me; it is to get them to speak in their world. I could spend many hours weekly to get them to speak to me, but that would be limited to once or twice a week, and I need them to be talking to people in their daily life, which doesn't include me. Focusing my therapy on getting them to speak to me seems a waste, since it will not generalize to others. Even when these kids are very comfortable, they often still communicate nonverbally. The TRAINOR Method places the focus on helping selectively mute children to speak by working with their parents. Their parents, whom they love, want to please, and are most comfortable speaking to, hold the key to their recovery. Parents can be the bridge to them speaking to other important people in their lives. My role is to guide their parents. This is Liza's story, which I have learned through working with many selectively mute children and their parents.

"I hate when Mommy and Daddy talk to me about talking. I hate it when they ask why I don't talk. I hate when they tell me to talk when we go places. I can't and I won't! It feels too bad. I don't know why it feels bad to talk. I guess I just don't want to feel those bad feelings. It's easier to not talk. Why do I have to talk? Maybe I'll talk when I go to first grade or when I'm six. I just want everyone to leave me alone about this. It's too hard."

Liza was a smart little girl, and like most selectively mute children, she had no specific answer to "Why don't you talk?" This often perplexes adults, who believe there has to be a reason. The reason is anxiety. Most of us can remember anxious moments when we were younger, or even as adults. Remember how bad anxiety feels? Hot and red in the face, shaking, scared, heart beating, trouble breathing? That is how Liza felt when asked to talk. She truly did not know why. She just knew she didn't get those bad feelings when she didn't talk, so silence seemed the way to go.

Her parents knew better. They knew that talking was not optional, and they worried about the future if she did not get over this. Once I explained that cognitive behavioral therapy (CBT) would help change the way Liza thought about talking and help change her speaking behavior, they knew they wanted this treatment for her.

But first, I met with Liza's parents, without Liza present, for several good reasons, including those I have mentioned but want to emphasize:

- Liza hated people talking about her talking. It made her feel embarrassed and angry.
- I was a stranger to her. Why would she want a stranger to know about this?
- Liza needed help talking in her world of school and teachers, peers and relatives. More important than her talking to me was my guiding the family to help her talk in places where it would make a difference in her life.
- Most important, Liza spoke freely to her parents. They were a link between her talking world and her silent world. They needed guidance to help her break through this anxiety. Working with Liza's parents and helping them apply the TRAINOR Method was the most effective approach to help Liza.

Step 1: Target Anxious Thoughts and Behaviors

First, we had to identify the thoughts that supported her anxiety. Remember, we look for thoughts that support the common defenses of denial and avoidance. For Liza, these thoughts included the usual denial—"I don't have to talk"—and avoidance—"It feels bad to talk and good to not talk, so I'm not talking." Her parents heard this reasoning from her all the time.

Liza's parents quickly learned that it was important for them to have a consistent and firm message to Liza that challenged her denial and avoidance and, at the same time, normalized her struggle. They learned to tell her things like "All children must talk, and you will also talk. You just need help to talk. It's not an option to not talk. Talking is hard for you, just like riding a bike is hard for some kids (you're great at that!), and with practice, you will talk like all the other kids. You're not shy; you just need help with talking." This message was firm and supportive, exactly the tone her parents needed to use to help her overcome her phobia of speaking.

Liza's parents made a list of all the situations where Liza did not talk and all the people in her life she did not talk to. When it came to talking, how was Liza different from other kids her age? Here is their list:

Liza does not talk

- at school
- at gymnastics, swimming lessons, or any summer camps she has attended
- at the bus stop
- to people who talk to her when shopping with her parents
- to her aunt Beverly or uncle Jim
- to Aunt Cindy
- to Uncle Peter
- to her doctor or dentist

Liza does talk

- at home with her family members
- with Annie at Annie's house and at Liza's house

- on other play dates at her house
- in restaurants, most of the time
- to her grandparents
- to her siblings' friends when they are at her house

Step 2: Rate the Anxious Behavior

Liza's parents talked to her about how difficult it would be for her to talk in these different situations. She, of course, did not want to talk about it, but her parents encouraged her, introducing the prizes she could earn by cooperating.

Since she was so young, we kept the rating system simple: Easy; Hard; Very Hard; Very, Very Hard. Here are her ratings:

Talking:

- at school
  Very, Very Hard
- at lessons and camp
  Very, Very Hard
- at the bus stop   **Hard**

- to people who talk to
  her when shopping   **Very Hard**
- to her aunts and uncles   **Hard**
- to order her food in
  restaurants   **Easy**

Step 3: Agree on Challenges to Work On

Liza's parents had a good idea of how hard all these speaking challenges would be for her—very, very hard. We discussed breaking the challenges down to be more manageable.

Talking at school was a big priority, so we listed several options:

- Liza talking to her parents as they get closer to the bus stop
- Mom taking Annie and Liza away from the large group of kids at the bus stop and playing a quick game with them where they have to talk, such as a guessing game
- Having more play dates at her house with the children from her class so that they hear her voice, and she experiences herself talking to them
- Having one of her parents play with Liza and Annie in the classroom after school so that she can experience herself talking in the classroom

- Once Liza has mastered talking in the empty classroom with her friend, introducing the teacher gradually into the room, so the teacher hears Liza's voice while she is playing

This list was a start to help Liza become desensitized, step by step, to talking. Because Liza talked freely with her parents, we hoped that they could introduce this list to her when she felt relaxed at home.

Liza's parents left my office with the challenging task of talking to her about these goals and getting her agreement on what to work on first. They needed her to buy into this plan, because she had to do the work of practicing these steps. I reminded Liza's parents to reinforce her speaking behavior and give her incentives for any time she speaks in a way she never spoke before. She needs to get the message that the more she speaks, the more she gains. She has a phobia of speaking. It makes her extremely anxious, and she would like to simply stay silent. As a little girl, she doesn't understand why this is not a choice she can make. She needs a lot of encouragement and a strong consistent message from her parents:

- She can do this.
- It will get easier as soon as she talks.
- Worrying about talking is a "silly worry"—we laugh at those worries and push ahead.

Since Liza is a little girl, we decided to call the steps a "talking game," so she would want to play. I reminded her parents to be firm, supportive, and positive. Liza felt scared, like she could not talk in difficult circumstances; they could help her by making sure the goals were challenging but not overwhelming. By keeping a positive "You can do it" attitude, Liza's parents could help her learn to talk back to the fear and push herself past it. She could learn to "just do it!"

Liza agreed to talk to her parents as they neared the bus stop. She also agreed to work on having more play dates with two girls from her class, Keesha and Jamie. And she would play with Annie after school in her classroom with her father present, when no one else was there. This was a great list of starting goals.

Step 4: Identify and Teach Strategies to Practice

The cognitive strategies involved reinforcing the same message to Liza: "You can talk. All kids must talk. You will talk, and we will help you. You can do this. It will get easy for you." The message also included the idea that she's not shy. Some selectively mute children get the idea that it's okay not to talk because they are shy. Liza's temperament was not quiet. At home, without anxiety, she was a chatterbox who wanted to be an actress. She needed to learn that her anxiety about speaking was something she had to push through. The behavioral strategies involved doing this step by step. Liza learned that she needed to push herself to do it—"Don't think about it, just do it!"

Step 5: Note and Chart Progress Made

I encouraged Liza's parents to make a "talking chart" of her speaking challenges and have her color and decorate it. Even at 5 years old, she needed to take charge of this process because she needed to do the work. Her chart listed the goals she had agreed to and had spaces for bonus stickers. Her parents explained to her that she could earn bonus stickers if she did any "new" talking behavior. Her parents said they would carefully notice when she spoke in a situation where she had not talked before, and later, they would reward her with a bonus sticker. This gave her the message that every time she fought her fear of talking, she won at the talking game. Her talking chart was done. It looked pretty, all decorated by Liza. She felt excited, but we all realized that fighting her fear of speaking would be hard work for little Liza.

Step 6: Offer Incentives to Motivate

We asked Liza to work hard at fighting her anxiety. She started with the attitude that she liked her pretty chart but didn't want to do this and really saw no reason she should. She was not motivated to work at this talking game. Incentives would motivate her. Liza knew that her parents were getting a big prize box with presents for her to pick from every time she did a new speaking behavior. In the prize box were coupons for special time with Mom or Dad, craft items she enjoyed, puzzles, books, and hair bows—all things she loved.

By playing this talking game, she would win stickers and prizes. Every new speaking behavior meant a prize. Practicing that behavior earned her a sticker, and three stickers won another prize. The first time she talked with Annie at the bus stop, she would earn a prize. After practicing it three more times, she would earn three stickers and another prize. With practice, talking to Annie at the bus stop would be natural.

What first felt uncomfortable quickly became easy. Once something on the list is easy, it is crossed off with much praise, and the next challenge is worked on. Step by step, Liza learned that fighting her anxiety is difficult at first, but that it quickly gets easy and feels good.

As part of this process, everyone helping Liza with her talking needed to remember several things. First, when she talked, no one should react. No praise for her. Liza would be anxious in that moment and would not want any attention on her. Teachers and others needed to act as though she had always talked like this. That would reinforce for her that talking is no big deal—she could do it! Later that day, long after her talking accomplishment, she would get her prize and praise, and she would feel happy and proud. Not praising is counterintuitive for most teachers and parents. Teachers are so eager to praise a child who makes progress. For children with this disorder, however, it is their nightmare that people will make a fuss about their speaking and draw attention to it. So everyone has to act like speaking has no importance. Then after, when the child is home, praise and incentives can be offered and readily accepted. In addition to rewarding Liza for reaching her goals on her list, whenever she did a new talking behavior that was not on her list, she would earn a prize.

For example, when Liza talked to a child at the playground, her mother noticed that was something she had never done before. It was not on Liza's list, but when they returned home, she received a bonus prize. She knew that the next time she talked at the playground, she would get a sticker; three stickers equaled another prize. Her parents paid close attention to the prize process, which reinforced Liza's speaking progress. She learned that the more she spoke, the more prizes she would get, and the easier speaking would become.

Step 7: Reinforce Progress and Increase Challenges

I continued to meet and guide Liza's parents every few weeks as they helped Liza talk more and more. Once a talking behavior became easy, we raised the goal. Liza's teacher was in daily communication with Liza's parents, reporting on progress at school so she could get her prize and stickers when she came home. Daily feedback was essential because quick reinforcement was important for Liza. If she was not rewarded until Friday for something she had done Monday, she would not even remember doing it.

Liza worked hard, and it took time, but she learned to push herself. She and her parents eventually added another anxiety-producing behavior—using the bathroom at school. Many selectively mute children do not feel comfortable using the school bathroom, even when they can nonverbally ask to go. Since first grade would mean full days at school, her parents felt concerned about this. The first step Liza agreed to was to go to the bathroom after school with her mother and then work up to using it during school. Liza's progress with pushing herself when fearful built on itself. She talked more and more, earning her prizes; gradually she became cured of selective mutism.

Some children with selective mutism simply have a phobia of speaking, just as some adults with minimal anxiety have a single irrational phobia—for instance, flying or snakes. These selectively mute children tend to be popular in preschool, even though they don't speak. I have worked with children like this who show no other signs of anxiety once they overcome their selective mutism, including one child who went on to speak on national TV!

Other children with selective mutism also have additional symptoms of anxiety, including perfectionism, separation anxiety, or obsessive compulsive symptoms. These children may need to manage different symptoms of anxiety in the future. The strategies they are learning to overcome their selective mutism will be useful for other anxiety issues, include recognizing the anxiety, setting goals, and not letting anxious feelings cause them to withdraw and avoid challenges.

Next Steps

Liza continued to make progress and even had breakthroughs. She seemed to make baby steps and then, when she was ready, big steps.

She was increasingly talking to her peers and her teachers. Her teachers learned to create opportunities for her without pushing her. They supported her being engaged with peers she liked but didn't put pressure on her to speak. Knowing she would get rewarded at home helped Liza push herself. Her teachers learned to give daily feedback to Liza's parents about her talking progress, but not to give Liza any praise in the moment. This was hard for them, because they clearly saw her progress and instinctively wanted to praise her. They learned that paying attention to Liza as she moved into the talking world would only cause her more anxiety. Together Liza, her parents, and her teachers were very pleased with her continued progress.

Social Anxiety

Social anxiety is one of the most difficult forms of anxiety to identify and to work on, especially when it is not very severe. Parents often don't notice it at first. They have a child who "likes" to stay home and "doesn't like" to do extracurricular activities, play dates, or other social activities. These children avoid as much social interaction with their peers as they can. They often feel more comfortable with younger children or adults. Peer interactions are more anxiety producing. These kids are not on the autism spectrum; their main problem is anxiety.

According to the fifth edition of the *Diagnostic and Statistical Manual of Mental Disorders* (DSM-5), kids on the autism spectrum have difficulties using communication for social purposes, struggle with changing communication to match the needs of the listener, find rules of conversation difficult, and can be very literal in their understanding. They experience these difficulties even when relaxed in the context of familiar situations.

On the other hand, children with social anxiety display none of these difficulties when they are in a relaxed setting. By avoiding social opportunities, however, they are missing out on experiences needed for social development and may appear less mature than their peers. Girls I have worked with who have social anxiety are often very attached to their mothers and to the TV. Boys are usually more involved with computer games, and their only social outlet may be playing games.

Here is one young man's story of how he used the TRAINOR steps to work on his social anxiety. Patrick was 13, and his parents, Lori and David, felt concerned because he did not seem to have many friends and spent most of his free time playing video games.

Lori and David's Story

The first day Lori and David came to see me, Lori told me that they'd had Patrick tested because she had started to worry that he might be depressed, have a learning disability, or have social problems. They had searched for answers for more than a year, trying to figure out how to help him. She said that the testing had shown that he was bright and should be doing better at school. It also said he had anxiety. The neuropsychologist who did the testing recommended that he get cognitive behavioral therapy (CBT), which led his parents to me. "That is why we're here," she said. "Can you work with him?" So I asked them to tell me about Patrick.

"Patrick is a great kid," Lori began. "Maybe we're wrong to worry, but he is home alone so much, it doesn't seem right. He's a decent student. I mean, he's no star student, but he passes all his classes. We always thought he was a really smart kid, but in the last couple of years, his grades have dropped. Instead of getting A's, he now gets B's and even some C's. We know he's capable of more. He seems happy, but it just doesn't seem normal for a 13-year-old boy to have no friends."

She paused, then continued. "We tried talking to his school counselor about this, but she said he seems fine, is always with other boys, and there's no problem. No problem? He comes home every day, does his homework, and then goes on the computer to play video games. He barely stops for dinner and then goes back to playing games until bedtime. The phone never rings. He never gets invited anywhere with friends. We never hear about any friends. Weekends he plays video games by himself or tries to get us to entertain him."

Lori hesitated, looked briefly at her husband, and went on. "David gets angry with him and tells him to get off those darn games and go outside. But that doesn't work. David sometimes has no patience with him. I feel sorry for Patrick; it must be lonely for him. He used to have friends when he was little; in fact, he was rather popular."

David spoke up. "I do get angry at him, and I know I shouldn't, but sometimes I think maybe he's just lazy and needs a kick in the pants. That testing said he has anxiety. Frankly, I'm confused. Watching him at home, he seems pretty relaxed, happy as a clam in front of that computer, playing games, drinking soda, and eating chips. Anxiety? I just don't see it. I suffered from anxiety, had panic attacks as a kid. I know anxiety. Patrick doesn't seem nervous about anything. Stubborn, yes. Spoiled, maybe, but I don't see him as nervous at all. I think the kid just may be lazy."

David's view clearly upset Lori. "This is where we disagree. You think he's lazy, but there has to be more to it than that. Patrick has never been a kid to do much outside of the home. He went through just about every sport. We would sign him up, and after a few practices, he would say he hated it and quit. He doesn't like sports, I guess. Then we thought music. We got him piano lessons, but as soon as someone mentioned a recital, he begged us to quit. We even told him he didn't have to do the recital. We couldn't get him to change his mind. No more music lessons. He says he hates music. We can't force him to do things he doesn't like. Frankly, I dread the summer. He refuses to go to camp. Says he hates camp. I imagine him at home, alone, all summer playing those games. He's gained ten pounds over the last six months, and he's starting to look chubby. I worry about that, too. This isn't normal. We need to help him."

Patrick's Story

Patrick came in to meet with me, and he was clearly angry, no, furious, about being in my office. I found out later that he had exploded at his parents when they'd told him about this appointment and had told them he would not say a word to me. Of course, I understand that even meeting with me challenges his denial, and he doesn't want to move an inch out of his comfort zone. The stronger the resistance, the stronger the anxiety. His anger did not silence him, however; he told me quite a lot. I am sure he was hoping he could convince me to tell his parents to leave him alone.

"I don't know why my parents make a big deal about this. I wish they'd just leave me alone. I like playing video games, and I'm good at them. What my parents don't get is that I play with my friends. We play together. They always want me to do more things. I've tried playing sports. I don't like it. It feels awful. And music lessons? No way. I would hate to have anyone listen to me play. I'm not good at it. My parents keep asking me to have friends over. I would never want to invite a kid over. I wouldn't know what to do. What if he hated it and had a bad time? What if I asked someone and the answer was no? I would feel like a real idiot. And I really don't want to go to someone else's house. It would feel so weird. No thanks. I'm most happy at home, playing my games. My dad explodes at me once in a while about being on the computer too much, but I just ignore him and play my games and he forgets about it. My mom yells at me about eating too much, but hey, I get hungry playing. Can't you just tell them to leave me alone? I don't need to see a doctor. I'm fine. The problem is they keep taking me to doctors.

"I also dread teacher conferences. My parents always come home and grill me about why I don't talk more in class. 'Raise your hand more. Your teachers want to hear what you have to say.' Yeah, right. I would probably say the wrong thing, and everyone would laugh at me and think I was a real dork. I'm happy staying quiet. They also get on me about my grades. I do okay. I wish they would leave me alone. I don't want to be the smartest kid in the class, and I'm not in any trouble at school. I do fine."

By the time he was done, I knew that Patrick didn't want my help. From his point of view, he felt no distress. In fact, just the opposite: he felt quite comfortable living his life the way he did. Meeting with Patrick—unless I wanted to play video games with him—would be a dead end. He didn't think there was a problem. He didn't feel anxious—just the opposite. He felt relaxed eating chips and playing video games.

Patrick's parents, however, felt worried, frustrated, and at times, angry and disappointed in Patrick. Mostly they felt helpless and at a loss for how to help him. In addition to having him tested for learning disabilities and ADHD, they read about Asperger syndrome and thought maybe he had that, or maybe he was depressed. I reviewed the testing, and it showed Patrick to be a happy boy, very bright, with social anxiety. In fact, he seemed to have all the classic symptoms of social anxiety. His primary defense against his anxiety was denial and avoidance. He didn't feel anxious because he avoided all situations that would cause anxiety. He participated in no extracurricular activities and said he hated them.

I have never known a kid with social anxiety to say, "I don't want to play soccer because it makes me feel scared and uncomfortable." They feel scared and uncomfortable and decide they hate soccer and quit. This confuses parents because they understandably think they should not force their children to do an activity they don't like. When they don't like *most* things, however, it is a clue that the anxiety is talking. And you never want anxiety to be making choices for your child.

A need for motivation was the biggest issue here. He was a smart kid whose world was growing smaller and smaller because of his anxiety. He experienced strong denial ("I'm happy at home; what's the problem?") and avoidance ("I don't like doing those activities"). Kids like Patrick will often avoid all activities that involve social interaction and performance.

I had already determined that meeting alone with Patrick would get me nowhere fast. I also knew that meeting with Patrick and his parents would be a disaster. His parents would bring up their concerns: "You have no friends, you play too many video games, you don't work hard enough in school, you eat too much junk food, and you're getting fat." Patrick would feel angry and criticized and swear he would never come to therapy again. And if I happened to mention that perhaps there should be some limits on his computer usage, well, I would just become the enemy in Patrick's eyes: "That doctor is an idiot—what does she know? We're not going back there. Are we, Mom? Please tell me we'll never go back there. She's so mean. Please. I'm fine. I don't need any help."

In that scenario, Patrick's parents would likely feel defeated once again and would not want to drag him back kicking and screaming. Understandably, many therapists might also say that if he didn't want help, therapy would not work. Given the way Patrick had set things up, he wouldn't want help any time soon.

So, I met with his parents. They held more power than they realized. They needed validation that, yes, their parental instincts were right. They had reason to be concerned about Patrick, even though his school thought he was fine, and even though he believed there was no problem. (I tend to think parents know best.)

Kids with social anxiety live in smaller and smaller worlds, and because they are in many ways high functioning, with so many strengths, they are at high risk for depression due to their social isolation. Patrick could complete high school longing for friends but feeling excluded. Or he could find other "outsiders" to hang with who might have deeper problems than his. He was also at risk for substance abuse, because most substances feel really good to anxious kids. In addition, he was at great risk for underperforming because he would not compete and take risks, even though he was very smart. He earned low grades despite his ability, and his grades were hurt by his lack of participation. He was involved in no extracurricular activities because he avoided social challenges. This smart, talented guy barely looked average. He seemed "okay" because he drew no attention to himself and was not a problem at school. He got by. In fact, if he had been the smartest in the class, that might have drawn attention and made him feel uncomfortable. Being an average student helped him blend in, unnoticed. This is how anxiety, in a subtle way, leads to underperformance.

His parents needed to understand that Patrick was a kid. He would choose what felt comfortable, not what was best for him. Knowing what is best for him is his parents' job.

Unlimited time on the computer is not healthy. Patrick could not regulate himself. The more computer time he had, the more he wanted. This felt good; doing anything else felt bad. As long as the choice included staying home and playing video games, he would stay home and play video games. Anxiety made these choices for him—deny and avoid.

Step 1: Target the Anxious Thoughts and Behaviors

Patrick did not have thoughts related to anxiety because he denied there was a problem and avoided situations that would make him feel uncomfortable. So the thoughts that needed to be challenged involved his denial, and the behaviors that needed to be targeted included his avoidance.

The first step was a tough one. His parents needed to set limits with video games. I advised them not to associate this with the therapy or we would lose any possibility of his cooperating with a behavioral program. I often recommend parents set these limits around natural transitions: "It's spring/summer/winter/fall/back to school/end of school/vacation/end of vacation, and we need to change the rules about being on screens." His parents needed to assert themselves and set the limit.

Most experts agree that the daily maximum for all screens for kids should be two hours during the week and three hours on weekends. Screens include TV, computers, and phones. That meant a major lifestyle change for Patrick. Both Lori and David had to agree on a limit they felt they could follow through with. Patrick would not be happy with this, so they needed to be ready for a fight and ready to follow through. They discussed it and agreed on three hours during the week and four on the weekends to start. They had the tough job of enforcing this, so their agreement was crucial.

Before we get to how that tough change went, let's look some more at Patrick.

Patrick believed it was okay to avoid situations that felt uncomfortable. This had to change. Summer was coming; it could not be an option for him to stay home alone with no plans and no supervision on his screen time. He needed to become active and connected with other kids his age. Isolation would only strengthen his anxiety. Choosing the right activity for Patrick was important. He could not, for example, be thrown into a baseball camp when he did not know how to play. It had to be an activity where he could feel fairly comfortable with his skills. He would have a high level of anxiety entering a situation like this if he also had to worry about not knowing what to do or not being good at the activity. He would feel completely overwhelmed. Remember, these kids fear embarrassment, failing, and being made fun of by other kids. He needed to enter a situation that was a good match for him.

Patrick's parents mentioned that he was a strong swimmer. A swim team would help him get exercise and be with kids his age. That seemed like a great match for him. Swimming is a comfortable sport for many anxious kids because they just get in the water and it's pretty clear what they have to do—swim to the other side. It is a team sport but a noncontact sport, with clear, predictable expectations.

Now the hard part—motivation. Patrick would not want to do this. He wanted to stay home all summer, play video games, and eat ice cream. His parents needed to be firm and supportive. Targeting his anxious thoughts and behaviors meant that staying home doing nothing could not be an option.

Step 2: Rate the Anxious Behavior

Patrick didn't acknowledge anxiety, but his anxiety became evident, in the form of oppositional behavior, when his parents spoke with him about doing an activity over the summer. He protested loud and clear. Keep in mind that anger is often fueled by anxiety, and this is what was happening with Patrick. So his parents needed to make it clear that he had choices, and his choices helped rate his anxiety. Swim team was one choice, attending a local summer camp another, and being a counselor in training at a camp for much younger kids another. He was not interested in the camp options, so they could be considered too high on his anxiety scale. He considered the swim team to be the least of all evils but still very difficult. He knew a boy on the swim team, so that helped. He still insisted that he was doing nothing all summer, but his parents clearly heard what would be possible for him this summer and what was too hard. His parents knew then that the swim team was a place to start, even though he insisted he was not doing it.

Step 3: Agree on Challenges to Work On

Joining a swim team seemed overwhelming to Patrick, who continued to say he wanted to just sit home all summer, but his parents held their ground. When a goal is too difficult, break it down. How could we make this easier for him? One way was to arrange for him to meet the swim team instructor. Or maybe he needed to take swim lessons to boost his confidence. Another option was to watch the team practice. We broke it down into steps he could agree to. Even though he didn't yet understand that process was about anxiety, his parents knew that as his comfort level increased, he would be ready for the next step. This was not easy for his parents; they needed a lot of support because Patrick kept fighting, convinced his parents would give in to him. The more his parents understood that this struggle was so strong due to his anxiety, the more they realized how important it was not to give in. He needed them to be strong and firm.

Step 4: Identify and Teach Strategies to Practice

At this point, it became important to discuss what made this so difficult for him. Meeting with me made more sense. His parents reminded him that I was someone who worked with lots of kids who struggle with doing things outside the house. They normalized his experience and meeting with me as much as possible. They presented me as more of a coach than a doctor for "crazy weird" kids. Patrick would not want to feel different or weird.

We suggested that Patrick choose whether he wanted to meet alone with me or with his parents. He chose to meet with me alone. At first he complained about the summer plan and even blamed me, so I told him about other smart, "normal" kids I have worked with. I shared with him what some of their feelings were and how they were able to push past them and ultimately feel better about doing more things outside the house. Their feelings had included being embarrassed, feeling like everyone would be looking at them and making fun of them, being afraid of messing up, and so on. I spoke about how they were able to challenge those feelings and replace them with more realistic thoughts. He listened, but I did not ask him to acknowledge that he had any of those feelings.

I confirmed that this was work and not easy. We then moved on to talk about incentives and rewards, and what he wanted to earn by doing this work. I told him that his parents had agreed to work out incentives and rewards with him. When we discussed what he might get out of all this, it brightened his mood. Of course, his parents would have to agree to his wish list.

Step 5: Note and Chart Progress Made

Because of Patrick's resistance to doing this work, emphasizing his rewards, plus negotiating what he was willing to do to get started, was crucial. His initial list of goals included making a chart. It also included coming to therapy to work on his anxiety. In addition, he agreed to meet with the swim instructor. His chart was small to start, with a strong emphasis on rewards, but it was a start.

Step 6: Offer Incentives to Motivate

Motivation is the most difficult aspect of helping kids with social anxiety. We were asking Patrick to move out of his comfort zone and feel uncomfortable feelings. We knew that as he did these things, they would become more comfortable, and he would experience great benefits. He did not yet know this, however. So incentives became very important. What would motivate Patrick to do this work? You guessed it: more computer time and computer games. Why would we reward his efforts with the very thing we wanted to get him away from? Because that was what would motivate him, ironically, to get away from the computer, get exercise, and connect with other kids. So we set up a system with Patrick: for each step he took, he earned points that he could cash in for more computer time or to use toward games. His parents were concerned that they would be manipulated and that he would take the rewards and then stop working on the issues. I guided them to remember that they were in control, and though money had been spent, they could remove new games or extra time if he did not continue with his steps. I also reassured them that most young people do not manipulate as soon as they start experiencing better feelings about leaving the house.

Step 7: Reinforce Progress and Increase Challenges

We then set up a second chart, listing Patrick's goals and the points rewarded for meeting those goals. When he met with the swim instructor, he received 5 points for that, resulting in four extra hours of screen time or ten dollars toward a game. That may seem like a lot, but the first steps are always the hardest. He now knew that this was not so hard, and he wanted more screen time and games. He was on board and working with us, so we could more fully develop the chart. He was willing to do the steps. Next step was to take swimming lessons. One hour of screen time for each lesson, or three dollars toward a game. Next, he would watch the team practice. One hour of screen time for each time he watched, or three dollars for a game. Next, he would join the swim team for a computer game or six hours of screen time. Once he joined, each practice meant one hour of computer time or three dollars toward a game. The first of everything was the biggest incentive, and then doing it again and again earned him less because it became easier for him. This was all charted with his points. We also included a bonus in his chart: if he joined a social activity, invited a friend over, or went to a friend's house, he earned a game or six hours of screen time.

Patrick was able to continue step by step and meet his goals because he was motivated. His parents did a good job of keeping track of his progress and gave him what he earned. As he reached one goal, he moved up, with goals always increasing.

If it had not worked, we would have had to reevaluate. Are the goals too high? Do we need to break them down into more steps? Are the incentives strong enough? Patrick needed to be motivated to do this work, and his parents had to stay united and firm in setting limits, as well as be supportive in providing him rewards and praise.

As Patrick continued to make progress, his parents were pleased with his reduced anxiety. By the middle of summer, he had experienced success in swimming, participating in the team as well as in team matches, even winning a ribbon now and then. We expected him to build on this. As summer came to an end, we established new goals for the fall, including extracurricular activities, increased class participation, improved grades, and continued swimming on the school's swim team, where he had some friends now. We met regularly together, sometimes all four of us, to negotiate with his parents these new goals and incentives.

Patrick had started to break out of his comfort zone of computer games and chips, but his parents had to learn to understand his anxiety, provide reasonable goals, and support his progress. In this process Patrick was experiencing success, which builds on itself. The swim team was a start, a first of many steps for Patrick.

Next Steps

Patrick continued on his journey. With limits set on his screen time, he was more motivated to do other things, especially with the incentives. His parents learned to pick their battles but to be firm in their expectation that he participate in activities and not withdraw. They also learned to give him the support he needed so that the goals were not too challenging for him.

Kids like Patrick are so anxious about trying new things that they need their skills to be strong. Often that means preparing them before they join a group activity so that they have confidence in their ability. Just signing them up for something they *should* be good at isn't enough; they need to go into the activity with confidence, so they only have to battle their social anxiety. If they have to feel their social anxiety on top of worrying about not doing well and not knowing what to do in an activity, that's far too overwhelming. Patrick's parents understood this, so Patrick was able to feel successful when he did his swimming, and this success led to more confidence, which led to more success.

DSM-5 Guidelines

Social Anxiety Disorder (Social Phobia)

The *DSM-5* identifies the diagnostic criteria necessary for a diagnosis. The assumption is that many readers will have children who meet some but not all the criteria.

A. Marked fear or anxiety about one or more social situations in which the individual is exposed to possible scrutiny by other. Examples include social interactions (e.g., having a conversation, meeting unfamiliar people), being observed (e.g., eating or drinking), and performing in front of others (e.g., giving a speech).

  Note: In children, the anxiety must occur in peer settings and not just during interactions with adults.

B. The individual fears that he or she will act in a way or show anxiety symptoms that will be negatively evaluated (i.e., will be humiliating or embarrassing; will lead to rejection or offend others).

C. The social situations almost always provoke fear or anxiety.

> **Note:** In children, the fear or anxiety may be expressed by crying, tantrums, freezing, clinging, shrinking, or failing to speak in social situations.

D. The social situations are avoided or endured with intense fear and anxiety.

E. The fear or anxiety is out of proportion to the actual threat posed by the social situation and to the sociocultural context.

F. The fear, anxiety, or avoidance is persistent, typically lasting for 6 months or more.

G. The fear, anxiety, or avoidance causes clinically significant distress or impairment in social, occupational, or other important areas of functioning.

H. The fear, anxiety, or avoidance is not attributable to the physiological effects of a substance (e.g., a drug of abuse, a medication) or another medical condition.

I. The fear, anxiety, or avoidance is not better explained by the symptoms of another mental disorder, such as panic disorder, body dysmorphic disorder, or autism spectrum disorder.

J. If another medical condition (e.g., Parkinson's Disease, obesity, disfigurement from burns or injury) is present, the fear, anxiety, or avoidance is clearly unrelated or excessive.

Specify if:

Performance only: If the fear is restricted to speaking or performance in public.

American Psychiatric Association. "Social Anxiety Disorder (Social Phobia)." In *Diagnostic and Statistical Manual of Mental Disorders*. 5th ed. Washington, DC: American Psychiatric Association, 2013.

Chapter 5

Where Are You, Mom and Dad?

Separation Anxiety

Separation anxiety is both normal and healthy when babies are between 8 and 14 months old. In fact, if babies don't experience both an attachment to their parents and a fear around strangers at that age, it's cause for concern. Sometimes anxiety about being away from parents continues in a milder form for several years. Separation anxiety after the age of 6 years old, however, is a cause for concern.

Children with separation anxiety often become very worried when they're not close to a parent and sometimes also to their home. They often worry something bad will happen to their parents if they're away from them. This may lead them to feel as if each separation could be a final one, which is the cause of a panic reaction. Parents leaving their screaming child with a babysitter will often be frustrated and say, "We're only going to the movies. We'll be back in a little while." But saying that over and over again makes no difference. To the child, clinging and screaming, "Don't go!" it's as if Mommy and Daddy will never come back.

This is another good example of how irrational anxiety is. When in this anxious state, children can't hear what's being said to them. They are in panic mode over what seems to be nothing to their parents. To these children, this feels like the last time they're seeing their mom and dad, so of course they're screaming, "Don't go!"

Some kids with separation anxiety don't worry so much about something bad happening to their parents; they worry that, without their parents, something bad will happen to them. They don't feel safe in the world unless they're close to their parents. Whatever the worry—that something bad will happen to their parents or to them—the anxiety is the same.

They feel most safe and comfortable being close to their parents, often one parent, usually their mother.

Kids with separation anxiety are the kids who have trouble being left at birthday parties, play dates, after-school activities, and, at its worst, school. They want their parents to stay with them, even when all the other kids are glad to have their parents leave. This can feel embarrassing, because now the clinging and screaming is happening in public, with other kids and parents looking on. When kids are flooded with this anxiety, they often don't care who sees them out of control, to their parents' surprise. Again, they're not thinking; they're only feeling overwhelming fear. They are reacting to this intense feeling of danger if their parents don't stay with them.

Separation anxiety disorder can be a small component of generalized anxiety disorder or a part of other anxiety disorders. Sometimes, however, separation anxiety disorder stands alone. Either way, the strategies for reducing this anxiety are the same: the step-by step method of establishing goals to change the thinking and behavior associated with the fear of separating from parents.

Kids with separation anxiety often complain of physical symptoms: stomachaches, headaches, and other pains of unknown origin. Do they really feel the pain caused by their anxiety? Or are they saying they're in pain to avoid the separation? Does physical pain become a more acceptable and effective way of communicating emotional pain? Though we will never know the answer to this, my guess is that it's probably a combination of all of the above. Kids are smart and learn pretty quickly that saying, "I'm scared; I don't want to go" will quickly be dismissed, often with annoyance, by their parents. Saying, "I can't go; my stomach hurts so much—it hurts, it hurts" will not be so easily dismissed. In fact, often the opposite occurs, and it becomes their pass to both stay home and get sympathy. We also know that when severely stressed, people commonly develop stomach pain and a lack of appetite.

Some kids, when anxious, get headaches, which may be in response to the stress. Headaches and stomachaches can be symptoms of anxiety. They can also be an excuse for a child to say, "I can't do this." We will never know how many kids really feel pain and how many use this as an expression of their anxiety. They may be "faking it," but they are doing that for a reason. They feel too overwhelmed by their fears.

Kids with separation anxiety, like other anxious kids, often have a hard time sleeping independently. Sleep often feels like the ultimate separation. They may cry and scream unless a parent stays with them until they go to sleep. They can have what look like panic attacks if they are left alone at night. Often they won't even go to their bed. They have to sleep in their parents' bed. Or if they fall asleep in their bed, with their parent with them, they may then wake up, panic, and run into bed with their parents. This makes sleeping a big issue for the whole family. Parents frequently give in, for many good reasons. They want everyone to get their sleep, including siblings, who could waken if the anxious child starts throwing tantrums in the middle of the night. Everyone has to go to school or work the next morning, and sleeping with Mom and Dad could mean everyone sleeps, albeit at a cost.

When an anxious child is in the parents' bed every night, some parents find themselves being "kicked out" of their bed and end up sleeping on a sofa or in the child's bed. Some parents give up and just put a mattress on the floor next to their bed for their child to sleep on.

Parents can be surprisingly accommodating to kids with separation anxiety. Why? Because it's so much easier than struggling with their child, fighting battles they can't seem to win. These kids, at any age, may throw huge temper tantrums when pushed, and parents naturally learn how to avoid these major struggles, often by enabling the anxiety. When patience is gone, however, parents often react with anger and frustration. A mother of a 12-year-old said, "When she won't go to sleep and keeps coming out of her room, and it's later and later, I am not at my best. I have had it, and I yell at her. I have to get to sleep, and it's just too much. I'm angry, and sometimes I lose it. It is not my best parenting moment, but there's only so much I can take! I give in. We all have to sleep."

Separation anxiety, like all forms of anxiety, can be very difficult to live with, but families like those described below can learn how to help their children manage their anxiety.

Casey and Kenneth's Story

Casey and Kenneth came to get help with their daughter, Kara.

Casey started. "Kara is 7 years old, and a delight. She's a happy little girl, but she's always had trouble leaving me. In preschool they had to peel her off of me, screaming, every morning. The teachers always said that once I left, she was fine. I can't tell you how many times I would be crying in my car as I drove away. It was so hard to see her like that. By the last year of preschool, she seemed fine and able to go to school, no problem. Then came kindergarten, a new school, new kids, new teacher, and it started all over again—the tears every morning and again not wanting me to leave when I dropped her off.

"Every night, getting her to sleep was a battle, with her crying about school. Her teacher was amazing, so nurturing and understanding. She would meet me and quickly whisk Kara into the classroom and get her involved in an activity. She said Kara was fine after that."

She continued. "First grade, the same thing happened, but it only lasted several weeks and then she was okay. This year she's in second grade, and in the beginning of the year, again it was rough, but now she goes to school with no major problem."

Kenneth added, "She really likes school, and she's smart, has lots of friends. She can be shy sometimes, but she's a happy little kid. Sometimes I think my wife's making too big a deal about this. I think she'll outgrow it all if we leave it alone. She's a very normal kid. Casey, you have to agree."

Casey got defensive. "I agree, she's normal most of the time, but it's not normal to need me to go to birthday parties. She's the only kid who can't be dropped off at these things. If I try to leave, she starts crying. And soccer practice, other parents don't have to stay there the whole time. She panics if she thinks I won't be there. The same with everything she does. You don't see it, because you're at work, and she's not the same with you. She always needs me with her, and frankly, it's starting to get embarrassing. None of her friends need their mother or father with them at all these activities. She may outgrow it, but in the meantime, she literally has a panic attack if I try to leave her. That can't be good for her, and that's not normal."

Casey took a breath and continued. "And we both know her sleeping with us isn't right, but we've just gotten used to it. It used to be in our bed, but it was so uncomfortable, we just put a cot next to our bed. So now, our 7-year-old sleeps in a cot next to our bed. This isn't normal. Kara has never been able to sleep independently."

Kenneth interrupted. "That's not true. Remember last year? She slept in her own bed for months."

Casey disagreed. "Yes, but who had to stay with her until she fell asleep? And when she woke up in the middle of the night, almost every night, where did she end up? In our bed. Let's face it, that's not normal behavior for a 7-year-old. Also, she still has temper tantrums like a 2-year-old. It often happens when I need to leave her, but it's ridiculous. She's too old for all of this."

The stage was set for me to meet with Kara and her parents.

Kara's Story

Kara spoke first. "I need my mom to be with me. I don't know why. I worry, 'What if something happens to me and she's not there?' I feel safe with my mom being close. I feel all alone and scared if she's not with me. At school, now it's better, I'm used to it, and I don't feel scared anymore. But birthday parties and soccer and dance, she can't just leave me there all alone. I get scared and need her to stay and not leave. I need her to stay with me.

"At night I can't sleep unless I'm close to my mom and dad. I just get scared. I don't know what I'm afraid of. I just can't do it. I feel cozy and safe when I'm sleeping in my mom and dad's room. Their bedroom is so warm and comfy. My room feels too scary to sleep in. I need to be with them at night."

I encouraged her to continue.

"My mom gets mad at me sometimes because of this. I can't help it. I just need to be with her. When she gets mad, it makes me mad, and it makes me cry more. I just need to be with her. I need it. I don't even want to talk about it. I just want everyone to leave me alone. It's the way

I am, and there's nothing wrong with it. It's not that bad."

Kara is like most anxious kids with separation anxiety. She's healthy in so many ways and seems happy and relaxed until she has to be in a situation without her mother. She doesn't worry that something bad will happen to her parents; she worries that something bad will happen to her, and her parents won't be there. She feels alone and vulnerable without her parents being close, especially at night. Sleep represents a major separation for many kids, and being without Mom and Dad feels very dangerous and scary for Kara.

Also like many anxious kids, Kara wants no part of any therapy that will force her to separate from her mother. She's convinced she can't do it, and she's angry that anyone would try to make her. She wants everything to stay the same, and she's very happy in her comfort zone with her mother and father staying close to her. She sees no need to change and doesn't even want to discuss it. In short, while Kara came to meet with her parents, she made it clear she didn't want to change anything. Talk to her about anything else, however, and she's a cute, charming girl.

Step 1: Target Anxious Thoughts and Behaviors

Kara stressed that she was angry at her parents for talking about her anxiety. I realized that forcing her to participate and asking her to talk about her anxiety would only create more anxiety and more distress and opposition.

Knowing that she needed to feel as comfortable as possible, I asked her parents to draft a list of her anxious thoughts and behaviors. The understanding was that if they got it wrong, she would correct them.

Her mom started with a list of her conception of Kara's thoughts:

- I always need Mom to be with me. (Hearing this, Kara looked up and got defensive. "Not all the time, just sometimes.")
- If something bad happens to me and my mom and dad aren't there, I'll be in danger.
- My room is too scary at night.
- I am only safe at night if I'm with my parents.

Her mom then looked at Kara and said, "I know what you're thinking right now . . . This is not a problem. I don't need to change this, and I can't change this without feeling too scared."

Kara added, "Yes, it's too scary, so why do we even have to be here? I want to go home now. How long do we have to be here? I hate this. I told you I didn't want to come here. Why did you force me? Take me home. I'm leaving!"

Her father then jumped in. "Kara, STOP THIS. We're not going anywhere. The appointment's not over yet."

Kara folded her arms and stared at him but said nothing. She was clearly angry.

Her father looked at me and apologized. "She's not usually like this. She's usually a very polite girl."

I knew that talking about these fears was making her anxious, and when she got anxious, she could quickly become angry. Many anxious kids get angry and oppositional when confronted with their fears. Understanding Kara's mindset, I offered her candy, which I always have in my office. She perked up when I gave her a lollipop. Sucking on the lollipop contained her anxiety for the moment by providing a pleasant distraction.

Next, I wanted to list her anxious behaviors. Kara still refused to talk, so her dad then began listing her anxious behaviors:

- Sleeping in our room
- Having her mom stay with her at birthday parties and all after-school activities
- Crying and not wanting to leave her mom every year when school starts
- Not wanting to go to camp because her mom can't be there
- Needing her mom to go on school field trips with her
- Needing to sit with us at school events instead of sitting with friends

He then reassured Kara. "See, that's not a long list. Just a few things we need to work on. You can do this!"

Kara still did not look happy, but her arms weren't folded anymore.

She picked up one of my toys and started fiddling with it, although she still had no interest in participating.

Optimistic nevertheless, I suggested moving on to the next step.

Step 2: Rate the Anxious Behavior

Kara again wanted no part in this step, but her mother explained to her that she's the only one who knows how hard these things will be.

Slowly, we persuaded her to help us with the rating system:

- Staying at birthday parties without her mom   **10**
- Going on field trips without her mom   **10**
- Sitting with her friends, not her parents, at school events   **10**
- Going to after-school activities without Mom   **10**

- Not crying every year when school starts   **10**
- Going to camp   **10**
  "I'm never going to camp, and you can't make me!"
- Sleeping in her room   **10**
  "I can't do that! Don't even say that to me!"

With Kara rating everything at least a 10, or impossible, we weren't doing very well. To make things worse, not only was Kara angry with us, but her parents were angry with her.

Kenneth was exasperated. "I knew this wasn't going to work. She needs us. I'm sorry, but she's just not ready for this."

Casey then looked annoyed at both Kenneth and Kara. "Who's the boss here anyway?" she said. "This stuff has to change. Kara, you have no choice in this. It's not normal to need me all the time, and your friends are going to start making fun of you and calling you a baby. This isn't 7-year-old behavior. You're too big for this now. Like it or not, you have to change this. I'm not putting up with this anymore." Kara started crying this time, really loudly.

It was apparent how much power this little girl wielded in this family and how her anxiety caused so much conflict. Casey was determined to force Kara to be more independent and was angry because she felt no support. Kenneth and Kara wanted no part in this.

Quickly, the family dynamics unfolded: Dad gives up and wants to avoid conflict with Kara; Mom fights with Kara and threatens her; Kara cries and screams until everyone gives up and feels hopeless.

The root of this was that Kara felt very anxious and was fighting to stay in control. So we were stuck in this cyclical family experience. Anxiety was winning this game, and nothing was about to change. But the good news was that the family dynamics playing out illuminated what life was really like at home. It became clear how stuck they felt and why they needed help.

At this point, I knew the direction had to be changed quickly since everything was moving toward anger and hopelessness. I started asking about what Kara could earn by doing all this work. I also let Kara know that she didn't have to make all these changes right away. We could break it down into steps, little steps for her. I told her I wouldn't force her to do something that was too hard for her. I told her she could be the boss of this work, but that we had to work together.

That reasoning caused her to look up and stop crying. As I considered the approach going forward, I knew she wanted to be in control and was desperately afraid of being forced into feeling those horrible scared feelings. Up until now, it had seemed like there were only two choices: keep everything the same and stay comfortable and close to her parents or be forced to do things she ostensibly couldn't do, that made her feel overwhelmed. Clearly, she needed to be the boss and feel like she had control of her out-of-control anxious feelings.

The more I reinforced that she would be the boss, the more relieved Kara looked. But she was not quite a believer yet.

Casey picked up on Kara's change in attitude and said, "Kara, you can do this, and we'll help you, and you'll earn prizes. Maybe you could earn getting a manicure, or a trip to the arcade with your friends, or getting a frozen yogurt with your dad. And you know what's coming soon? That new movie you want to see. I bet we could take a couple of your friends to see that with you."

Dad smiled and added, "I'll even let you get some candy at the movies." Kara looked surprised, like that was a big deal, and said, "My dad is a health nut and makes us give out raisins for Halloween."

Kara demonstrated how her mood could quickly shift, as with most kids. Once she felt she had regained her control, she could relax, and it was like all that crying had never happened.

Okay! Now we had to talk about the work ahead.

Step 3: Agree on Challenges to Work On

Together we looked at the list of anxious behaviors.

We decided to start with after-school activities, because they happen every week. Practicing challenges makes the activity easier, so frequency is important. Kara didn't have another birthday party to go to for a while, but soccer had two practices a week, and she went to dance once a week.

At all of Kara's activities, her mother couldn't leave; she had to stay right where Kara could see her. I suggested we start with Mom going to the bathroom and coming back. Kara would know this was going to happen—no surprises. Her mom would go to the bathroom, and if Kara saw that her mother wasn't there, she would know that she was coming back in a few minutes.

Casey immediately said, "I never thought of going for just a few minutes. I thought the goal would be I just drop her off."

I asked Kara to rate how hard it would be if her mother left for a few minutes to go to the bathroom or get a drink of water. She thought about it and said, "She's not going to get in her car and leave?"

Her mom reassured her that she would not leave in her car. Kara then said it was a 6. I reminded her that she would earn points for doing this, toward her prizes. We then agreed that her mother would do the same thing during her dance lessons. Kara said that this would also be a 6. I reminded Kara that there would be no tricks, no surprises. If we say that her mom will go to the bathroom, she won't leave instead.

Next, we looked at school field trips. There was one in two weeks to the science museum. Kara immediately got upset and said to her mom, "I need you to come, or else I won't go."

Casey responded, "You have to go. You don't need me there. You can do this. Don't think you're staying home from school because of this silliness."

Kenneth looked away, and Kara started crying. Here we go again. Kara felt like she couldn't do this, Mom was angry and frustrated, and Dad wanted nothing to do with the fighting between the two of them. I reminded them that when this happens, we have to break it down. It seemed like it should be easy, but for Kara, it felt too hard. I suggested that Mom go on the field trip as planned, but not sit with Kara, and that Mom lead a group that Kara wasn't in. So Mom would be there but not close to Kara during the trip. Kara looked relieved and said that would be a 5.

That didn't sound like much of a change to her mother, but Kara needed baby steps to build her confidence. If the goal felt too hard, we were creating a battle that couldn't be won. Kara had to be engaged in this process for it to work. Now we had a plan for the after-school activities and the field trip.

Again, I reminded Kara that she would earn points for all this work. I also reminded Mom and Dad that we had to work together. If we set the goal too high, everything would blow up.

And so the (baby) steps continued with number four.

Step 4: Identify and Teach Strategies to Practice

For this step, we looked at Kara's thoughts. Her primary thought was that she couldn't be alone in these situations without her mother because she thought something bad would happen to her, that she would be in danger. We all spent some time challenging that thought. Kara needed to be actively involved in this discussion. Talking at her would not be effective. She would just tune that out. So we started by asking her what she thought would happen. She didn't know. Like many kids with anxiety, she wasn't necessarily aware of her anxious thoughts. So I suggested we brainstorm. What could happen if Mom was not there?

"I could get sick," Kara said. "The coach could get sick. It could start raining on the soccer field, and we wouldn't be able to practice. I could get hurt at dance. I could get lost at a field trip and not know where to go. Some bad guy could come." Kara admitted that the chance of anything like this happening was very small. But what if it did happen?

I asked Kara to explore each scenario and what she'd do if her mom wasn't there. Her responses:

- If I got hurt at dance or soccer, the teacher or coach would call my mom and she would come.
- If I got sick, I could tell the grownups, and they would help me until my mom came.
- If I got lost on a field trip, I would go to a police officer and ask for help.
- If a bad guy came, I would run to my teacher or my coach and scream for help.

We all reinforced the fact that her parents only leave her in safe places. She was reminded that she was always with responsible adults, whose job it was to take care of her.

Her dad joked, "Kara, you act like we are dropping you off in the middle of a jungle with lions and tigers and bears all by yourself. We're talking about Miss Lucy's Dance Studio and soccer practice with Mr. Williams and Mr. Cooper. They're not lions and tigers and bears." Kara laughed, which is always a good sign.

We then discussed the need to talk back to the anxiety when she gets these fears. She could laugh like she just did, remembering she's not in a jungle. We asked what she could say to herself when she gets anxious. She smiled and said, "I'm safe. I'm not alone with lions, tigers, and bears."

So a little humor led to progress.

Step 5: Note and Chart Progress Made

We then discussed making a chart, which Kara, the artist, wanted to decorate.

- She would earn a point for each after-school activity her mother was able to leave for a few minutes.
- She would earn 5 bonus points if her mother left five times in a row and she was fine.
- She would earn 5 points for going on the field trip and not in a group with her mom.
- She would get 10 bonus points if she stayed away from her mom the whole trip.

I also explained that bonus points could always be awarded if she did something else she hadn't done before that allowed Mom to separate from her. After she did these brave things, she had to rate how hard it was for her on a scale of 0 to 10.

On to the incentives.

Step 6: Offer Incentives to Motivate

We discussed the prizes. She really wanted to go to a movie with three of her friends and get that candy, so we agreed that she needed 20 points for that prize.

- Going to a movie with three friends and getting candy   **20**
- Going to the arcade with a friend   **10**
- Getting frozen yogurt with Dad   **5**
- Getting a manicure with Mom and a friend   **50**

It was gratifying to see this going in a positive direction.

Step 7: Reinforce Progress and Increase Challenges

We met three weeks later to review results. Kara was successful at letting her mom leave her activities for a few minutes and now rated that a 1. She also did very well on the field trip and earned her 10 bonus points. She went to the movies with her friends and is now working toward the manicure.

So what's next? We discussed Mom leaving activities, driving away in her car to get a cup of coffee and then returning. Kara rated that a 7. She would get 2 points every time she did that, because it felt hard, and 10 bonus points for five times in a row of her mother leaving her at her activities.

We also discussed bedtime. This felt like the hardest for Kara but was the one thing her parents wanted most to change. Taking the cot out of her parent's bedroom and having her mom or dad stay in Kara's room until she fell asleep in her bed seemed like a good first step. The first night she did that would earn an automatic 10 points and a special prize in the morning. The next night 9 points, then 8, then 7, and so on. The first night is always the hardest, and then it gets easier. She would get 5 bonus points for five days in a row.

I emphasized the importance of consistency and suggested she listen to music in her room. We also reviewed how she needed to talk back to her worries.

Finally, Kara seemed ready to make a giant leap, and her parents were ready to support this.

"Things are getting better," her mom said, "but we still have more work to do."

Next Steps

Kara continued to work on her goals. Her parents learned to break the goals down and then gradually increase them. They understood the concept of challenging Kara but not overwhelming her. They worked on the sleep issue and were surprised at how quickly she was able to sleep independently.

This is common with sleep anxiety. The idea of sleeping alone is more anxiety provoking than the reality. When the child and the parents all agree to the goals, and parents are able to follow through, the step-by-step approach should work.

I often recommend doing this, the way Kara did, over a long weekend to start. Planning and agreeing when to start this is important. Parents have to be willing to set the limits, which can include doing things that affect their sleep, like bringing the child back to her bed.

Starting this on a long weekend when sleep was not an issue, having a good incentive, and using music quickly worked for Kara. As a result, her parents understood that under no circumstances should she go back into her parents' bed. This should not be thought of as a "treat" or something to do when Dad was traveling. Even if Kara is sick, Mom and Dad need to get their sleep and not take her into their bed.

Keep in mind: if kids go back to their parents' bed, this anxiety can easily return.

Dallan and Brendan's Story

Dallan and Brendan came into my office and started to tell me about Mary, their oldest of four kids. "She's 12," Dallan began, "and she's always been a very happy girl, but change has always been hard for her. She reminds me of what I was like as a child. We're here because it's hard to know how much of what she's going through is just normal 12-year-old stuff, and how much we should be concerned about. I was also sensitive as a child, and I never got help. I want Mary to learn some strategies to help her.

"Last year, going to school was often hard for her, and many times she'd go to the nurse with complaints of stomachaches, and I'd pick her up. In the back of my mind, I'd think she wasn't really sick. I'd get the call from the nurse usually when Mary was anxious about something. I tried to explain to her that her belly aches are really the worries, and she's not sick. She would cry in the nurse's office, begging me to take her home. She could literally scream about the pain in her belly. It broke my heart, so of course I would take her home."

Brendan interrupted, "She's a drama queen, Dallan. Let's face it. You get sucked right in."

Dallan responded, "You know that nurse. She always insisted I take her home. When I would say, 'Keep her in school,' they acted like I was being neglectful or something and demanded I take her home. And the nurse would always insist. Sure enough, when we got home, she always said her belly still hurt, but she sure didn't act like it. She could always eat anything and was usually hungry for lunch. She seemed very happy playing on the iPad or watching TV. When I'd ask her about her belly, she would say, 'It still hurts really bad.' If I tried to confront her about this and say, 'I don't think your belly hurts so much,' she would immediately scream about how bad the pain was. I know she likes drama, but what am I supposed to do? What if it really does hurt?"

Dallan described what they had already tried. "We took her to doctors, and she had all the tests. Everything's normal. They said it's just anxiety. She needs to be put on medication for her anxiety. So we started her on Prozac, but so far, it's not working, and she's starting to look like she's more distracted and a bit hyper. Medicine worries me; there has to be another way to help her. I secretly wished they'd find something wrong that we could treat, and all this would go away."

Mary's parents needed help understanding how treatment and medication can work together to help reduce anxiety. Yet knowing what kind of treatment is helpful and when to add the right kind of medication can feel overwhelming and confusing to parents.

"We took her to another therapist, and they did play therapy," Dallan continued. "I'm not sure what they did, but she loved going because they played games. Sometimes the therapist only had times to see her during the school day, so I took her out of school. She loved that. Every week we went there, but I have no idea what went on. I talked to her therapist, who was nice. She said they were working on her anxiety. But after all these appointments for over a year, and all this money, she's still crying at school, and I didn't see any change. She's been taking the Prozac now for a couple of months. My husband and I just felt we had to look at something else."

I asked Dallan to reflect on her own experiences.

"I remember feeling like she feels at school when I was her age. It was like a wave would sweep over me. It was very physical. I would feel hot and shaky and just feel like I had to go home. She says the same thing. I remember it like it happened yesterday. Change was hard for me too, but I never got help. I just had to deal with it."

I then asked Dallan to provide more details about Mary's experience at school.

"This year Mary started middle school, and I thought she'd be fine. She took a tour of the school last spring, and all summer, she seemed excited to go. The first week or two was fine, but then it all started again, only worse. She cries every night, saying, 'I can't do it. I can't go to school. Please don't make me go!'

"Then she cries in the morning and says she can't eat breakfast, her stomach hurts. Now she's breaking down and crying in school. I'm sure her getting to sleep late because she's so upset, and not eating breakfast, is only making everything worse. Everyone at school has been wonderful. When she gets anxious and starts to cry, she can go to the school counselor and stay there until she's ready to go back.

"This past week she had a couple of days where she didn't cry at school. I keep telling her she can cry at home, not at school, but then I don't want her thinking she can get attention for crying at home. It seems like she gets home from school and immediately talks about how hard it was and starts crying. I don't know what to do."

Dallan seems exasperated. "Did I say the wrong thing to her? It's so hard to know. I wonder, did I create this? But her sister, Julie, who's a year younger, is just the opposite. She's so independent. She has no anxiety. She'll go anywhere and do anything, not a care in the world. I think to myself, is this girl mine? It's great to see. I'm so proud of her. But, wow, she's so different from me. I guess she's more like her dad. My husband has zero anxiety. He is clueless when it comes to all this."

Brendan, who had let his wife do most of the talking, jumped in. "Mary is like you, and Julie is like me. I never had anxiety. I was always excited to go places. I went to camp all summer when I was a kid, every year. I love my parents, but I had a blast being away from them. I never missed them. I think both our kids should go to camp too, but this is where we disagree. I think we should just force Mary to get over this nonsense."

"Camp?" Dallan said. "Maybe Julie for a couple of weeks, but Mary hates camp. She went to day camp for a week and cried every morning, and after two days she stopped going. All that money we paid for it, down the drain. She likes staying home in the summer. Her cousins live close, and she plays with them. We go on vacation as a family, and she's fine, no stomach problems. She has a great time in the summer. She's just not a camp girl. She can't even do sleepovers with friends."

Brendan looked annoyed. "How are we going to help Mary if she can't do sleepovers? All her friends do it, and she always has to come home early. Remember last year when her class went away for two nights, and she cried every night, wanting to come home? She made it through, but other kids weren't crying like that. Maybe sending her to camp would cure her of this. She'd cry in the beginning but then settle down. I remember when I was a kid, there were always a few kids who were homesick in the beginning, but then they'd be fine and have a great time in camp. We have to get her over this."

Dallan raised her voice. "I can't do that to her! That would be torturing her. We can't just force her to go to sleepaway camp." She took a deep breath and continued. "I know we have to do something. I know when I went away to college, it was so hard for me. I ended up home the first year. I couldn't do it. I don't want that to happen to Mary. I know that's far off, but we have to help her and give her strategies. In so many ways, she's this happy, active kid, but this is a problem. Sometimes, I think I should just homeschool her. Then she wouldn't have to deal with all this stress. Don't you think kids are so overscheduled and pressured now? Homeschooling might give her relief from all this."

Brendan rolled his eyes and said, "I can't believe you're saying this. You two would kill each other if you had to homeschool her. Look at how much you fight now. Homeschooling would be the worst thing for both of you."

Then Brendan appealed to me. "We really have a great marriage. Honestly, it seems like Mary is the only thing we argue about. We're all fed up with this. Even her sister is angry and upset with Mary over this."

Brendan looked at Dallan, then back to me. "We need to tell you about the questions. She needs to know where we are every minute of the day. Every morning she grills us about when we're going to be home. If we're not going to be home, she needs to know where we'll be and for how long. I always tell her I'll be at work and that's the end of it, but with my wife, it can go on and on. Mary panics if we don't tell her."

Dallan chimed in. "Because I work from home, she's worse with me. It's like she wants me home all day when she's in school, and if I have to go into the office or even to the store, she gets upset and wants to know when I'll be back. It's like she worries about us if we're not home or something. Then the same panic happens when I have to pick her up somewhere. She needs to know what time I'll get there. Then she watches the clock, and if I'm a few minutes late, she panics. Now I've been trained to be perfectly on time with her or there'll be a crisis. I find myself getting anxious if I hit traffic or something."

Then Dallan's phone beeped. Brendan looked at me and said, "I guarantee you that's Mary. This happens constantly. When they're not together, the texting is constant."

Dallan quickly texted back. "Yup, that's Mary. She texted 'I love u, where r u?' She knows where we are. She has to check. If I don't return her texts, she panics. I always have to keep my phone on. I know she also expects me to text her when we're on our way home. He's right—it's constant. I guess I'm used to it. I don't think about it anymore, but it's actually stressful for me. I always have to be available to her, because I don't want her to get stressed. I know what that feels like, and I don't want her to have those feelings.

"I don't know if this is part of the change thing, but it's like she's younger than her friends. She's popular, and she does a lot of activities, but more and more, it seems like she doesn't want to grow up. It's like she hates the idea of puberty. When she got breast buds, she actually cried. Every time I try to talk to her about wearing a bra, she wants nothing to do with it. I think she wants to stay a child. She still sleeps with her doll. Her sister, Julie, on the other hand, is a year younger, but not only does she want a bra, she's bugging me about wearing makeup and shaving her legs. These two couldn't be more different."

Brendan nodded, but then said, "I know we've been talking a lot about Mary's anxiety, but wait till you meet her. She's popular, athletic, smart in school, and she's kind. She's the first kid to notice when another kid is sad or hurt. She's very sensitive. She's got the whole package, and ironically, in some ways, she has no anxiety. She had the lead last year in the play. She was Annie. She can sing and perform in front of a huge crowd of people, and she loves it. She's even running for student council. It makes no sense."

Brendan shook his head. "I can't figure it out. Here she is, crying at school and, at the same time, preparing her speech for student council and talking about tryouts for the next play."

Dallan agreed. "That's what's so confusing. She's so normal, and we know in a month or so, the crying will be totally gone, and she'll be fine. It's just that she shouldn't have to struggle like this every time there's a change. She needs strategies. I don't want her to go through life like this. We've provided her with a very stable life. Our family's great. We're really very fortunate, but her life can't always be like this."

I told the parents that Mary's life didn't have to be like this. They nodded hopefully, and we made plans for me to meet with Mary.

Mary's Story

As Mary settled in with her parents, she was a little hesitant but then began to express herself, echoing much of her parents' concern: "I don't know why I sometimes get so upset about school. It just feels so different being in middle school. I liked my other school, and I felt so comfortable there. This feels so big and loud, and I just get these strong feelings like 'I have to get out of here. I have to go home!' I get really hot and feel sick. My stomach hurts, and I get this shaky feeling, and I can't help crying. Sometimes when it's really bad, I feel like I can't get enough air. I can't breathe. My heart beats really fast. It's scary.

"I'm afraid all these bad feelings are going to come again. Sometimes I just feel like I have to get home. I can't stay in school another minute. I have to see my mom. Once I'm home, these feelings totally go away. When I'm with my family, I feel so happy. That's why I love summer so much. We're all together. I get to stay home. Everything's great. No worries."

She catches her breath. "Then school has to start, and we're not together. That's so hard to get used to. I don't worry something bad will happen to me. I worry something bad will happen to my mom and dad . . . I worry they'll be in a car accident, or something terrible will happen and they'll die. I know that sounds weird, but I worry I won't see them again."

I ask her to tell me more.

"When my mom's picking me up at my activities, I get so stressed out. I keep worrying until I see her, then I relax. And if she's late, I panic. I think the worst, and I can't help it. My mom doesn't understand this, but I like it better when we carpool and my friend's mother picks me up. I have no worries then. When it's my mom, it can be really hard. I also need to know where my parents are going to be every day. If my dad travels, until I know he's landed in the plane, I worry the plane is going to crash, so he has to text me when he gets on the plane and when he gets off. I wish my mom would just stay home all day. If she leaves home, I need to know when she's leaving, and she needs to text me when she gets home. I need to know she's okay. If she doesn't text me right back, I start to worry. I think something must be wrong. So I keep texting her until she texts back. She needs to keep her phone on when we're not together."

Mary continued. "I love the way things have always been. I have such great memories. I never want to lose my memories. My mother wanted to change my room because I'm getting older. I told her I liked my room just the way it was. She thought it was babyish. So she 'surprised me.' I came home one day, after being at my friend's house, and my bedroom was totally different. She got me all new furniture. I was so mad at her. I cried. I wanted my old furniture back. I begged her to get it back. She said it was gone. I couldn't believe it. I'll never see that furniture again. I got so angry, and then she got angry at me. She said I wasn't grateful. She thought I should be happy. But I never wanted new furniture. It makes me sad just thinking about it. I wish I could get my old room back. I hate surprises. I'm still so mad she did that."

Dallan was silent as Mary continued. "The other thing my mom does that drives me crazy, she wants to talk about my body changing. I don't want to hear about it. I want her to stop and leave me alone. I get mad at her every time she brings it up. She doesn't understand. I hate all these changes. I wish my body could just stay the same. I don't want to talk about it."

I asked her about her sister.

"Julie acts like she's a big teenager or something. She's so annoying. She acts stupid with makeup and all that. I don't want to hear about it. When she wants to put makeup on me, I get really mad at her. We used to have fun playing together. Now, especially when she's with her friends, she acts so different. They talk about boys and crushes. I hate it.

"My dad doesn't understand. He thinks I should be doing sleepovers like Julie does. I can't. I need to sleep with my parents. I know most kids don't, but I do. I would get too scared being in someone else's house. I need to be close to my mom and dad at night. That's just the way I am." She sighed as this session came to an end.

Mary was like a lot of kids with separation anxiety. She seemed happy and, in many respects, normal and well adjusted. When she was in her comfort zone of being with family and not coping with changes, she was free of anxiety. When triggered by some separation from parents or unexpected changes, however, panic could overtake her, seemingly out of nowhere.

Though her dad may not have accepted this yet, Mary was in crisis. What we all acknowledged was that this was very disturbing for the whole family. Even when things settled down and the anxiety abated, it returned with the next change.

In between periods of high anxiety, parents often learn to accommodate the lower level of separation anxiety by not challenging their child to do things they know will trigger panic. They accept things like texting with Mom, not wanting to sleep away from home, not wanting parents to leave home, asking questions about safety issues, and some clingy behavior, more the way a younger child acts. Parents assume this is "just the way she is" or that "she'll outgrow this."

In this case, Mary's mother had experienced many of the same feelings as a child and didn't want her daughter to go through what she had gone through.

So we were all ready to tackle strategies that I expected would help.

Step 1: Target Anxious Thoughts and Behaviors

Mary started by reiterating her worry that something bad would happen to her mom or dad. When asked about what bad things she thinks of, she paused, then said, "I worry they're going to get into a car accident or something like that. I worry they're going to die, and I'll never see them again." Her eyes welled up, and she started to cry. "Sometimes when I'm really worried, and I have to leave them, it feels like this is the last time I could see them, and I get so upset. I don't want to leave them."

Her parents looked surprised at the intensity of her feelings. They hadn't realized she was quite so worried about them dying. But of course it made sense, in a way. Why else would she become so hysterical at separation?

Mary continued. "I think I have to know where they are, just to make sure they're okay. I wish they would just stay home all the time, but if they go places, I need to know when they'll be home. If they're late, even by a few minutes, I start to worry, and that's when I get so scared and upset."

Then she looked at her parents and said, "That's why I need to know when you're coming, and you can never be late or it freaks me out."

Her parents seemed to begin to appreciate the depth of Mary's feelings as she continued to talk about how she hated change and aging, and the scariest inevitability of death.

She stated what we all realized: "I don't want to grow up. I want things to stay just the way they are."

Then she restated her fears about often not wanting to stay in school. "When I go to the nurse, I really do feel sick. I know my dad doesn't believe me. I hate when he makes jokes about me faking it. My belly really does hurt. At school I have to text my mom to make sure she's okay, and if she doesn't answer, I call her, and if she doesn't pick up the phone, I keep calling her until she does. I hate these feelings."

I explained that we could isolate those feelings and confront them.

Step 2: Rate the Anxious Behavior

Mary needed to identify her anxious thoughts and change them so she could "talk back" to her anxiety. Her thoughts about her parents' safety fueled her anxiety, so she really had to work hard at challenging her anxious thoughts.

How hard was it for her to talk back and challenge her anxious thoughts? How hard would it be to ignore these anxious thoughts when they came?

She rated her worries accordingly:

- Worrying that something bad will happen to my parents when I'm at school   7
- Worrying something bad has happened to my mom when she's late picking me up   10
- Worrying something bad has happened to Dad when he's traveling   6
- Feeling sad and upset about changing things in the house   5
- Worrying something bad has happened to my parents when they go out together   4
- Worrying something bad has happened to my parents when they go out together and are not home on time   10
- Worrying about changes   5
- Worrying something bad has happened to my mom when I know she's gone into the city   6

Then she rated how hard it would be not to do her anxious behaviors:

- Not knowing where Mom and Dad are each day 8
- Not texting Mom when I'm at school 7
- Not texting Mom when she is not at home 8
- Not texting Mom if she's late at pick-up 10
- Not texting Mom when I don't know where she is 8
- Not texting Mom when we're both home but in different parts of the house 3
- Not getting upset about changes in the house 3
- Talking about body changes 5
- Staying home when mom runs errands 5
- Not going to the nurse when I feel worried 8
- Not going home when I feel really scared at school 6

Step 3: Agree on Challenges to Work On

Mary looked at her list, and together we talked about what she could work on.

Everyone wanted to focus on her anxiety at school, since that was causing so many problems right now.

She agreed to work on five goals:

- Not going to the nurse at school
- Not calling or texting Mom from school
- Not texting Mom when she's not home
- Not asking Mom and Dad every day where they'll be
- Challenging her thoughts at school about her parents' safety

Next, we agreed it was time to begin the implementation stage.

Step 4: Identify and Teach Strategies to Practice

We discussed talking back to the worries and realizing that her worries about her parents were silly worries. She didn't like the term "silly worries"; she thought it meant she was being silly. So we talked about what she wanted to call her worries, and she decided to group them under the name "Brain Trickster," because they tricked her brain into believing false things and worrying.

We reviewed the reality: her parents were not sick, and they didn't do dangerous things, so the chances of something being wrong with them were very slim. So she needed to learn to talk back to the Brain Trickster: "My parents are fine. I will see them later. I am not going to be bothered by these worries. I am going to focus on being here and everything that's happening around me in school now. I am not listening to what the Brain Trickster is telling me. I will not be tricked. I need to ignore these worries, watch them fly by in my head. I can focus on being with my friends, learning from my teacher, doing my work at school, having fun at home. I can switch the worry channel off in my head because I'm the boss of my brain. I am smarter than the Brain Trickster, which lies to me when it says something bad happened to my Mom and Dad. I can listen to music and focus on happy things and not the worries. I can do this!"

She agreed to make a calm-down playlist of music she can listen to and sing with to help calm herself. After all, she is a little actress and loves to sing, so this was perfect for her.

She also made a calm-down list of things she can do that help her relax. At home:

- Draw
- Write stories
- Read
- Listen to music
- Sing and dance
- Do yoga stretches
- Play in the backyard
- Play games
- Watch TV

At school:

- Use her squeeze toy
- Focus on the teacher and her friends

- Remember they are brain trick worries
- If she needs to, take a break and get a drink of water
- Doodle on her doodle pad
- Talk back to the worries and let the thoughts fly out of her head

Step 5: Note and Chart Progress Made

Mary and her parents worked on making a chart and recording progress.

Her dad worked in computers, so he used a spreadsheet that included the date, her goals, her ratings, and her points. They agreed to keep it in the computer, and every evening they created a new spreadsheet with a flowchart showing progress. At this time, they would review her goals and her progress and add up the points she'd earned.

Step 6: Offer Incentives to Motivate

Mary's point system included more points for firsts as well as bonus points for repeated success:

- She would get a point every day she didn't go to the nurse at school, with a bonus 5 points when she didn't go five days in a row.
- She would get 2 points every day she didn't call or text Mom from school.
- If she called or texted and Mom said, "Talk back to the worries," Mary would get 1 point if she remembered to be in the here and now, use her calming list, and not call or text anymore.
- She would get a bonus 10 points for five days in a row of no texting or calling Mom from school.
- She would get 2 points when she didn't call or text Mom when Mom was not home.
- She would get a point every day she didn't ask Mom and Dad where they would be all day, with 10 bonus points for five days in a row.

Using points for days in a row of changing behavior is a powerful way to make the change stick. Mary was excited when we talked about her prizes. Based on her point system, her parents decided how many points she needed to get her prizes. Together they made the list.

- Go roller skating with friends **50 points**
- Go to the movies with friends **50 points**
- Have a sleepover **60 points**

- Make brownies **20 points**
- Go out to breakfast with Dad **25 points**
- Choose what Mom will make for dinner **10 points**

She was excited to begin working to get her prizes.

Step 7: Reinforce Progress and Increase Challenges

Mary came back two weeks later with her parents, and they had printed out their chart from her dad's spreadsheet. She was making progress.

She had earned points for not texting or calling Mom from school but had not yet gotten five days in a row. That had gone down from a rating of 7 to 5. She had gone four days in a row, so she was close. We discussed what had happened on the day that triggered her to text. Mary thought about it and then remembered: "In health class, we talked about diseases, and I started to worry that my mom might get a disease. I just had to text her to make sure she was okay." We then discussed how she could handle that if it happened again. I asked her what she could say to herself. How could she talk back to that worry? "I know my mom's healthy. She's not sick. I know it sounds silly now that I was so worried. I could have let the worry pass, ignore it, and focus on school and my friends. I also could have taken a break and gotten a drink of water. I just went right away to my phone to text her."

She had done a great job of not asking every day where her parents would be. That was down to a 2. She was proud to say she'd only been to the nurse once since we'd met, and she had been there for only a short time and returned to her classroom. Her parents praised her for this, and she earned a lot of points. Not going to the nurse was down to a 2, almost gone as an issue.

Not texting Mom when she wasn't home and Mary was home was still hard. She had some days when she didn't text and others when she texted once but didn't keep calling or texting. She rated that a 6. She still had to work on that one.

We looked back at her list, and she decided to work on some other goals since she was doing better. We added "Not texting Mom when we're both home but in different parts of the house," which was a 3. She also added to her list "staying home when Mom runs errands," which was a 5. She would get a point for each day she worked on those and 5 bonus points for five days in a row.

Mary was also excited to tell me she had already earned some prizes. She had gone out to breakfast with Dad, and she had chosen her favorite dinner, macaroni and cheese. She was also very close to having one of her bigger prizes.

All of us were happy that we were moving in the right direction. Her parents talked to the doctor who prescribed her Prozac, and they decided that since she was making progress, they would wean her off the Prozac. Her mother said, "We really don't think it's doing anything for her, and she now knows strategies and is able to work on managing her anxiety. We want to see if she can be okay without it."

It was agreed that they would continue doing the CBT every day without the medication. Mary was very happy not to be taking the medicine, which she said "tasted awful." For her, that was another reward for working on her goals.

Next Steps

Mary continued to make progress. When we discussed her "fighting" the anxiety, this was hard for her. Her parents were eager for her to "get angry at the worries."

She explained that she had a hard time doing that because she's not an angry kid. She really had no personal experience getting angry at anyone or anything in an extreme way. So getting angry at the worries was hard for her. What she found works was imagining a cartoon character running around getting all excited in her head, and she could say back to that character, "Calm down. I know you want to protect me, but everything is fine, so don't get so excited. Everything is fine!"

Talking back to her worries that way really worked for her. This is a good example of how the approach needs to be individualized. It's certainly not one size fits all. This example also shows how kids teach us what works best for them. We have to learn to ask them and listen.

Mary had one week when her anxiety was high, and she felt exhausted. Her parents considered putting her back on Prozac, but the following week was better, and Mary has continued to get better. After several months of CBT, Mom called with very good news: Mary was doing very well, and they saw no need for an appointment at that time.

Mary's story is a good example of how anxiety can go up and down. Learning how to manage anxiety takes time and practice. It also demonstrates that many children don't need to be medicated if they engage in CBT. The need for medication depends on the severity of the symptoms and the ability of the child to respond to treatment. It is not a black-and-white situation. Although Mary may continue to do well, she may also need a "tune-up" in several months or even years from now.

DSM-5 Guidelines

Separation Anxiety Disorder

The DSM-5 identifies the diagnostic criteria necessary for a diagnosis. The assumption is that many readers will have children who meet some but not all the criteria.

A. Developmentally inappropriate and excessive fear or anxiety concerning separation from those to whom the individual is attached, as evidenced by at least three of the following:

   1. Recurrent excessive distress when anticipating or experiencing separation from home or from major attachment figures.

   2. Persistent and excessive worry about losing major attachment figures or about possible harm to them, such as illness, injury, disasters, or death.

   3. Persistent or excessive worry about experiencing an untoward event (e.g., getting lost, being kidnapped, having an accident, becoming ill) that causes separation from a major attachment figure.

   4. Persistent reluctance or refusal to go out, away from home, to school, to work, or elsewhere because of fear of separation.

5. Persistent and excessive fear of or reluctance about being alone without major attachment figures at home or in other settings.

6. Persistent reluctance or refusal to sleep away from home or to go to sleep without a major attachment figure.

7. Repeated nightmares involving the theme of separation.

8. Repeated complaints of physical symptoms (e.g., headaches, stomach-aches, nausea, vomiting) when separation from major attachment figures occurs or is anticipated.

B. The fear, anxiety, or avoidance is persistent, lasting at least 4 weeks in children and adolescents and typically 6 months or more in adults.

C. The disturbance causes clinically significant distress or impairment in social, academic, occupational, or other important areas of functioning.

D. The disturbance is not better explained by another mental disorder, such as refusing to leave home because of excessive resistance to change in autism spectrum disorder; delusions or hallucinations concerning separation in psychotic disorders; refusal to go outside without a trusted companion in agoraphobia; worries about ill health or other harm befalling significant others in generalized anxiety disorder; or concerns about having an illness in illness anxiety disorder.

American Psychiatric Association. "Separation Anxiety Disorder." In *Diagnostic and Statistical Manual of Mental Disorders*. 5th ed. Washington, DC: American Psychiatric Association, 2013.

Chapter 6

Tap, Check, Count, Wash, Repeat

Obsessive Compulsive Disorder (OCD)

Obsessive compulsive disorder (OCD) is an anxiety disorder that causes people of all ages, including children and teens, to have distressing thoughts, or worries, that they cannot control. These worries cause them to feel an urgent need to perform certain rituals or rigid routines. The worries are obsessions, and the things they feel they need to do are compulsions. Children often feel they have to do these compulsions or something bad will happen.

Fortunately, OCD is very treatable, and there is much research supporting CBT as the most effective form of treatment. Specifically, the preferred approach is called exposure response prevention (ERP), which means the child practices being exposed to the OCD trigger and does not do the compulsion. With ERP practice, the feeling of needing to do the compulsion gradually disappears. This is how to become free from OCD.

One of my patients didn't know about OCD; she called her compulsions her "have to do's." Children with OCD usually think the "bad things" that could happen involve harm coming to themselves or their family members. These compulsions provide immediate relief from anxiety temporarily, but then soon they have to do them again and again. This cycle of obsessions and compulsions may take up hours of a child's time each day. OCD causes great distress and is confusing for children because they know they shouldn't be doing these compulsions, but they can't stop—the behavior feels out of their control.

Common obsessions are the fear of dirt or contamination, the fear of hurting others, the fear of thinking evil or sinful thoughts, intrusive violent or sexual thoughts, the need for symmetry or exactness, excessive doubt, and the need for reassurance. Common compulsions are repeated washing or showering, using excessive soap, repeated checking, avoiding touching things that are "dirty" like doorknobs or sticky substances, counting, arranging things, repeating tasks or words, making others repeat things, rereading, rewriting (writing over letters), rituals involving the keyboard or the Internet (having to go back and redo when typing, for example, or having to do certain things when the computer is turned on or off), touching, tapping, mental rituals to cancel out "bad thoughts," hoarding useless things, and seeking reassurance. The Children's Yale-Brown Obsessive Compulsive Scale is a useful reference to see a complete list of the OCD symptoms kids may have. It's also used as a reliable measurement of how severe the OCD is.

Up to 4 percent of children and adolescents have OCD, and most are diagnosed in childhood. That represents over one million children and teens. The disorder is often genetic, with one or both parents or other relatives having it. Usually by the time children are diagnosed, they report having had OCD symptoms for years. Many of these children and teens are high-functioning kids, good students, and athletes, popular, kind, and sweet. They are high functioning in every way, except they have OCD. Sometimes these kids resist treatment because having a "disorder" and needing help is a huge contrast with their self-image as normal, successful kids.

Some children have a sudden acute onset of OCD, sometimes accompanied by severe anxiety and motor or vocal tics. This type of OCD is thought to be caused by strep or another bacterial infection, known as PANDAS (pediatric autoimmune neuropsychological disorder associated with strep). This is controversial since the research is conflicting, and certainly more research is needed. There is no doubt, however, that a subset of kids with OCD very suddenly develop severe symptoms.

OCD can be extremely painful for children, making them feel trapped in a cycle of obsessions and compulsions that are overwhelming and confusing. For parents, family life can be much disrupted because OCD, like other anxiety disorders in children, can greatly affect the whole family, often turning day-to-day family living upside down.

With this as a backdrop, I present two illustrative case studies based on my patient experience.

Willy and Anna's Story

Anna called my office sounding desperate. She left a voicemail that ended with her in tears. She wanted my soonest available appointment because she felt so worried about her young daughter, Atalaya. I met with her and her husband, Willy, as soon as possible. They arrived early to the appointment, and once they came in, they began talking rapidly.

Anna started. "We are here because of our 7-year-old daughter, Atalaya. Something is really wrong, and we don't know what it is. She seemed fine up until ten days ago. Then she suddenly began worrying about germs and washing her hands all the time, saying things were dirty over and over again. We tried to talk to her about it, but it was like she couldn't hear us. We thought it would just go away, but instead it has gotten worse. We called you because it got to the point where she is now having a hard time using our bathroom. She woke up in the middle of the night and had to pee but she was hysterical about the toilet being dirty, the sink, the doorknob. She was crying that everything in the bathroom was too dirty. The poor thing ended up using the toilet squatting so she wouldn't touch the seat. She has never been like this before. She was the kid I used to have to remind to wash her hands."

Willy, looking concerned, added, "It is not just the germ thing. I get her and her sister up and dressed in the morning and take them to school. Getting her dressed has become impossible. She keeps saying nothing feels right, and she breaks down crying. I hate to say it, but she has worn the same loose t-shirt and loose flannel pants to school for the last week. She says these are the only clothes she can wear. She looks like she is wearing pajamas to school. I'm sure the kids and teachers are going to start to notice. In addition she is worried about her fingerprints. She feels like she has to wipe off her fingerprints. I know this sounds weird, but she is frantic about it."

Anna added, "I wash her clothes every night. I try to get her to wear different clothes, but she just panics and cries. She also told me that now she can't use the bathroom at school. She is holding it in all day. And she thinks even our bathroom is contaminated. She's washing her hands so much they are red and chapped. She asks a lot of questions over and over again, and my husband realized now she's trying to get us to repeat things. At first I thought she wasn't hearing us, but she keeps asking us to say the same things again and again. What has happened to our little girl?"

"She also asks the weirdest questions," Willy added. "It feels like it's all day long now. She says things like, 'I touched the chair and then I touched my mouth—is that okay? Should I wash my hands?' I say, 'No, don't wash your hands,' but she runs into the bathroom and washes them anyway. Lately, and I know this sounds disgusting, but she has started spitting, thinking she is getting rid of dirt in her mouth. If I don't answer her questions, or if I tell her to stop spitting, that there is nothing in her mouth, she gets really angry and melts down. Putting her to bed has become a nightmare, between the questions and the washing and what I need to say to her eighteen times before she lets me leave her. It's taking almost an hour just to get her into bed. She has these things we have to say to her over and over, and she has to wipe her fingerprints, and she is doing things over and over again. She is getting to sleep so late, and we are all exhausted."

Willy looked down at his hands. "I admit I get angry at her. I just want her to stop this. She has a younger sister, and it feels like she's being neglected because all our time is being spent with Atalaya. We are so worried and don't know how to help her. She was never like this. She was a happy, normal child. A month ago I was thinking she could grow up to be the president. Now I worry she may never be . . ." Willy suddenly stopped, and his eyes watered up as he said "normal."

Anna took Willy's hand and said, "We just don't know how to help her. I don't know what's going on, but she is getting slower and slower. Willy is right. It's such a struggle. I dread bedtime. My stomach gets tight once dinner is over, knowing what we face. By the time she gets to bed, it's so late, I know she must be exhausted. I'm exhausted and angry. I know I shouldn't, but I feel so angry. She says such mean things to me when she's like this."

"And she wakes up in the middle of the night and ends up in our bed," Willy said. "Then I end up in her bed. It's crazy! She was always such a good sleeper. We used to just tuck her in at night, and she would go off to sleep. In the last two weeks, everything has changed; we don't know what to do. We feel either sorry for her or angry at her or both. We don't know whether to punish her or just comfort her. It's so confusing. None of us are sleeping, and her sister is wondering what's going on."

Anna then said, "We started reading about OCD on the Internet, and we think that's what she has, but what do we do about it? I worry about what's happening at school. I can't imagine that she's not worried there, too. I don't want to tell her teacher. We don't know what to do. We just want to help her, but instead of it getting better, it seems to be getting worse."

I could see on their faces how hopeless and defeated as parents they felt, not being able to help their child. We agreed that the next step would be to meet with Atalaya.

Atalaya's Story

Atalaya began to relate her concerns: "I have so many worries all of a sudden. I don't know what's happening to me. I think everything is dirty, and I have to wash my hands a lot. I keep thinking about germs, like they're everywhere, and now everything is germy. Bathrooms really scare me now because everything feels so dirty in the bathroom. It feels like pee is everywhere. Sometimes I have to change my pants because I think there is pee on them. Sometimes I want to wash my leg after I use the bathroom because I think maybe pee is on my leg, but I know it isn't. At first it was just the school bathrooms that were dirty, but now even my bathroom at home feels germy. I wish I never had to use the bathroom ever again. I try to hold it as long as I can, but then I have to go. I hate taking showers now; it feels like I have to do more and more to get clean. Sometimes I feel like as soon as I am clean, something happens to make me dirty again. It makes me so mad. I just want to scream. Nobody understands how bad this feels!

"Then I have the worry about fingerprints. I feel like I have to rub them off. Someone could be seeing my fingerprints and will then try to hurt me. Everything I touch, I have to rub."

It was easy to feel Atalaya's pain as she continued. "I also have a really hard time getting dressed. None of my clothes feel right. I try to put them on and have to take them off because they feel so, . . . so uncomfortable.

I can't stand it. I don't know why, but I have only a few clothes that feel 'right.' The rest I can't wear. Mommy and Daddy don't understand. I can't help it. Sometimes I just cry and cry because it feels so bad. I can't wear the clothes I used to wear. I just can't. Everything takes so long now. I am always late, but I have so many things I have to do in the morning now, and my parents keep yelling at me to hurry up. I can't go any faster. I have to make sure everything is right, and I have to wash."

I asked Atalaya about bedtime. "At night my worries get worse," she said. "I hate bedtime. I have all these things I have to do before I go to bed. Turn the light switches on and off, fix my stuffed animals a certain way, close and open my drawers, check the closet and close the door, and then brushing my teeth is a big deal, and the washing. Then when finally I get into bed, I feel like my parents have to keep saying, 'Good night. I love you. Everything is okay. See you in the morning. I love you. I love you.' Four times, or if that doesn't feel right, six, eight, ten times. Last night they had to say it sixteen times. It can't be an odd number, because I know that is bad luck, and something bad will happen. They get mad at me sometimes, and then they have to start over. If they won't do it, I can't get to sleep. I can't. Something bad will happen if they don't do it. They have to say this before they leave me at night. I don't know why this is happening to me."

Clearly feeling exhausted, Atalaya wrapped up her story: "At school sometimes I can forget about it all . . . until I have to go to the bathroom, or I touch something that's dirty, and then I get worried all over again. There are two boys in my class who are really dirty. One of them picks his nose, and the other picks at his ear. I can't even walk by them without feeling like I have to wash my hands. Sometimes even just looking at them from my desk makes me have to wash. I am so glad there's hand sanitizer in the classroom. I keep using it over and over again. Some kids asked me why I was wearing my pajamas to school. I couldn't explain to them. I didn't know what to say. I don't know why. I told them it wasn't pajamas and walked away. Sometimes I worry I must be going crazy. I want this all to stop."

I explained that if we worked together, we could begin to make it stop. I explained the seven steps, starting with Step 1.

Step 1: Target Anxious Thoughts and Behaviors

What are Atalaya's anxious thoughts (obsessions)? Atalaya and her parents made a list of all her worries.

- Germs and pee and poop getting on me
- Feeling really dirty, so dirty it just sticks on me and won't go away
- Not being able to get clean enough
- Getting poisoned by putting the wrong thing in my mouth
- Wearing clothes that feel so uncomfortable and that yucky feeling won't go away
- Fearing something bad will happen to me or my family
- Fearing someone will get my fingerprints and hurt me

What are Atalaya's anxious behaviors (compulsions)?

- I have to wash my hands a lot, with at least four squirts of soap over and over, or use hand sanitizer.
- I have to spend a lot of time in the shower. I have to wash every part of my body over and over again an even number of times and tap the soap.
- I can't turn the shower on or off; I need my parents to do it because the shower handle is too dirty to touch.
- I can't use the school bathrooms. They are way too dirty.
- It is getting really hard to use the bathrooms at home. There is only one that I can use now, and I can't sit on the toilet. The seat is too dirty. After I use the toilet, I have to wash my hands and sometimes my legs because I worry I got pee on me.
- Sometimes if I think something touches my mouth, I need to ask about it to make sure it is okay. And then I usually have to wash my hands and sometimes even spit to get the dirt out of my mouth.
- When I touch some things at school, I have to use the hand sanitizer. I always have to use the hand sanitizer if I go near two of the boys in my class who are really dirty.
- I sometimes have to ask my parents if they washed their hands, especially when they are cooking.

- I can't wear most of my clothes. They don't feel right.
- My parents have to say good night to me in a certain way and a certain number of times or else I can't go to sleep.
- I have a lot of things when I brush my teeth. I have to put just the right amount of toothpaste on the brush, then tap it against the sink four times. Then I have to brush each side top and bottom an even number of times. When I'm done, I have to spit an even number of times and then tap the toothbrush against the sink and then I'm done.
- I have to wipe all my fingerprints away, especially at night, because that's when bad things happen.

Atalaya's parents listened patiently as she made her list. Before it was over, her mom had tears in her eyes. I asked Atalaya to leave the room as I could see her mother was starting to cry. Her mom broke down. "It's so hard. I'm exhausted. I get mad at her. None of us has gotten enough sleep. We haven't told anyone about this. Her sister keeps asking what's wrong. We don't know what to tell her. When she's up at night doing all these things and I get mad at her, she starts crying and screaming and wakes her sister up. Our whole family feels like it's been turned upside down."

We discussed how OCD is really a family illness, because everyone becomes affected. We also discussed telling the other kids that their sister is not feeling well and is having a lot of worries that she can't control. They needed to know that she was getting help and this would get better. I reassured Atalaya's mom that getting angry is a normal reaction, and that we would soon be working together to fight the OCD, which would make things feel more positive at home instead of a struggle with each other.

Atalaya came back and joined us as we talked more about how we would work together to get rid of her OCD. Atalaya looked relieved that she had shared all her worries and felt, perhaps for the first time, that her parents understood, and that she really wasn't going crazy—she just had this thing called OCD. I let her know that lots of great kids have OCD and that she would learn how to "kick it out" of her head. Since she is a good soccer player, this made her laugh.

She was ready to do the work and go on to the next step.

Step 2: Rate the Anxious Behavior

Next Atalaya read through the list and rated each compulsion or behavior on a scale of 0 (easy) to 10 (impossible) based on how hard it felt to not do what OCD was telling her to do.

- Not washing my hands when I feel they are dirty   9
- Using two squirts of soap when I wash instead of four   7
- Washing only once in the shower, not over and over again   5
- Turning the shower on and off myself   7
- Using the school bathroom   10
- Going into the school bathroom   8
- Using my parents' bathroom without sitting on the toilet   3
- Sitting on the toilet   7
- Using the bathroom downstairs   8
- Not washing my legs when I think I got pee on them, even though I know there is no pee there   4

- Not seeking reassurance about getting something dirty in my mouth   6
- Not spitting when I feel like I have dirt in my mouth   4
- Not using hand sanitizer when I think I touched something dirty at school   4
- Not using hand sanitizer when I come near the dirty boys   5
- Not asking my parents to wash their hands   3
- Wearing clothes that feel uncomfortable   8
- Not doing the bedtime rituals with the lights and stuffed animals   8
- Not having my parents say good night to me that certain way   9
- Not doing the tooth-brushing things   8

Since sleeping had been such a problem, as it often is in children with anxiety, we decided to add it to our list.

- Going to bed by myself, without needing Mom or Dad to stay with me   8

- Staying in my bed throughout the night and not going into Mom and Dad's room   10

With the identifying and the rating accomplished, we were ready to work on certain challenges.

Step 3: Agree on Challenges to Work On

I explained that we needed to pick some things that she could work on to fight OCD. Atalaya was beginning to learn that OCD needs to be seen as something outside her that she can fight and get rid of. The more she fights OCD, the weaker it gets, and the stronger she gets. I explained to her that OCD is a liar, telling her to worry about dirt that isn't there and telling her she has to do things she doesn't have to do. She can say "no" to OCD, and that is what will make her better. I also reinforced that lots of kids have OCD; she was not alone, she was not going crazy, and she would get better. I told her she was going to kick OCD really hard right out of her head.

Thinking about what to work on was something we all did together. Atalaya became fidgety and suddenly seemed to look like a much younger child as she leaned into her father. She was scared, afraid it would be too hard to do this. We focused on the things on her list that were not rated too high. I reassured her that I wasn't going to force her to work on something she didn't feel ready to work on. She could choose with us what she'd work on, and I would help her with making her OCD go away.

Her hands were not only cracked but also had been bleeding from so much washing. I knew that hand washing had to be brought to the top of the list. Her little hands really hurt. I was also concerned that they could become infected. I let her know that whatever she decided to work on, she would be earning points toward prizes for doing this work. She was excited about the idea of prizes. I listed everything that was not too hard, and Atalaya led us in choosing what she'd work on.

Not washing when she felt her hands were dirty was rated very high, but we needed to help her with her cracked skin. She agreed to try to work on it, but how? We needed to break it down into steps that were not rated so high. With hand washing, sometimes kids' hands look red not because they are frequently washing their hands but because when they do wash, they use too much soap, or they don't dry them because they don't want their clean hands to touch the towel. Atalaya was both washing too frequently and using a lot of soap, which explained why her hands looked so bad. Plus it was winter, and the cold air made them even drier.

She agreed to use two squirts of soap instead of four. She rated that a 7, very hard. Because her hands looked so sore, however, we encouraged her to work on this.

She agreed to work on exposures concerning the hand washing. We made a list of "dirty" things that she agreed to touch without washing her hands afterward, and she rated them:

- Doorknobs in her house (but not the bathroom doorknobs, which was too hard). She thought that would be a 6.
- Not washing after she touched the TV remote, the computer mouse, and her iPad. That was a 7.

She understood that to do an "exposure," she needed to practice touching these things over and over again and not washing, until she felt like she didn't want to wash. Her anxiety level would go up at first, but then it would go down. This is the work of fighting OCD. I explained that it is called exposure response prevention and that it's the greatest tool in overcoming OCD.

She also agreed to a few additional goals:

- Not wash after each meal and snack. She rated that a 5.
- Not use hand sanitizer when she looked at or walked by the boys in her class that OCD was telling her were dirty. She rated that a 5.
- Work on wearing different clothing. This was a priority because of the obvious social effects. Again we had to break it down. She agreed to wear one shirt that she had not been wearing because she thought it was uncomfortable and didn't feel right. She rated that a 6.

Next, although she was most anxious about bedtime compulsions, we needed to talk about them since they were so disruptive to the family. Also, kids with OCD and anxiety need their sleep. If they don't get enough sleep, their symptoms can be much worse. We agreed to start with her limiting the bedtime verbal ritual with her parents. Her parents were extremely frustrated with having to say these bedtime phrases over and over again. She agreed that they could say them twice instead of four, eight, or twelve times. She rated Mom and Dad saying the bedtime ritual twice as a 6. We also discussed her listening to an audiobook of her favorite story. She loves *Diary of a Wimpy Kid*, so listening to that made her feel good. She agreed that her parents could leave her with the book on a timer, to turn off automatically, and that she could turn the book on again if she woke up in the middle of the night. We talked about "silly worries" and her need to focus on the book and remember that she is safe in her bed. We also added an additional bonus reward she could get in the morning if she stayed in her bed all night. Dad agreed to make M&M pancakes. That was a great treat for Atalaya.

We agreed we were making progress and proceeded to the next step.

Step 4: Identify and Teach Strategies to Practice

The first strategy is to label the OCD and recognize that OCD is something she can fight and not give in to. Learning to recognize that her worries were OCD would help her see them as things she needed to "boss back." She liked the idea of thinking about it as a game she could win and OCD could lose. When OCD was telling her she had to do her compulsions, she had to learn to say "No" and remember that she is the boss of her brain. She needed to change the way she was thinking about these obsessions and compulsions. Her parents were also learning how to help her with this. Their role became like coaches, encouraging her to fight OCD and supporting her efforts through praise and incentives.

The second strategy is to resist doing the compulsion. She had to practice not doing what OCD told her she had to do and realize that nothing bad happens. This was hard work for her and felt very uncomfortable at first, but she learned that it got easier and easier the more she practiced. We talked more about how to do exposures, where she intentionally triggered OCD and then resisted doing the compulsions, again and again, until she no longer felt like doing them. Some of her behaviors, like getting dressed, were difficult to do exposures with since they happened only once a day. She was starting to understand that any time she could do exposures, they would help her fight the OCD.

Willy and Anna had to learn strategies that could help them parent

Atalaya through this difficult time. They needed to be reminded that this was a process and would take time. They had also researched more about PANDAS and had taken Atalaya to her pediatrician. While waiting for the strep test results, they were learning how to stay focused on the agreed-on goals and how to coach Atalaya to fight the OCD and reinforce this work with positive incentives. Having a plan of action made them feel optimistic, less helpless, and ready for the next step.

Step 5: Note and Chart Progress Made

Charting is extremely useful for several reasons. First, it gave structure to Atalaya's CBT plan. The chart would list specifically everything we had agreed that Atalaya would work on, so the goals would be clear. Second, the chart would remind Atalaya to work on her goals. She was a busy girl. With school, homework, sports, and other activities, it might be easy to forget about the need to *fight* her OCD and not just give in to it. Looking at the chart reminded everyone, including Atalaya's parents, of the work that needed to be done every day. Third, it gave Atalaya an opportunity to chart not only the work she was doing, but more importantly, her progress. By keeping track of how hard these things were, using our 0-to-10-point scale, she would see how that number goes down as she practices, until it is a 0 and she can cross it off the list. Having such a clear measurement of her progress as she did this work would help keep her motivated and positive about the process. And last but not least to Atalaya, her chart would help her keep a running total of the points she had earned toward her prizes.

Her chart needed to be simple and easy to work with for both Atalaya and her parents. Together we discussed how to do this. She would list what she was going to work on each day, check it off when it was done, and rate how hard it was. Atalaya would work with her parents to design the chart. They also discussed where they would keep it. Atalaya didn't want her friends to see it when they came over, so they decided to put it in her drawer next to her bed. They also decided on a time each day to review the chart together. After dinner made the most sense, so they agreed to do it then.

Now, on to the all-important incentives.

Step 6: Offer Incentives to Motivate

Every day that Atalaya worked on her list and recorded her anxiety rating, she earned a point. Since she was working on eight things, she could earn up to 8 points a day. If her parents noticed that she was fighting OCD on things that were not on her list, or if she told them she fought OCD, she could earn bonus points. For example, the first week of doing this, not only did she wear a different shirt, but she earned bonus points for wearing different pants.

But what did she want to cash her points in for? This was the fun part. Atalaya and her parents discussed what she would like to earn and came up with a fun list. They then figured out how many points she needed to get to earn these prizes. Given her young age, she needed to earn prizes quickly to keep motivated.

Her point and prize list:

- Gift card for bookstore **50 points**
- Breakfast out with Dad **35 points**
- M&M pancakes for dinner **25 points**
- Baking with Mom **15 points**

- Sleepover and movie with two friends **50 points**
- Ice skating with a friend **20 points**
- Swimming at the Y with a friend **25 points**

Atalaya was now very excited to fight the OCD. She was ready to show results.

Step 7: Reinforce Progress and Increase Challenges

After a couple of weeks, Atalaya was proud to show off her chart. In the meantime, her test for strep came back positive, and Atalaya was diagnosed with PANDAS. She started taking antibiotics. She made progress with her goals and was proud to show me that her hands were looking much better. We reviewed her chart, and she had gone beyond her goals. She was now earning points for one squirt of soap when she washed, since after a few days, two squirts became easy (rated a 0), so she reduced the soap even more. Touching the remote, iPad, and mouse and not washing were now 0, so we crossed that off her list. Doorknobs were still difficult, so she needed to keep working on that. Touching them without washing was a 3, and we wanted it to be 0. She was able to walk by the "dirty boys" without sanitizing her hands, so we crossed that off her list. Not washing her hands after eating was still a 3, so she needed to keep working on it. Having Mom and Dad do the bedtime ritual twice was easy, so we discussed not having them do it at all. She said that would be a 6, but she was ready to work on it.

Since we had crossed off things that she was no longer worried about, we needed to add some more things. We agreed to start tackling some of the bathroom difficulties. She agreed to take faster showers (fifteen minutes or less) and to turn the shower on and off herself. She said that was now a 7. She also agreed to sit on the toilet in her parents' bathroom, rated a 6, and to use the other bathroom in the house, a 7. She now understood the power she had to fight OCD and was excited to talk about the prizes she had earned.

Anna and Willy were pleased. Anna said, "It is still hard. She is making progress, but we have more work to do. We are fighting with her less and so proud of her because we see how hard she's working. I never in my wildest dreams thought we would have to go through something like this, but having a plan and seeing the progress gives us hope."

We agreed to meet again in a few weeks to monitor her progress and increase the goals.

Next Steps

Atalaya was able to make very quick progress. She went from experiencing acute onset OCD to feeling completely better within weeks. Her mother said, "We have our daughter back!" Her parents are convinced it was the antibiotic that made a huge difference for her, and they are now firm believers that their daughter has PANDAS. They also realize that no matter what the cause, OCD responds very effectively to CBT. They know to be aware that if her symptoms come back, it may again be strep. We all hope that she will not have a relapse, but they know to call me if she does. Atalaya now refers to her OCD as "the time when my brain went crazy" and is so glad it's gone. She has also learned that if the symptoms return, she needs to immediately start working step by step to control them.

Don and Lori's Story

Don called me with concerns about his son's increased worries, and he seemed eager to meet as soon as possible.

"My son Barry is 14 and really struggling," he began. "He is doing weird things, and he came to me and his mother last week and announced that he has OCD. I was frankly shocked, because he is an athlete and loves nothing more than being covered in dirt. And if you looked at his bedroom . . . to put it nicely, he's a slob. I always thought OCD was about hand washing and keeping clean. That's not my son. He insists he looked OCD up on the Internet, and he's convinced he has it. His mom and I are divorced and share custody. She was as surprised as I was by this, although we both have been worried about him. We researched OCD, and I guess it can include a lot of different things. I don't know if he has OCD, but I know my son needs help."

I agreed to set up an appointment with Barry's parents. They agreed that they could easily meet together. Although some divorced parents prefer separate meetings because they have strong conflicts with each other, these parents thought it would be better to meet together.

Both arrived on time and explained that they had been divorced for almost ten years and shared custody. Lori, Barry's mother, started. "I have known something has been wrong for years. He has always been a worrier and had these weird things he had to do at night and things he made me say at bedtime. I talked to my pediatrician about this several times, and she always said that if it doesn't interfere with his functioning, leave it alone. Well, now it's interfering. My son's suffering with lots of weird things he feels he has to do over and over again. And his guilt . . . he's guilty about everything. Not only that, but he's now spending hours on homework. Nighttime is so difficult, with him spending so much time doing God knows what, but he's not getting to sleep until very late. Then getting him up and to school is such a struggle. He also asks questions over and over again: 'Is this okay, is that okay?' It feels like he is constantly seeking reassurance even about silly things. As much as I try, he's been late to school, and I've been late to work. This has to change!"

Don added, "I see the same thing. I try to talk to him, and it doesn't work. He's going to bed later and later, and mornings are a struggle in my house, too. When he said he has OCD, I don't know if that's what it is, but he's right, something's very wrong, and we need help. He's been so irritable, and when I see him up way past his bedtime in the bathroom, I try to get him to bed, and he screams at me and says, 'Now I have to start all over again.' I have no idea what he's talking about. Nothing I do seems to work. Last night he was crying and saying, 'I have to do this. Leave me alone. I have to do it.' It was after midnight. I have no idea how to help my son, but I know he needs help."

It was clear that I needed to meet with Barry as soon as possible.

Barry's Story

Barry seemed to welcome the opportunity to express his thoughts: "I finally told my mom and dad what's been going on in my head, but I didn't tell them everything. I've had this thing in my brain that tells me to do things for a long time, but lately it has gotten so much worse. I have to count just about everything now: the steps I take, brushing my teeth, chewing my food, opening and closing my locker, everything has to be in multiples of four.

"It's so annoying. I can't stop it. If I don't do it, it feels like something very bad will happen. It could be that I will fail a test or worse, something bad could happen to my parents. I thought I was going crazy until I looked it up on the Internet and found out that it's OCD. I read stories about other kids who count and have to read over things again and again, and they worry just like I worry. I thought I was the only one who had all this stuff going on in my head. What a relief to read other kids saying they do exactly what I do."

Barry described worrying about everything. "Sometimes I think I did something bad, like cheat on a test. I know I didn't cheat, but then I worry that maybe I did. It's crazy. I feel guilty about all the things I did wrong in the past. I can't get them out of my head. It's all worse at night. I keep asking my parents all these questions to help me stop worrying. I know they're getting frustrated with me, but I can't help it! They yell at me in the morning because I'm so slow. I don't mean to be slow, but I have to do all these things over and over again. Nothing is easy anymore. And at night it takes me a long time to get to bed and finish my homework. I have to read things over and over again. I used to like to read, and now I hate it. Then in bed, I sometimes get these bad thoughts. I get the thoughts during the day too. Thoughts that I am going to stab someone like my mom or dad or even my dog. I am afraid of knives, scissors, anything sharp. I feel like I might do something bad. I need help. I can't get this stuff out of my head. My parents don't understand. I hate this OCD!"

Barry agreed to meet with his parents and me so we could all work together to help him.

Step 1: Target Anxious Thoughts and Behaviors

Barry made a list first of his worries (obsessions) and shared it with his parents.

- Something bad will happen to me or my parents if I don't do things a certain way or in multiples of four.
- I will go crazy and become a mass murderer.
- I did something very bad.
- I will do something very bad, like stab someone or my dog.
- I'm a bad person.

Then he made a list of his anxious behaviors (compulsions), which he would later rate based on how hard it would be to resist doing them (0, easy, to 10, impossible).

- Counting and doing things in multiples of four, including:
  Brushing my teeth

Washing my face

Having to wash everything at least four times in the shower

Turning lights on and off

Opening and closing doors and drawers

Opening and closing my locker and backpack

Chewing

Stepping (I have to always start with my left foot, and I can't stop walking unless it has been an even number of steps.)

Rereading

- Seeking reassurance when I think I did something bad or when I doubt what I'm supposed to do:

From my dad

From my mom

From my teachers

From my friends

- Avoiding:

Sharp objects (knives, scissors)

Reading

As is often the case, while his parents listened to him make his list, they were surprised and saddened by the burden Barry was carrying. His father said, "Barry, I can't believe you're still able to do everything you're doing with all this in your head."

His mother agreed. "Now I understand why you were doing these weird things and why homework has been such a struggle. It all makes sense now."

With this heightened understanding, we moved on to Step 2.

Step 2: Rate the Anxious Behavior

Barry next assigned rating codes:

- Not counting and doing things in multiples of four   **8**
- Brushing teeth   **7**

- Washing face   **3**
- In the shower   **6**
- Turning lights on and off   **7**

- Opening and closing doors and drawers **5**
- Chewing **8**
- Walking **5**
- Rereading **8**

- Opening and closing locker and backpack **6**
- Not seeking reassurance **8**
- Not avoiding sharp objects **10**
- Not avoiding reading **6**

Next, it was time to address the challenges.

Step 3: Agree on Challenges to Work On

Barry and his parents had already started learning about OCD. Barry needed to change the way he was thinking about the disorder and realize that it was something he needed to fight and not give in to. Barry knew that there was no special power in doing these things, but he felt he couldn't stop because not doing them made him so anxious. We discussed how difficult everything was for him due to his OCD and focused on the most important obsessions and compulsions to work on. Getting to bed earlier and getting to school on time was very important to Barry's parents. Don said, "Barry, you're being so selfish. Don't you realize you're making your mother and me late for work because of all this? We are all so stressed in the morning. It's not fair!"

Barry looked sad, and tears swelled in his eyes. "Selfish? I'm sorry, Dad. Don't you realize it's because of you I have to do these things? I feel that if I don't do them, something terrible will happen to you or Mom. I can't stop it."

I explained that this is OCD, and that Barry is not intentionally causing these problems; he feels out of control. Our goal was to get him back in control and rid him of the OCD.

Barry agreed to work on several behaviors:

- Not rereading. Even though he rated his rereading compulsion at an 8, it was important that he reduce this because of the effect it was having on his life. He used to be an avid reader, but now that had stopped. Homework was taking so long because of his rereading. He was frustrated by it and wanted it to stop.
- Not seeking reassurance from teachers. Barry was a good student and was

aware that his questions to teachers were starting to annoy them. He liked his teachers and wanted them to like him, so he was very motivated to stop this. He knew the questions he asked were silly, like asking over and over again what the homework was or when the next test was. He was also aware that even his friends in class were getting frustrated with him. He asked these questions because he kept doubting himself. Obsessive doubting is a common OCD symptom.

- Not seeking reassurance from his parents.
- Taking less time in the shower. This was important to him because his shower compulsions made his morning routine take too long. He had been late for school and was making his parents late for work.
- Not opening and closing his locker four times. He wanted to stop this because he was worried kids were starting to notice, and it was weird.

As Barry bought into our approach, he was more prepared for the next step.

Step 4: Identify and Teach Strategies to Practice

The first thing that Barry needed to learn was that OCD was lying to him, telling him he had to do these things when he didn't have to. He needed to strengthen his insight into the fact that these behaviors had no special power to prevent or cause bad things. Life doesn't work that way. He needed to take the power out of OCD by seeing it as something outside himself that he had to resist. He also needed to be reminded that many great kids have OCD. He wasn't losing his mind, and he could get rid of his OCD. He also needed to learn to "talk back" to OCD when he doubted himself and wanted to seek reassurance. He needed to remind himself that he knew the answer and didn't have to ask more questions. Then he needed to focus on the here and now and not on his obsessive thoughts. This is how mindfulness helps with OCD: focus on the experiences in the moment, not on the OCD thoughts—let them go.

His parents also had to understand the disorder so that they could help him. They had to learn that trying to be rational with him when he is stuck with OCD only escalated his anxiety. They also had to remember that as hard as all this was for them, it was harder for Barry. These behaviors can have a great impact on the whole family, and sometimes it's hard to remember that OCD behavior is not your child's choice; it's something they feel they "have to do." Barry didn't want to be doing these things; he felt he had no choice. Working together as a team, we would change that.

Rereading is a very common OCD symptom. Sometimes it's driven by just having to read something a certain number of times; sometimes the anxiety is that everything has to be understood perfectly, so the rereading occurs until it just feels "right." This is not to be confused with children who have ADHD or a reading learning disability, who really need to reread because they do not understand the content of the material. Barry felt he had to reread until he understood everything perfectly. But he needed to change the way he was thinking about this. He didn't have to know it all perfectly. All the details aren't important. There are a few strategies to help with rereading. One is listening to audiobooks and reading along with them. Barry needed to remember that the longer he went without rereading, the easier it would be. He had to read and listen to the book without rewinding the audio. When an audiobook was not available, he could try reading out loud to help him resist rereading. He could make a game of it, by trying to see how long he could go without rereading and then trying to go longer the next time. He was a very competitive kid, so this seemed like a great strategy. When he rereads, he needs to think that OCD wins, and he loses. This was a strategy that clicked with Barry. Because he's a boy who always likes to win, OCD didn't have a chance against him.

To help Barry work on not seeking reassurance from teachers, we needed more information. How many times was he asking teachers questions to seek reassurance? Reassurance questions are those he knows the answer to but that his obsessive doubting makes him feel he needs to ask again and again to make sure he's right. Barry said he easily asked four or five questions in each class, with less in math, usually one or two, and science more, up to about eight questions sometimes. He sheepishly admitted that yesterday he had asked the science teacher four times when the next test was. The fourth time he asked the same question, the teacher was clearly angry. He also noticed, for the first time, that some kids were rolling their eyes and laughing as they started to notice.

The strategies he used included remembering that the questions were OCD, and that he knows the answers. Then he needed to limit himself to a certain number of reassurance questions per class. He agreed to no questions in math, three questions in science, and two questions in all the other classes. Knowing he had a limit and keeping track of it would make him more aware of each question, and he would want to think a lot before he asked because he wouldn't want to use up his questions too fast. This would help him ask fewer questions, and eventually we would work on him asking no OCD questions in school.

For not seeking reassurance from his parents, it was agreed, since this was so frequent, that he would have two times during the day when he could seek reassurance. The first was at breakfast, and the second was after dinner. When he wanted to seek reassurance at other times, he needed to postpone his questions until the designated times. This was easier than saying he couldn't seek reassurance at all. That was too hard for Barry right now. When Barry's reassurance time came, he most likely would not need to seek reassurance, because his urge for it will have passed. This is a good step toward no reassurance seeking.

For the shower, he agreed to wash himself twice, not four times. Talking back to OCD meant reminding himself, "I am clean enough."

For the locker, he agreed to opening and closing twice instead of four times to start, telling OCD "No" when he got the urge to do it more.

Step 5: Note and Chart Progress Made

Barry agreed to keep a simple chart in his phone for his OCD work.

For the rereading, he would keep track of how long he went without rereading. To keep it simple when he's reading, he would just record the date and then how long he was able to read without going back and rereading (two paragraphs, one page, three-quarters of a page, etc.), and at the end of all his reading for that day, he would rate it based on how hard it was not to reread, from 0 (easy, no rereading) to 10 (couldn't resist at all), with 5 meaning he reread about half the time.

For the shower, he would record just the date and how many times he washed, keeping it simple for him.

For school, he decided to use a laptop that he had with him all the time. Using a notes program, he would record how many times he asked

OCD questions and how many times he opened and closed his locker. This would keep it easy for him to remember as well as private.

Barry also agreed to use a point system.

For the shower, he would get 5 points if he washed only once, 3 points if he washed twice, and 0 points if he washed more than twice.

For the OCD questions at school, he would get 2 points if he asked no OCD questions in math, 0 if he asked one or more questions; for science, since that was his hardest, he would get 5 points for no OCD questions, 4 points if he asked one, 3 points if he asked two, 2 points if he asked three, and 0 points for more than three. For all the other subjects, he would get 3 points if he asked no OCD questions, 2 points if he asked one, and 1 point if he asked two—any more than two, and he would get 0 points.

For seeking reassurance from his parents, he would get 5 points for seeking reassurance in the morning only at the designated time, which they identified as five minutes after he eats breakfast, and 5 points for saving his later questions for the five minutes after dinner they had agreed on. If he slipped and asked an OCD question, his parents would quickly say "OCD" and not answer the question. If he was able to refocus on something else not related to the OCD and resist continuing to seek reassurance, he would still get his points. We also agreed, however, that if he absolutely needed reassurance and couldn't resist, his parents would reassure him, but he would not earn any points.

For his rereading, he would get 5 points every day he worked on it and showed less rereading overall than the day before, 4 if it was the same, 1 point if he tried and was using the strategies, and 0 points if he didn't try.

Since his parents were divorced and he went back and forth, keeping the chart in his phone, which he always had with him, made this simple. Every evening, they totaled up his points for the day.

But what about incentives?

Step 6: Offer Incentives to Motivate

Barry was excited to get in on this discussion. We realized what hard work this was going to be for him, and his parents wanted to offer him rewards for his effort in fighting his OCD.

Barry quickly announced what his parents already knew, that he wanted new basketball sneakers. He also wanted to go to sporting events with his dad and maybe a friend. His father makes his favorite meal, homemade pepperoni pizza, so he put that on his list too. With Mom, he loves her carrot cake and enjoys going to breakfast with her.

It was decided:

- Sneakers   **50 points**
- Tickets to college basketball games with a friend   **30 points**
- Ticket to a professional sporting event with Dad   **100 points**
- Pepperoni pizza made by Dad **20 points**

- Carrot cake made by Mom **20 points**
- Breakfast out with Mom **20 points**

And now on to the final step . . .

Step 7: Reinforce Progress and Increase Challenges

After three weeks, Barry and his parents were ready to meet again. He had been working hard and making progress. He had earned his sneakers, breakfast with Mom, and pizza from Dad.

His chart showed progress, with his numbers of difficulty down. These numbers were important because they told us how hard it was for Barry to resist these compulsions. His most recent daily chart showed the following numbers.

- Reassurance morning, 0. He no longer needed reassurance in the morning. Great accomplishment!
- Reassurance evening, 6. He still needed to seek reassurance in the evening. The urge was still there.
- Shower, 0. He no longer felt the need to keep washing, but he was still doing it twice.
- Rereading, 5. He was still struggling with this one; it had improved, but he needed to keep working on it.

- Teacher reassurance, 3. This was much better but still needed more work.
- Locker, 2. This was almost done, but occasionally he was still doing the opening and closing.

Next we had to increase the challenges.

- Reassurance seeking in the evening, which he wanted to keep working on, 6. It now seemed easy for him in the morning but still difficult in the evening.
- Shower, washing only one time, 3. It was easy to wash only twice; now the goal was to wash only once.
- Teacher reassurance, 3. Decreasing his reassurance seeking was much easier than when he had started, so it was time to increase the goal. The goal now was no reassurance in his classes except science, which was the hardest, so he is allowed two OCD questions in that class only.
- Rereading, 5. Not rereading continued to be difficult, so we decided to keep those goals the same.

Now he also wanted to add some other OCD goals, including not counting steps. Since it always had to be an even number of steps, he would do an exposure of intentionally walking an odd number of steps. We did that in the office: he got up and took five steps and then sat down. His anxiety level went up to a 7, but after ten minutes, he was at a 0, no anxiety. He agreed to practice this every day and rate it. To chart not counting steps throughout the day could be too tedious, so we agreed that he could just rate himself at the end of the day. If he didn't count at all, that would be a 0; if he counted all the time and didn't resist, 10; if he counted about half the time, 5. At the end of the day, he would earn 10 points for not counting steps at all, 9 points for not counting most of the time, 7 points for counting half the time, 3 points for trying and resisting many times, and 0 for not trying or for resisting very little. He was on the honor system, but it was clear that Barry couldn't lie about this since he feels too guilty. He was an excellent reporter. We now planned to meet again in a few weeks, but he was really making excellent progress and reducing his OCD symptoms.

Next Steps

Barry continued to work on his OCD. After a couple of months, he was clearly making progress, but it was slow. Even though we attempted to work on his intrusive violent thoughts, to take the power out of the thoughts, he still couldn't do any exposures to sharp objects. He avoided all knives and scissors and was greatly bothered by these thoughts. In addition, he felt his anxiety was really interfering with his ability to concentrate at school. So he had a consult with a child psychiatrist, who added medication to his treatment (I refer patients for medication when appropriate but don't prescribe myself). With medication, his progress doing this work was much more rapid. He was better able to apply the skills he had learned and was feeling less anxious. We continued to meet once a month to review his progress and to agree on new goals.

His father said, "He is much better, and we are so proud of him. The work he has done to manage this OCD has been so hard. He really is a strong kid!"

DSM-5 Guidelines

Obsessive-Compulsive Disorder

The *DSM-5* identifies the diagnostic criteria necessary for a diagnosis. The assumption is that many readers will have children who meet some but not all the criteria.

A. Presence of obsessions, compulsions or both:

Obsessions are defined by (1) and (2):

1. Recurrent and persistent thoughts, urges, or images that are experienced, at some time during the disturbance, as intrusive and unwanted, and that in most individuals cause marked anxiety or distress.

2. The individual attempts to ignore or suppress such thoughts, urges, or images, or to neutralize them with some other thought or action (i.e., by performing a compulsion).

Compulsions are defined by (1) and (2):

1. Repetitive behaviors (e.g., hand washing, ordering, checking) or mental acts (e.g., praying, counting, repeating words silently) that the individual feels driven to perform in response to an obsession or according to rules that must be applied rigidly.

2. The behaviors or mental acts are aimed at preventing or reducing anxiety or distress, or preventing some dreaded event or situation; however, these behaviors or mental acts are not connected in a realistic way with what they are designed to neutralize or prevent, or are clearly excessive.

Note: Young children may not be able to articulate the aims of these behaviors or mental acts.

B. The obsessions or compulsions are time-consuming (e.g., take more than 1 hour per day) or cause clinically significant distress or impairment in social, occupational, or other important areas of functioning.

C. The obsessive-compulsive symptoms are not attributable to the physiological effects of a substance (e.g., a drug of abuse, a medication) or another medical condition.

D. The disturbance is not better explained by the symptoms of another mental disorder (e.g., excessive worries, as in generalized anxiety disorder; preoccupation with appearance, as in body dysmorphic disorder; difficulty discarding or parting with possessions, as in hoarding disorder; hair pulling, as in trichotillomania [hair-pulling disorder]; skin picking, as in excoriation [skin-picking disorder]; stereotypies, as in stereotypic movement disorder; ritualized eating behavior, as in eating disorders; preoccupation with substances or gambling, as in substance-related and addictive disorders; preoccupation with having an illness, as in illness anxiety disorder; sexual urges or fantasies, as in paraphilic disorders; impulses, as in disruptive, impulse-control, and conduct disorders; guilty ruminations, as in major depressive disorder; thought insertion or delusional preoccupations, as in schizophrenic spectrum and other psychotic disorders; or repetitive patterns of behavior, as in autism spectrum disorder).

Specify if:

With good or fair insight: The individual recognizes that obsessive-compulsive disorder beliefs are definitely or probably not true or that they may or may not be true.

With poor insight: The individual thinks obsessive-compulsive disorder beliefs are probably true.

With absent insight/delusional beliefs: The individual is completely convinced that obsessive-compulsive disorder beliefs are true.

Specify if:

Tic-related: The individual has a current or past history of a tic disorder.

American Psychiatric Association. "Obsessive-Compulsive Disorder." In *Diagnostic and Statistical Manual of Mental Disorders*. 5th ed. Washington, DC: American Psychiatric Association, 2013.

Chapter 7

....

Scared to Death

Specific Phobias

All children have fears, and many of these fears are normal. Young children are often afraid of the dark or supernatural creatures, like ghosts or witches, and older children often fear bad things happening to them, like natural disasters. When a child develops a phobia, it's typically severe and persistent and affects normal life. Rather than getting better or growing out of it, kids with phobias often feel more frightened and avoidant over time, not less.

Children having a phobic reaction are in a "fight or flight" sense of panic. Their bodies respond as if they're in great danger when they are not. Their muscles become tight, and adrenaline is released, often causing physical symptoms, including rapid heart rate, nausea, chest pain, dizziness, and shortness of breath. Children having a panic attack like this may also become disorganized in their thinking and have difficulty processing what's happening to them.

Talking to a child in this state of intense anxiety is usually not helpful and can actually make things worse. They can't take in what is being said to them, and they are highly sensitive to being criticized. This is not a teachable moment—they are too far over the top with anxiety to process rationally what is being said to them. The best thing to do to help them is to focus on relaxation strategies and to rationalize only after they have calmed down.

Although all cases of phobia are unique, the examples in this chapter are representative. They focus on phobias related to dogs, thunder and lightning, and bugs.

Suma and Larry's Story

Suma and Larry came to my office very concerned about their daughter. Suma explained, "We are here about our 8-year-old, Ellen. We have three kids, all girls, and she's our middle child. She always seemed so happy-go-lucky, and in many ways, she's a normal kid. I would have never thought we'd find ourselves getting help for her, but here we are. Ellen has developed a severe, intense fear of dogs. She is petrified of them. In our community, this is a major problem. Most of her friends have dogs. Most of our neighbors have dogs. Dogs are everywhere. So she's severely limited by this fear. Ellen can't go on most play dates because there are dogs. Riding her bike is now out of the question. She can't even walk to the bus stop. She is basically housebound because of her fear."

At first, Suma hadn't wanted to accept her daughter's condition and would force her to go out and do normal activities. "That was until two weeks ago," she continued, "when we were bike riding together. It was a beautiful day, and we were talking and laughing side by side until she saw a dog. It was a little tiny dog, on a leash, all the way across the street from where we were riding. Ellen freaked out. She started screaming and crying and actually fell off her bike, she was so scared. I realized this was now a safety issue. I could imagine, God forbid, her running into traffic if there was a dog around. She becomes totally out of control, reacting and not thinking at all. Later, she feels so bad about it she cries. She knows it's irrational. Now I feel like I can't take the chance of having her outside if a dog might come around. I don't trust her to stay safe."

Suma then mentioned another fear that was also getting out of control: "She's afraid of thunder and lightning. She was always sensitive to noise, but instead of this getting better, it's getting worse."

She then looked at her husband and said, "I worry Larry is making it worse by praising her for her great knowledge about weather. I think it's gotten way out of hand."

Larry looked defensive and quickly jumped in. "She loves the computer, and it's a great learning tool. Our little girl knows more about weather patterns than a meteorologist. I got her lots of books on the weather, and she devoured them. She checks the current weather conditions and the forecast on the computer several times a day. If you want to know anything about the weather in this area for the next seven days, she has it memorized. She even did her science project on the weather. How can all this knowledge be a bad thing? Who knows, she may grow up to be a famous meteorologist on TV."

Suma interrupted. "Larry, it hasn't helped. If anything, she's worse." Suma then turned to me and said, "My husband is a scientist. He likes to think Ellen's following in his footsteps. I know knowledge is good, but this is out of control. The more she learns and studies weather forecasts, the more frightened she becomes if a storm is coming. If there are clouds in the sky, she doesn't want to go outside. On cloudy days, I literally have to struggle with her to go to school. Now with all her 'knowledge,' it could be sunny out, but if she thinks a storm could be coming, she's afraid to go outside. Her teacher says that if it's cloudy out, she spends a lot of time looking out the window and is distracted. On sunny days, she's fine. It's just like with the dogs. When there's thunder and lightning, she goes into a complete panic. She runs into the basement, huddling in a corner, away from any windows, covering her ears, often crying until it's over. In the middle of the night, if there's a storm, she runs into our bed and stays there, scared to death. Soccer season is starting, and she loves soccer, but I know, as soon there's a cloud in the sky, she's not going to want to leave the house. And what are we going to do about summer camp? Keep her home every time there's a chance of rain?"

Suma caught her breath and stated the obvious: "We clearly need help with this."

Larry added, "Don't get us wrong. She is a sweet kid and a joy. Other than this, she's our easiest kid; I can't believe she's gotten so extreme with all this. She has lots of friends, and her teachers love her. She's very smart and does well in school. Maybe she's too smart? I thought more information would help her to be less afraid, but maybe my wife's right. It certainly has gotten worse. I don't know the answer. We just need to know how to help her."

This sense of frustration led these caring parents to ask their daughter to meet together with me.

Ellen's Story

Ellen seemed mature and poised as she started to express her feelings: "I know dogs are cute and all, but they really scare me. I don't know why. I get so scared when they are near me. I just freak out. I can't help it. I guess I think they're going to hurt me, bite me. I feel like dogs can just get so out of control. I can't explain it. I just really get so scared. Even if they're on a leash, they might get off the leash. I just don't feel safe. I don't think dogs like me. Three of my friends have dogs, and I can't go to their houses to play. Even if they put the dog in another room, I'm still scared it will get out."

She took a deep breath before continuing. "When I was riding my bike the other day, all of a sudden I saw a dog being walked across the street. I started crying and screaming and got so scared, I lost control of my bike. I jumped off the bike and scraped my arm and leg. I can't ride my bike now because there are too many dogs around. I wish there were a place where no dogs are allowed, but I don't know of any place like that. I wish there were no dogs in this whole world, and then I would be fine. I don't hate them really. I just can't stand being anywhere near them."

Ellen then elaborated on the other big fear: thunder and lightning. "I get really scared that maybe there could be a tornado or a hurricane and we'll all die. That's how it feels when the sky starts to get dark, like we could die. People do die from lightning and tornadoes and hurricanes. I've read about all the damage they can do. It could happen to us. It's possible. When I know there's a storm coming, I feel like it's going to happen, that this could be it. I just get so scared. Nature can be unpredictable, you know. If there's thunder and lightning, forget it. I can't be outside. I have to go down in the basement and cover my ears until it's all over. Of course you never want to be near a window if a storm is coming. I think about this every day. That's why I always check the weather. I need to be prepared. If there are clouds in the sky, I check the weather reports again, and if there's a storm coming, I need to know when and how bad it's going to be and for how long. I've learned all about the weather and how to track storms, sometimes before I even see the weather report.

"If I had three wishes," she concluded, "there'd be no dogs ever, no storms ever, and every day would be sunny. That would make me so happy."

After hearing Ellen's words, I explained my recommended strategy, to use the seven steps. We agreed to set up the next session together to start working on Ellen's fears.

Step 1: Target Anxious Thoughts and Behaviors

First, we specified the different phobias, starting with the fear of dogs.

Ellen's anxious thoughts were hard to identify because she quickly moved from 0, being relaxed and happy, to 10, being in a panic. It seemed she instantly became filled with paralyzing fear. Rationally, she knew that dogs may not want to hurt her, but when she was faced with a dog, her thinking changed. She needed to first become more aware of her anxious thoughts about dogs, so she could challenge them before she automatically jumped to panic, oblivious to rational thoughts.

Ellen's anxious behaviors included:

- Total avoidance of friends' homes if they had a dog
- Not walking or riding her bike outside
- Avoidance of any setting where there could possibly be a dog, which in her community meant almost everywhere
- Crying, screaming, and running away in a panic if she saw a dog

Next, we addressed the phobia of thunder and lightning.

Again, she was uncontrollably afraid that something terrible could happen when a storm approached. Her fears included a hurricane or tornado that would kill people, or lightning that would strike her or her family. Although she was convinced that every storm could be fatal, she needed to understand that these were irrational thoughts that shouldn't trigger panic. We needed to work on greater clarity regarding these thoughts so that she could "talk back" to them and replace them.

Her anxious behaviors included:

- Checking the Internet to monitor the weather every morning, afternoon, and evening

- Avoiding being outside when clouds were in the sky and she feared a storm might be coming
- Not wanting to go to school on a cloudy day
- Seeking reassurance from others that a storm was not coming
- Reading everything she could about weather, storms, and other weather-related topics such as natural weather disasters
- Frequently looking out the window at school, making sure no clouds were in the sky
- Not being able to sit near a window at school, for fear lightning could strike her
- Not being able to go outside when it rains, for fear she's in danger

When a thunderstorm actually struck, her anxious behaviors included:

- Hiding in the basement away from windows
- Holding her ears
- Sometimes crying in fear
- Needing to sleep in her parents' bed
- Being unable to go outside

Next, it was time to address our rating system.

Step 2: Rate the Anxious Behavior

We went through all the behaviors on her list and asked her to rate how hard it would be, from 0 (easy) to 10 (impossible), not to do these things. She listened and then folded her arms, looking straight at her parents. "I'm sorry," she said. "I can't do any of this. It's too hard. They are all a 10. I can't change the way I feel. I'm too scared. Isn't there some medicine I can take to make this go away?"

At this point, it was very important to calmly assess the situation. I reassured Ellen that although there was no magic pill for this, we could make these scary feelings go away by working together. We broke down her challenges one at a time. First we looked at the dog phobia. I asked her parents if they knew of anyone who had a nice, sweet, mellow dog that we could work with. It should not be an active, playful puppy. It had to be a dog that they could see often, ideally daily, to work with. Ellen and Larry thought about it and then came up with a friend's dog, Sophia. She was 10 years old, very calm, and loved kids. Perfect. Ellen also knew Sophia, and she didn't used to be scared of her, but since this dog phobia had taken hold, she was even afraid of Sophia.

Ellen needed to challenge her irrational thoughts about dogs, but first she had to recognize them. This was hard for her, but she needed to know that these false beliefs fueled her anxiety.

She began to list these fearful thoughts:

- I am going to be attacked by Sophia.
- The leash could break, and Sophia will run after me.
- Sophia is going to hurt me.
- Sophia is going to bite me.
- Sophia is going to jump on me and knock me down.

We then discussed whether it was likely that Sophia would do these hurtful things. Ellen didn't even have to think about it. She knew Sophia was a sweet, gentle dog and would never hurt her. Her mom joked that Sophia was not a hungry wolf on the tundra; she was a spoiled golden retriever that lived like a queen. Ellen laughed and was on the verge of understanding that these worries were "silly worries," not based on what's real.

She then repeated the rational thoughts that she needed to tell herself, what she had to say in her head to talk back to her silly worries:

- Sophia is a nice, gentle dog and doesn't bite.
- The leash is strong and won't break; even if it does break, Sophia won't hurt me.
- Sophia likes kids and likes me and is happy to see me. That's why her tail wags so much.
- Sophia is a cute, soft dog who always looks like she's smiling.

We discussed where we could start in desensitizing Ellen to dogs, but we needed Ellen to guide us. I asked her a few questions, and then asked her to rate the difficulty, how high her anxiety would be.

- Can we walk by Sophia's house and look at her behind their front door? Ellen rated that a **1**.
- Can we have Sophia's owner, Mrs. Lee, walk across the street with Sophia on a leash? Ellen rated that a **4**.
- How about you walk by Sophia when she is on a leash and sitting? Ellen rated that a **6**.
- How about petting Sophia when she is on a leash, sitting, and your mom or dad is right with you and you just quickly touch Sophia? Ellen looked serious and said immediately an **8**.
- Touching Sophia when her owner has her sitting, on a leash, and covers her mouth? **6**.
- Riding your bike across the street from Sophia when she is on a leash? **7**.
- Putting food in a bowl for Sophia and watching her eat when you are away from her? **7**.

Now Ellen had told us where we should focus with her dog phobia. A rating of about 4 in her anxiety level would be a good place to start.

Next we addressed her storm phobia. Again, Ellen said everything was a 10, and she felt totally overwhelmed by this fear. We worked on the cognitive aspects. She knew her fears were irrational. I asked her to tell me her anxious thoughts and together we would work on replacement thoughts.

She listed her anxious thoughts:

- I see clouds, and a storm is definitely coming.
- I need to know if a storm is coming so I can be prepared and protect myself.
- If a storm comes, I could get struck by lightning and die.
- If a storm is coming, it could mean a deadly hurricane or tornado, and we can all die or lose everything.
- These storms could destroy our house.
- The louder the noise from the lightning, the more dangerous it is for me. If it's too loud, it will hurt my ears, and it means something bad is going to happen.
- Being outside or near a window when it's raining is very dangerous, and something bad could happen to me.

Then she listed her replacement thoughts, or as we called it, "The Truth about Storms":

- Clouds are not a message that a storm is coming. Many times there are clouds and no storm.
- I don't need to check the Internet. If a storm is coming, I will be okay.
- I'm safe if a storm is coming, and I don't need to hide in the basement.
- The chance of getting struck by lightning is very, very small.
- The chances of a tornado or hurricane coming where I live are very small.
- If a major storm is coming, my parents and teachers would be notified and know what to do. It is not something I need to prepare for.
- The loud noise of thunder is not connected to any danger.
- The chances of being struck by lightning by being near a window or walking outside during a storm are extremely small.

Once she has challenged these thoughts, she has a better mindset for rating the behaviors:

- Not checking the Internet at all   10
- Checking the Internet only in the evening   5
- Not seeking reassurance when there are clouds in the sky   6
- Not going into the basement when there is a thunderstorm   7
- Not covering my ears when there is a thunderstorm   5
- Not going into Mom and Dad's bed during a storm at night   10

- Walking outside during a storm   9
- Walking near a window during a storm   7
- Not crying or screaming during a storm   4
- Not complaining about going to school when it is cloudy or a storm is predicted   5

Now we were ready to tackle the phobias head on.

Step 3: Agree on Challenges to Work On

Ellen reviewed all she had written about her phobias, and we looked at actions that were not rated too high.

For the dog phobia, she first agreed to work on walking outside and looking at Sophia from across the street, where Sophia would be on a leash. Ellen would need to practice with Sophia as much as possible to reduce her anxiety. After each practice session, she would rate her anxiety level on a scale of 0 (no anxiety) to 10 (I can't stand it). For each session, her anxiety would go up, but then it would go down. When her anxiety was down, she could stop the session. She was reminded that the more she practiced, the faster her fear would go down until she was no longer afraid. When this was no longer hard, we would increase the goal to getting closer to Sophia with Sophia still on the leash, until Ellen could eventually pet the dog.

For the storm phobia, Ellen agreed to try several goals:

- Check the Internet only once a day, at night.
- Not complain about going to school on a cloudy day.
- Not seek reassurance when it is cloudy.
- Not cry when there is a thunderstorm but challenge her thoughts.
- Not cover her ears when there is a storm.

In addition, she agreed to work on gradually exposing herself to the sights and sounds of storms. She would download the sounds of thunder and wind on her iPod and listen to them. She also agreed to watch YouTube videos of thunder and lightning. At the local science museum, there was an exhibit about thunder that created a loud noise, and Ellen agreed to go to that with her father and not cover her ears.

We were seeing results as we began to implement strategies.

Step 4: Initiate and Teach Strategies to Practice

Ellen was taught how to challenge her anxious thoughts, talking back in her head with her replacement thoughts. For instance:

- Use mindfulness to experience what was happening around her and not rush to catastrophic expectations about what would happen if there were a thunderstorm.
- Practice staying in the here and now, where she is safe and in no danger.

- Focus on the feelings of rain falling on her and the sounds of rain and even of thunder. Closing her eyes, she could imagine these sensations and feeling calm. In addition to challenging her thoughts, she could work on desensitizing herself to the sights and sounds of storms. She had to stop running away from the feelings they provoked.
- Use calming activities to help her relax, including music, drawing, and reading.

We were getting there.

Step 5: Note and Chart Progress Made

Ellen and her mother drew up a chart that listed her goals and her ratings of how hard it was to practice these exercises.

Step 6: Offer Incentives to Motivate

As is usually the case, Ellen was very excited about earning prizes for doing this work. We agreed on a point system where she would earn one point every time she practiced working on her goals and two points when she moved up her goal to the next step.

We then discussed what she wanted to earn. She was eager to earn craft supplies (she loves making bracelets), special time with Dad going out for breakfast, special time with Mom baking cookies, and having breakfast for dinner. (She loves pancakes and waffles, and having them for dinner is a special treat.)

Mom and Dad looked at her wish list and decided how many points she needed:

- Craft supplies **30 points**
- Breakfast with Dad **25 points**
- Baking cookies **20 points**
- Breakfast for dinner **15 points**
- Sleepover and pizza with two friends **50 points**

Ellen was eager to earn her points.

Step 7: Reinforce Progress and Increase Challenges

Ellen and her parents came to meet four weeks later, and we reviewed her chart. It was filled with decorations and lots of stickers. Each sticker equaled one point, and she had clearly earned a lot of points.

She had been working very hard with Sophia on the dog phobia. For instance, every day after school, she had a "play date" with Sophia. She had graduated, step by step, from walking across the street from Sophia on a leash all the way to petting Sophia and giving her a treat when she was sitting. They were fast becoming good buddies as Sophia had learned to expect Ellen's play date as well.

When Ellen was even more comfortable with Sophia, the next step would be to go out and be exposed to other dogs. Ellen rated this a 6, much better than when we had started. She said, "I think I'm not so scared of dogs anymore. Sophia is fun to play with."

With the storms, she had done well with checking the Internet only once a day. Our goal was to get her to stop checking it at all. I suggested she move to checking once a week. Ellen's smile disappeared, and she looked worried. "No, I can't do that," she said. So I suggested checking twice a week on Sunday and on Thursday. She agreed to that and said it would rate a 7 on her anxiety scale.

She'd been watching videos of storms, and that was now "easy." She had also been listening to the sounds of thunder on her iPod, and she had gone to the science museum to listen to storm sounds. She said that both were also easy.

She did well with not complaining about going to school when it was cloudy, but one day when it was raining, she had not wanted to go to school. So we needed to help her with that when it was raining.

Unfortunately, unlike with the dog phobia, exposure to her weather-related fears was dependent on when there were thunderstorms, which were not that frequent. There had been only two thunderstorms since we'd last met. The first storm had been harder for her than the second. During the first one, she hadn't covered her ears or gone to the basement, but she had cried and hadn't been able to go near windows. During the second thunderstorm, she hadn't cried and had been able to walk by a window. She was making progress, but there was more to work on.

Ellen was also proud to show me her list of prizes and seemed very motivated to keep progressing. Hopefully, there would be more nonthreatening thunderstorms and friendly dogs for her to practice with.

Next Steps

Ellen's parents were able to work together and help Ellen face her fears, and she continued to make progress. After the most recent rain shower, she emailed me with great pride: "I was outside in the rain and not afraid. Yea!"

We continued to meet once a month. She's learned not to run away from her fears but to practice facing them.

Lenny and Tara's Story

Tara and Lenny came to meet with me because of their concerns about their 13-year-old son, Sam. "Sam is a great kid," Tara began. "He has Asperger's, and I always say he's our gift from God, just the way he is. He's sweet, gentle, and kind. There's not a mean bone in this kid's body. He has his quirks, for sure, but we love that he's different. However, the one thing that is really getting in his way lately is his fear of bugs."

Lenny added, "Flying bugs, to be specific. Show him a huge furry spider, and he couldn't care less, but a little flying moth, and he's in a panic. Makes no sense. He has had different fears in the past, fear of the dark, fear of monsters in his room, fear of being left alone, but they all came and went. This fear of bugs isn't going anywhere. I think it's even getting worse."

Tara agreed. "He's so scared of flying insects that now he's avoiding lots of things. Every day, it's something new. He won't go outside to play with his friends in the neighborhood. He won't go out for recess at school. He won't play in gym class if it is outside—you name it, he won't do it. He has become a huge homebody, which is not like him."

Lenny continued. "At first I thought he was staying in just to play those stupid computer games, but no. I took the games away, thinking that would get him to go outside, and it made no difference. He still wouldn't budge. He refuses to go out of the house. He is so afraid of bugs, he runs like a maniac from the house to the car when we are going somewhere, and he does the same thing when we get somewhere. He's out of the car but running into shelter like he's being ambushed. I have even seen him flapping his arms to keep the bugs away. I tried to say, 'Buddy, you got to stop that; it looks really weird.' You know what he said? 'Dad, I have Asperger's. I don't care how it looks.'"

Tara was shaking her head. "This kid is smart as a whip, and he has an answer for everything. He's right. He doesn't care what anyone thinks, and I guess there's good and bad to that. Sometimes I wish I had Asperger's, so I wouldn't worry so much about what other people think."

"Tara, this isn't about Asperger's, or other people," Larry said. "I don't want Sam scared so much of the time. He used to love nature, hiking and playing outside. He was the kid who could play outside with a stick and walk around picking flowers in the backyard by himself for hours. Now, in seconds of being outside, he's in a panic. Sam needs to be outdoors. He needs the fresh air and exercise. Since this whole thing got so much worse several months ago, I'm sure he's put on weight. He stays home sitting and eating snacks, instead of being out, running around with the other kids. It's not healthy for him. I feel like I've tried talking to him till I'm blue in the face about bugs, insects, nature, you name it. He listens and seems to learn, but then he goes right back into fear mode when it comes to going outside. You would think our house was surrounded by killer bees."

It was time for Sam to see me.

Sam's Story

He began, "I have entomophobia, or insectophobia. Take your pick. It means fear of bugs. I have a very bad case of this disease. I hate bugs. You don't have to tell me about bugs. I know all about them. I have thirty-four books on bugs. I know their names, what they look like, how they mate, what they eat." He told me there are some nine thousand different kinds of insects in this country and 6 to 10 million species on the planet. He also reported that the evolution of winged insects is very controversial. Some researchers believe that their wings evolved from gills; others disagree. He believes in the gill theory himself, although he said that there's not conclusive evidence to support it 100 percent.

"Last year I did a science project on bugs," he told me. "I am the bug expert in my school and still I suffer from entomophobia. I don't think anyone is going to be able to help me. Therapy just won't work with me. I think it's okay if I'm afraid of bugs. There are worse things to be afraid of, actually. Do you know how many different phobias there are? I've studied that too. I love my mom and dad and my sister, Alice. That's really what's most important, right? There are lots of things I'm not afraid of too. So why don't we just leave my little fear of bugs alone, okay? So let's just forget about this therapy stuff, okay? I talked about it for months with another therapist, and it didn't help. I can accept that I have this phobia, but I wish my parents would leave me alone and not keep bringing me to therapy."

I encouraged Sam to continue. "I love the game Minecraft and can play it and not go outside. I don't really want to go outside. I just want to stay in my room and play Minecraft, okay? I really am fine with having Asperger's and entomophobia. No big deal. They kind of go together in my mind. Of course, most kids with Asperger's don't have entomophobia, and most kids with entomophobia don't have Asperger's, but I bet a lot have both I will have to look that up. I kind of like having both. I am the bug expert, remember?"

At this point, I discussed with Sam's parents how therapies can be very different and that cognitive behavioral therapy can be particularly effective with phobias. I also expressed how important it was for Sam's parents to be on the same page with each other and with the therapist about his anxiety. Clearly, if they just complied with what Sam wanted, there would be no progress.

Tara and Lenny agreed to meet again to discuss this and not keep things the way they were, even though there was pushback from Sam, . . . and even though Tara had mixed feelings.

"Well, it is clear Sam doesn't want to engage in this treatment," she said. "He wants nothing to do with these goals. He wants to stay at home, in his room playing Minecraft, and doing his own thing away from kids and away from bugs." She hesitated, then continued. "Maybe that's what he should do. Kids with Asperger's like to be alone, right? Should we impose our goals on him if he doesn't want to work on this? He needs to have his voice heard, right? He hated the last therapy. He finally said, 'Mom, why am I seeing that doctor? He knew nothing about Minecraft, and even after I taught him, how is this helping with my bug problem?'"

Tara said she'd had to agree that there had been no progress, so they had stopped therapy, and I could understand her frustration when she wondered if they were now pushing too hard to make him be someone he's not.

"We accept the Asperger's," she continued. "I think we need to accept that this is just part of it and stop pressuring him about it. I don't want him to start feeling bad about himself. He seems happy playing inside. Doesn't he have the right to make a decision about therapy? Since he really wants no part of this, can we drag him in here?"

Lenny sighed, looked at me, and said, "We have a good marriage, but honestly, this is the thing we fight about. I'm sorry, but I think my wife is way too overprotective of Sam. I know he's special, and he has Asperger's, but everyone agrees his Asperger's is mild, and his anxiety is the problem. That's what the school says, and that's what everyone who meets with him says: very smart boy—gifted, in fact—mild Asperger's, severe anxiety. So I think we have to help him with the anxiety. I can't see how letting him avoid situations is the right thing to do. I know that's what he wants. Let's face it, he will never work on his fears unless we push him."

He went on. "And we both have to agree it's the right thing to do. I've done a lot of reading about all this. I think cognitive behavioral therapy is the way to go, and we've never tried it before with Sam. I know he's almost 14 years old, and that's what worries me. We have a small window now to influence him and get him help. I don't want my son to grow up to be a man who's afraid to go outside because of bugs. What kind of life will that be for him? We don't want him living in our basement on the computer."

In a positive way, Lenny confronted Tara, saying that in the past, Sam had always known his mom would give in and let Sam avoid things.

"You're a great mother," Larry said, "but you never agreed on pushing him, so let's face it, we failed. His anxiety has gotten the better of us, and it's gotten worse with time, not better. He's way too comfortable isolating himself and acting different from his peers. I think he can be much more mainstreamed."

Tara shook her head. "I don't think this is fair. We need to hear his voice. If he doesn't want to work on these goals, we shouldn't force him."

Lenny now raised his voice in frustration. "His only hope is to get over this anxiety so he can reach his potential. I understand you don't want us to force him into goals he doesn't agree with, but what exactly are his goals? He wants to stay alone and play computer games. That can't be good for him. I know he said he wants no part of this therapy and says he's fine the way he is. Well, he's not fine. He should be able to go outside. He loves nature. He loves animals. He'd love to pet all those animals at the farm like he used to. Now he can't because of this bug thing. His life has become so limited, not by his Asperger's, but by his fears.

"If it takes incentives, bribes, limits, whatever, we need to get him over this. I think he can do it. He needs to be pushed, and we can push. If we don't help him out of this now, we will only have a bigger problem later."

Tara was still unconvinced and reluctant to force Sam back into therapy to get over his fears. "His mind doesn't work like everyone else's. How is this going to work anyway? What kind of rewards can we give him? He's smart, you know. He'll know we're just bribing him to do this."

Lenny was calmer now and simply said, "I will bribe him. I don't care what he thinks. I just want to be able to go outside and take a walk with my son, ride bikes like we used to, go into the city. Let's face it, this problem is affecting our whole family. Do you think our daughter hasn't noticed that we never do any family activities anymore? What do you think our vacation is going to look like this summer? Even if he goes to a computer camp all summer, I'm not having some kind of indoor computer vacation with my family. I know you may disagree, but this is our son, and our opportunity to help him is now. If we wait, it will be harder."

Tara listened intently and then finally said, "I guess you're right. I just find it hard to impose our values on him since he has Asperger's, and we need to respect that he's different."

"Hey, no one is trying to change the fact that he has some type of autism," Larry said. "But think about it. We're talking about helping him get free from his anxiety. If our daughter had this phobia, would we, for a minute, think we should let her avoid activities and not get over this fear? No. So the same should be for Sam. If we can help him to be less anxious, doesn't he deserve that?"

Thinking about it that way helped Tara to get on board with helping Sam.

It's not unusual for parents to disagree on how much to push their child to fight the anxiety and how much to give in to it. For one thing, giving in to it is easier in the short term. And it can be confusing sorting out how much of this is not anxiety but a feature of something else like Asperger syndrome or being shy or introverted. In the end, Tara and Lenny agreed to help Sam with his anxiety.

We discussed the steps and needed to have an initial discussion about the rewards and incentives first, before we started with Sam. Without powerful incentives that both parents can agree on, we would not even get Sam to the next appointment to start the work. Even though we would discuss the specific rewards and how he would earn them later in the process, Sam needed positive motivation to even get started with the therapy, so exciting him about the idea of earning prizes was needed from the start. Sam was a child who seemed to have everything, and since he was avoiding activities because of his anxiety, we were limited in our choices for rewards. His parents had to start a point system for Sam, and their first homework was to come up with a list of incentives that could motivate him to even come to therapy. They could then offer him points for coming to each meeting, in addition to doing the actual CBT. We also needed to be very positive with Sam about this process. The kids who are the most resistant to this work feel this way because they are so scared to challenge their anxiety; they are afraid it will be too hard.

After convincing Tara, it was time to help Sam realize he could do this . . . step by step.

Step 1: Target Anxious Thoughts and Behaviors

Sam and his parents arrived for their first session together with Sam. "Sam is not happy being here," Lenny said. "It was a struggle to get him to come."

Sam sat down and looked at his hands, where he was fiddling with a toy. He quickly announced, "I am only here for the points. I got fifty points for doing this."

His mother quickly reminded him that if he wanted his points, he also had to cooperate, and he reluctantly agreed. So we started with Sam making a list of his anxious thoughts about bugs:

- They could bite, and that would hurt.
- They feel creepy on my skin.
- The flying thing just scares me.
- They could fly into my mouth or my ear. Yuck, who knows where they could fly into?
- I have never been stung by a bee. What if I'm allergic? I could die!
- What if African killer bees come after me?
- The biggest thing I'm scared of is getting stung. I bet it hurts a lot. I never want to get stung.
- Bugs are interesting, yes, but really very gross.

We then challenged these thoughts. For example:

- Some bugs sting or bite, and it can hurt, but it is not unbearable—it is just a sting. We reminded Sam of how strong he was and how he had broken his finger once, which hurt much more than any bug bite.
- African killer bees are not in our area. They do not kill; they are just more aggressive.
- Bees usually sting us when they feel attacked, as a defense. Their primary interest is not to attack us.
- Bees are important for our food supply and to make honey.
- Bugs that land on our skin, like a fly, don't usually stay for long, and it feels like a tickle more than anything else. As soon as you move or swat the bug, it flies away.
- Bugs can be "gross," but some bugs are beautiful when you look at pictures of them up close.

Then we listed his anxious behaviors:

- Avoidance was primary.
- Not going outside unless absolutely necessary.
- Running to and from the car when I have to go anywhere.
- Not going to the bus stop.
- Not going outside at recess or gym.
- Not being able to look at a bug.
- If there is a fly in the house, screaming and running until someone can catch it and kill it.
- Checking around the house to make sure there are no flying bugs.

Okay, one step at a time.

Step 2: Rate the Anxious Behavior

Again we had to break down Sam's avoidance behaviors into small steps.

Sam was ready to rate 0 to 10. He called 0 "too easy" and 10 "Don't you dare ask me to do this!," which we changed to "Don't you dare ask me to do this *yet*!":

- Walking to and from the car, instead of running in fear   **6**
- Not screaming when there is a bug in the house   **4**
- Going out the back door and standing outside for five minutes   **6**
- Walking with Mom or Dad around the backyard   **8**
- Looking at a fly in a jar   **6**
- Going to a butterfly garden where butterflies fly around   **8**
- Looking at YouTube videos of bugs   **2**

It's one thing to rate behaviors, and another thing to agree on dealing with them.

Step 3: Agree on Challenges to Work On

Sam reviewed his list of what to work on:

- Looking at a bug in a jar ("You can't let it get out, right?")
- Not screaming when a bug is in the house
- Walking to and from the car without running
- Looking at YouTube videos of bugs
- Going out the back door and standing outside for five minutes

We all agreed that these were baby steps toward helping Sam feel less anxious about bugs and more able to be outside. Once he realized we weren't going to make him do something that was too scary and that he had control over what was expected of him, he became less resistant and more cooperative. Many kids are resistant because they don't want to feel that horrible panicky feeling and think that's what we are going to make them do. Understanding that he needed to challenge his anxiety but not be overwhelmed by it helped Sam feel like this could work.

We had to start where he was comfortable and build from there, and this seemed promising.

Step 4: Initiate and Teach Strategies to Practice

Sam agreed to write down and then read his challenges to his anxious thoughts. For instance:

- He learned "self-talk," where he reminded himself of what was real and that he was not in danger from bugs.
- He learned to pay attention to his breathing in the fresh air and to the pleasant smells, sights, and feelings of being outside. He needed to remember what he used to like so much about being outside and about nature, instead of hyperfocusing on bugs and reacting with fear.

We then did some focused relaxation exercises. Sam closed his eyes and focused on his breathing being slow and deep, in and out. I then guided him to imagine being outside, helping him focus on positive smells and sounds of the outdoors: the birds singing, the sound of the wind, the feeling of the cool air on his face. I helped him to think of a time when he had fun and enjoyed being outside and to remember what that felt like. He agreed to practice that at home.

We also did *imaginal exposures*, where I guided him to imagine being outside with bugs. Imaginal exposures can be a useful step in desensitizing a child when a real exposure may not be possible or is, at that point, too difficult. They can be a good first step.

Sam, becoming more engaged, closed his eyes, did his breathing, imagined being outside when everything was pleasant, and then added bugs to the picture. He was hearing the bugs, seeing the bugs, feeling the bugs, and looking at the bugs without fear—noticing the bugs rather than reacting to them. This was far more difficult for him to do, but with practice, he became better able to stay calm and keep his breathing even as he visualized being around flying insects. He also practiced this at home.

Step 5: Note and Chart Progress Made

Together, the family designed Sam's chart. Sam happened to be a great artist and got excited about drawing pictures of flying bugs all over his chart.

Step 6: Offer Incentives to Motivate

With Sam, this was the first step, just to get him to agree to work with us. So he continued to get points for coming to the therapy sessions but most important, he also earns points for doing the work he agreed on. What will he get for his points?

His parents had discussed this in advance with Sam and come up with this list:

- Gift certificate to bookstore
- iTunes gift card
- App for his iPad
- Extra time on the weekends for use of computer
- Choosing where the family will get takeout on Friday nights

- Staying up a half hour later on Friday or Saturday night
- New computer game

At this point, Sam's parents raised an important issue. Sam had a sister who was just two years younger. Allison already felt jealous of the attention Sam got. Tara asked, "What is Allison going to feel when she sees Sam getting these rewards for doing what she does every day? I bet she's going to feel angry about all this, or worse, feel like she has to have fears to get rewards. How do we handle that?"

This was a good question and is a common issue when there are siblings. The best option was to talk with Allison about what she could work on. This would help Sam to realize that everyone has something to work on; he's not the "problem child." And it helps Allison to share in getting positive reinforcement for working on her challenges.

It was agreed that Allison would get points for doing things that were hard for her. She had a hard time making her bed and cleaning up after herself, and she easily raised her voice with her parents. She made her own chart and was happy to be earning prizes too.

Step 7: Reinforce Progress and Increase Challenges

After three weeks, Sam came back to my office with his parents, and his mood was certainly much better than at our last meeting. He was smiling and glad to show off his chart and his progress.

We looked at his chart:

- Now walking to and from the car was **0**, so we crossed that off the list.
- After standing outside in the backyard, he was now able to sit outside on the deck. His parents had the idea of bringing a board game out there that he could play with his sister. He had been out there over two hours and said it was a **0** if there were no bugs, a **5** if he saw a bug flying around.
- Relaxation and imaginal exposures were now easy: **0**.
- Looking at the YouTube videos, easy: **0**.
- Not screaming if a fly is in the house couldn't be worked on because no fly had come into the house: **5**.
- Looking at a fly in a jar, easy: **0**.

Now Sam was ready for the next steps.

- He agreed to walk around the block with his mom or dad.   7
- He would continue to work on being in the backyard on the deck.   5
- He agreed to shoot baskets in the driveway.   7
- He agreed to go out for recess. **Rating 5.** The longer he stays out and doesn't come in the school, the more points he earns. We discussed what he could do outside, and his mom agreed to call his school to make sure he can be helped to join a group outside so he's not alone out there worrying about bugs.

At one session, Sam's sister, Allison, joined us and showed off her chart. She was working on making her bed and keeping her room clean, not leaving her dishes in the family room, keeping her voice down, and not screaming when she got upset. She had also earned points for a gift certificate at the bookstore and was working on points for a trip to the mall with her mom.

Next Steps

Sam was on his way, and although the progress had been slow, it was tangible, and Sam was proud of himself, despite all the original protestations.

Both his parents agreed to get a medication consultation to help Sam overcome his fears. Since starting on his medication, he has been less anxious and more able to move up his goals. We continue to meet monthly, and he has been able to go on a walk with his father for fifteen minutes. Next, he plans on visiting a local farm and petting the animals.

*   *   *

Both Ellen and Sam experienced anxiety in different ways, and their parents had different opinions on how to respond. Parents can be enablers of anxiety, especially when children seem very comfortable in their avoidance. Parents understandably want to avoid a struggle with their child. Many anxious children are very resistant to change, and although they are often not functioning up to their potential, they are still functioning.

Parents often experience conflicts about how to deal with an anxious child. Resolving these conflicts and getting parents to work together can be an important part of this process.

DSM-5 Guidelines

Specific Phobia

The *DSM-5* identifies the diagnostic criteria necessary for a diagnosis. The assumption is that many readers will have children who meet some but not all the criteria.

A. Marked fear or anxiety about a specific object or situation (e.g., flying, heights, animals, receiving an injection, seeing blood).

> Note: In children, the fear or anxiety may be expressed by crying, tantrums, freezing, or clinging.

B. The phobic object or situation almost always provokes immediate fear or anxiety.

C. The phobic object or situation is actively avoided or endured with intense fear or anxiety.

D. The fear or anxiety is out of proportion to the actual danger posed by the specific object or situation and to the sociocultural context.

E. The fear, anxiety, or avoidance is persistent, typically lasting for six months or more.

F. The fear, anxiety, or avoidance causes clinically significant distress or impairment in social, occupational, or other important areas of functioning.

G. The disturbance is not better explained by the symptoms of another mental disorder, including fear, anxiety, and avoidance of situations associated with panic-like symptoms or other incapacitating symptoms (as in agoraphobia); objects or situations related to obsessions (as in obsessive-compulsive disorder); reminders of traumatic events (as in post-traumatic stress disorder); separation from home or attachment figures (as in separation anxiety disorder).

Specify if:

Code based on the phobic stimulus:

300.29 (F40.218) Animal (e.g., spiders, insects, dogs).

300.29 (F40.228) Natural environment (e.g., heights, storms, water).

300.29 (F40.23x) Blood-injection-injury (e.g., needles, invasive medical procedures).

> **Coding note:** Select specific ICD-10-CM code as follows: **F40.230** fear of blood; **F40.231** fear of injections and transfusions; **F40.232** fear of other medical care; or **F40.233** fear of injury.

300.29 (F40.248) Situational (e.g., airplanes, elevators, enclosed places).

300.29 (F40.298) Other (e.g., situations that may lead to choking or vomiting; in children, e.g., loud sounds or costumed characters).

> **Coding note:** When more than one phobic stimulus is present, code all ICD-10-CM codes that apply (e.g., for fear of snakes and flying, F40.218 specific phobia, animal, and F40.248 specific phobia, situational).

American Psychiatric Association. "Specific Phobia." In *Diagnostic and Statistical Manual of Mental Disorders*. 5th ed. Washington, DC: American Psychiatric Association, 2013.

Chapter 8

When Bad Things Happen to Good Kids

Post-Traumatic Stress Disorder

Post-traumatic stress disorder (PTSD) is an anxiety disorder that is triggered by a terrifying event—directly experiencing it or witnessing it. The symptoms include intrusive memories of the event; the feeling of re-experiencing it (flashbacks); avoiding situations that are associated with the event; feeling numb or without feelings, especially right after the event; becoming hypervigilant, which can include being irritable; having trouble concentrating and sleeping; always being "on guard" due to a fear of being in danger; and becoming easily startled.

Young children with PTSD may experience more separation anxiety and have more trouble with toilet training, going to the bathroom, or bedwetting. Older children may act out the trauma through play, drawings, or stories. They may have more physical complaints and become more fearful and anxious. This anxiety could be expressed through avoidance, or aggressive behavior, or both.

Complex PTSD develops after the experience of prolonged trauma. Combat veterans and people who experienced child abuse have suffered many traumatic experiences. With multiple experiences of traumatic events, the treatment usually involves a multimodal approach, in which cognitive behavioral therapy (CBT) can be part of the treatment but is not the only approach. CBT can be most effective alone when the person has experienced only a single traumatic event.

This chapter walks you through two representative stories of children who have PTSD.

John and Carolyn's Story

These parents were distraught when they saw me about their daughter, 3½-year-old Molly.

Carolyn started the session: "Eight months ago, we were eating in a restaurant, and the waitress was pouring my tea and someone bumped into her from behind, and the waitress poured boiling hot water on Molly's shoulder and down her arm. It was horrible. Molly screamed. The waitress screamed. I screamed. It was chaos."

Carolyn started to cry and couldn't talk.

John jumped in. "I grabbed her out of her high chair and ripped her clothes off her as quickly as I could. She screamed so loudly. Someone called 911, and an ambulance came with the sirens and the lights, and she was rushed to the hospital. It was a nightmare; she was so hurt and scared. We were with her but couldn't hold her because of the burns. It was by far the worst day of my life. Since then, she's been back and forth to doctors, and amazingly, it's healed. Of course she has scars, and I'm not sure if they'll ever go away. But thank God, the pain is gone. We had to keep bandages on and change the bandages frequently to avoid infection. It never got infected. The doctors say she's now pain-free. But I know it must've hurt her so much."

Carolyn then spoke. "Our problem now is she's afraid of water. I mean any water that gets on her body. Giving her a bath is impossible. She screams like she's being burned all over again. I can't bear it. It brings it all back for me, seeing her looking so scared. So we take a cloth with soap and water and gently clean her. We know this can't go on. She has to get over this."

"Honestly, John added, "we thought this would all just go away with time. We hoped she would forget what happened, and she's so little. But her fear of water is not going away, so she must still be haunted. We know she has to be able to take a bath. We just don't know what to do. Now that summer's coming, we were hoping we could get her in a pool or go to the beach with her. That seems impossible now. We don't know how to help her."

I explained that I've seen other young and old people undergo similar traumas. We could deal with it methodically.

Step 1: Target Anxious Thoughts and Behaviors

Molly was so little, and she had experienced a significant trauma. Because of how young she is, she can't understand how to put this horrible burn in perspective. Her anxious thought is "Water will hurt me." Her anxious behavior is to avoid any water, and when she gets near water, to scream in fear as if she's about to be burned all over again.

So we needed to start with changing her thoughts and feelings about water. She would benefit most from graduated exposure to water to help her overcome her fear.

Step 2: Rate the Anxious Thoughts and Behavior

I suggested we start with a water table for her to play with water inside. Because she was so little, her parents provided the ratings based on their experiences with her.

- Standing at the water table and playing with toys in a little bit of water   5
- At the water table, putting a little water on her arm and shoulder where she had been burned   10
- Standing in a kiddie pool with water in it   5
- Sitting in a kiddie pool with water   8
- Standing in the tub   8
- Sitting in the tub with water   10
- Sitting in the tub playing, with no water   6
- Singing with parents and with music, sitting in the tub with toys and a little water   8
- Going to the pool and watching other kids playing in the water   7
- Putting her feet in the water at the pool   8

I suggested that they avoid touching her burn area with water since that triggers her to scream right away. She needed to feel more comfortable with water and build up to putting water where she was burned. That would be the last step. The parents agreed, and we went on to the next step.

Step 3: Agree on Challenges to Work On

Carolyn said, "I know this all makes sense. We have to gradually help her get used to water. But honestly, I get so nervous even thinking about this. I don't want her to be hurt and scared anymore, yet I wish she didn't have to go through all this."

I explained that if they weren't comfortable doing this with her, she would pick up on their anxiety and become more afraid. We could take small steps in exposing her to water, I said. We didn't want to overwhelm and retraumatize her. She would feel scared and uncomfortable at the start of each step, but then she would relax.

I stressed that they had to be willing not only to tolerate her discomfort, but to stay composed, and when she was afraid, to guide her through it. They needed to make it playful and be lighthearted with her to help her experience that water is not going to hurt her. It can instead be fun.

"You need to know," John said, "that my wife, I think, blames herself for all this. She thinks somehow it's her fault. She says things like 'I shouldn't have put the high chair there. I shouldn't have ordered tea, and we should have had dinner at home.' Some nights she goes on and on like this. No matter what I say, it doesn't seem to help."

We then turned the conversation away from Molly, and they spoke about what all this has been like for them. Carolyn said, "You're right, that's how I think sometimes, and I can't help it. It's been hard. I had nightmares. They've gotten better, but at first, I couldn't sleep at all. I kept dreaming Molly was suffering in all kinds of horrific ways, and I couldn't get to her. I couldn't save her. Every night, I dreaded going to sleep."

John put his arm around her. "For weeks after this happened," he said, "she'd wake up crying, and Molly would be crying. None of us got any sleep. I felt like I couldn't do enough to help them. I also still feel guilty, especially when I look at her scars. I'm her dad. It's my job to protect her. It's hard not to feel like I failed in some major way."

We talked about how, by witnessing this, they too were traumatized. If they didn't lessen their own anxiety, it would be hard for them to help Molly relax and recover from her experience. They agreed to see a couples' therapist who specializes in PTSD to help them recover as a couple from this trauma.

John felt strongly that he was able to start the exposure therapy with Molly. "I really think I can do this, and it will help me feel like I'm doing something to help her. So far I've felt helpless, not knowing what to do for her. We really have fun together. I love playing with her, and she easily laughs with me. I want to get started with this."

Carolyn looked relieved, knowing she wasn't ready to experience Molly's discomfort. Avoiding water with Molly, and trying to forget it ever happened, was her way of coping.

We all agreed that standing in a kiddie pool in the family room, where Molly loves to play, was the best way to start. She and her dad love to dance together in the family room with music, so putting on the music and dancing with Dad in the pool with a little water sounded like a good first step. We also thought putting new water toys in the pool might get her curious enough to want to play in the water. In addition to that, they agreed to set up a water table with new toys so Molly could stand and put her hands in the water to play with the toys.

We were on our way.

Step 4: Initiate and Teach Strategies to Practice

We agreed to the following strategies:

- Keep everything playful.
- Use music and laughter and keep her playing through the exposures.
- Talk to Molly over and over again about how great water is, to help her change the way she thinks.
- Use every opportunity to model what fun water can be. Let her see you having fun with water.
- Keep relaxed and confident. Remember you are guiding her through her fear of water. She needs to feel from you that she's safe doing this.
- Since she loves bubbles, have her blow them when she's anxious. This will help with her breathing.

Overall, we decided to go slowly with each step, being patient and following Molly's lead, since I expected that Molly would let them know when she was relaxed and ready for the next step. I reminded the parents not to overwhelm her by pushing her too fast.

Step 5: Note and Chart Progress Made

Though Molly can't rate her progress, her parents can based on her reaction to the exposures. John was confident that he could measure her discomfort based on observing her, and they would keep a chart with a simple rating of easy, hard, very hard, and couldn't do it. It was very important that they stay in the easy-to-hard range. She shouldn't become overwhelmed by the exposure; it shouldn't be too anxiety producing for her. We wanted it to be challenging but not overwhelming and as positive as possible. It's most important to be playful in this process, even if that takes longer to make progress.

Step 6: Offer Incentives to Motivate

As is often the case, positive reinforcement will be very important to make this work. Molly loves stickers and M&Ms, so that's what we went for.

Carolyn said, "It worked like a charm for toilet training. I bet it'll work for this too." Her parents would take her out to choose stickers and explain that she can get stickers and candy for playing the "water game" with Daddy. Her parents thought she would be very excited about this. She was really in love with princesses, so princess stickers would be great. I encouraged them to use a big sticker for when she did something new that she hadn't yet done with water, and smaller ones for practicing the same water activity. Similarly, they should give her more M&Ms for the first time she took a new step in increasing her exposure to water. The first time is always the hardest, and then it gets easier.

Step 7: Reinforce Progress and Increase Challenges

After a month, we met and discussed Molly's progress.

Carolyn started. "First I want to tell you, John and I have been seeing another therapist to help us with this. It's helped me realize how intense my feelings about all this are. I'm working on it, and even started working a little with John on the exposures with Molly. The exposures are really helping her feel less afraid."

John described what had been going on. "We started with the water table and standing in the pool. It was tough at first to get her to do it. But I kept being patient and offering more and more candy. Finally, she took the bait and went in. She looked scared, but I got her laughing and singing. We kept doing it, and she gradually became more relaxed. I couldn't figure out how to get her to sit in the water and play. I know this sounds ridiculous, and it sure looks ridiculous, but we bought a big kiddie pool, big enough for me to get in. I set it up in the family room, got in my bathing suit, filled the pool with some water and all her water toys, and I started playing in the pool. It was big enough for both of us to sit in it. She watched me and before long put one foot in, and then the next, and ended up sitting with me in the water playing."

Carolyn said, "When I saw that, I started to laugh and cry. Looking at my husband in that ridiculous pool, and seeing her sitting and playing in the water, it made me feel so happy. I know she's getting better."

Now it was time to talk about next goals:

- Taking a bath. Transferring her from the pool to the tub would be a challenge. We discussed first bathing her with fun bubbles in the pool and then gradually getting her in the tub with her dad.

- Going swimming in a real pool. We discussed taking her to the YMCA pool, where she could first watch kids play in the water, then gradually put her feet in the water, with Dad close to her. Next, Dad would play in the water while Mom stayed with her on the side, watching until she was ready for Dad to place her in the water. This would be a huge accomplishment and would probably take many visits to the pool.

- Exposing her burn area to water. Molly would still get scared and start to cry if any water touched the skin where she was burned. Doctors had reassured her parents that the burn was healed and that it no longer hurt her. It was her fear that was now causing her pain. We discussed gradually having drops of water fall on that area when she was in the kiddie pool and rewarding her right away, reinforce over and over that water would not hurt her. They would continue doing this, slowly having more and more water touch her burn area.

Through these exposures, Molly was starting to experience water as something fun. She was changing the way she felt about water and how she acted with water.

Carolyn said, "It's really working now. Before we learned how to do this, we were pushing her too hard to get into the water. Our goals were too high, and she couldn't do it. Then we created this cycle where she would get anxious and start screaming, and I would overreact, as if she was in pain, and quickly get her away from the water. We'd both be a mess after that and give up. We were stuck. If anything, that probably gave her the message again and again that water is dangerous."

Carolyn and John have since learned how graduated exposure works; they have also learned how they had to heal along with Molly to recover from the trauma they all experienced when she was burned.

We continued to meet monthly, and after seven months, Molly was doing really well in the water. Her fear had greatly diminished. Carolyn and John made good use of their couples' therapy, which helped them realize how traumatized they had been by experiencing Molly getting burned. They were healing as a family from the burn, which was not just physical but psychological for the whole family.

Next Steps

It took several months of just about daily water play, but Molly made consistent progress and is now able to go in the pool with her parents. Meanwhile, Carolyn and John have continued in their therapy and are working on healing their own PTSD. One of the things they realized in therapy was that deep down, not only did they blame themselves for what happened, they blamed each other. They had known they were often angry at each other since the accident, but they hadn't realized why. The more they accepted that they were not to blame for what happened to Molly, the better they felt. Unexpectedly to them, this process helped strengthen their marriage.

Maura and John's Story

Maura and John came to see me because they were worried about their 19-year-old daughter, Monica. As is usually my approach, I let the parents ventilate without interrupting.

Maura started. "Monica just finished her freshman year at college. She was always a happy kid. We never had any problems with her, beyond the usual stuff. In high school she had a busy social life but kept her grades up and worked hard. She got into her first choice school. It's a large university. We thought she might do better in a smaller school, but she wanted large.

"She always had lots of good friends," she continued. "I guess you could say she was popular. As far as I know, she drank a little at parties her senior year, and I imagine she smoked pot. She never had any problems with that stuff though. Twice she was late for curfew in her senior year, and we grounded her, and that was it. She usually respected our rules."

John looked impatient and interrupted. "The reason we're here is that she's coming home from school for the summer, and she told us she needs to see a therapist."

Maura continued. "I'm sorry. I didn't mean to get off track, but I wanted you to know a little about her. Anyway, John's right, she needs to see a doctor to talk to. She won't tell us why. That's the hard part. If only we knew, maybe we could help her. I'm worried sick. I know something's wrong. I just don't know what it is."

Nervously, Maura went on, "She had a great first semester at school. She was home at Thanksgiving and Christmas and seemed really happy. Her grades were great too. All A's except one B in math. She was making friends, had good roommates. Everything seemed fine. When she came home for March break, something had changed. She seemed . . . reserved, quiet, no emotions. I don't know how to explain it. Low energy, in her room, sleeping a lot, not herself, but every time I'd ask her, she'd say she's fine. She didn't want to see her high school friends, which was a big red flag for me.

"At night, sometimes, I could hear her crying in her room. We were always so close; she used to tell me everything. If she had a problem, she always came to me. I asked her older sister to talk to her and Monica said the same thing to her—everything's fine.

"Well, Monica went back to school after the break, and every time I'd talk to her, she seemed down, irritable, like I was bothering her by calling. At first I felt hurt, since she never acted like this toward me before. I wondered if I did something to upset her. So I backed off and stopped calling her so much. But she called me crying last night. Her semester is over, and she's coming home in a week. Her grades are down, all Cs and one B. I don't care about that, but she said she's not sleeping, and she's having panic attacks. She never had this problem before. Maybe this school is not right for her? I don't know . . ."

Maura became tearful. "I just wish I knew what was wrong and how to help her."

John took up the conversation. "She was always a happy kid. I don't get it. I hope she didn't take drugs or something like that. Could that cause this? I just keep imagining the worst. I don't know what got her in this state. But we have to decide if she should go back to school, or maybe she needs some time off. I always thought she shouldn't be so far away from home in such a large school. Maybe it's just too much for her. She's sensitive, you know."

John paused. "She's supposed to work this summer as a lifeguard. She's had that job for three years. I hope she can do it. Can you help us figure this out? Can you help her?"

It was clear that I needed to meet with Monica, and the fact that she had expressed needing to talk to a therapist was a good sign. So we arranged for her to see me without her parents.

Monica's Story

Monica came in looking scared and was hesitant at first. "I don't know how to do this. I've never gone to a therapist before. I just know I need help, and I promised my roommate I would get help over the summer." She then started to cry. "I'm sorry . . . I don't know where to begin."

I told her that she was in a safe place and that she could start by telling me what had brought her here. She regained her composure and continued: "I'm having trouble sleeping. I have nightmares. And sometimes I get panic attacks, like my heart is beating so fast, and I feel like I can't breathe, and I get hot and sweaty. I also sometimes can't concentrate. My grades have gone down this semester. I don't know how I got through it. I'm glad I'm home, and I thought being home would help, but I have the same feelings."

I asked her when this all started. "It was several months ago. Something happened to me. I can't really talk about it. I get too upset."

She stopped short and asked, "This is confidential, right? You're not going to tell my parents, are you?"

I reassured her that I would not. I reviewed with her that I would tell her parents only if I thought she was in danger of hurting herself or others.

"No, I'm not suicidal. It's nothing like that," she said.

I asked her to try to tell me what had happened since I couldn't really help without knowing the facts.

She again started to cry and said, "I'm too ashamed."

I explained that talking about it could help with those feelings, and she finally started to open up.

"I was at a frat party, and I was . . ." Her voice trailed to barely a whisper. "Raped. I can't tell my parents. They couldn't handle it. My dad, I swear he would try to track down and kill the guy. I'm serious. They can never find out. They would never let me go back to college. My mom would create a big scene at school. She'd want to sue them or something. She's a lawyer. They would be so disappointed in me. I don't want them to ever find out. I'm close to my mother, but she can never know this happened to me. I just want to stop feeling these feelings and be back to myself. I know I need help to get over this. I thought it would just go away, but it's not. I wish I could just forget about it."

I assured Monica that she wasn't alone and that I was confident our strategic approach would help her feel better.

Step 1: Target the Anxious Thoughts and Behaviors

It was hard for Monica to describe her thoughts, but it was time to get to work, and Monica tried to cooperate: "Most of the time I'm fine, but sometimes, I feel panic come over me, like I can't breathe. I feel like something bad is going to happen. I get even a bit paranoid. Like someone's going to jump out of nowhere and hurt me. Sometimes, while studying in my room, my roommate would walk in, and I would jump like a bolt of lightning."

She took in a deep breath and forged ahead. "I feel like I can't trust guys anymore. I'm sometimes afraid of them. I feel angry at myself now. How could I have let this happen to me? Sometimes I think I'm bad or dirty in some way. I know I'm not. It wasn't my fault, but it feels like I should have prevented it. It's confusing."

I asked Monica to elaborate.

"I have nightmares over and over again, the same kind of dreams. I'm always helpless, and bad things, violent things are happening to me and I can't stop it, until I wake up crying and in a sweat. It feels so real. I wake up, and I feel exhausted."

I explained to Monica that she had post-traumatic stress disorder (PTSD), which was common after being raped. I encouraged her to learn more about PTSD.

She said, "No, I'm sorry. Usually I like to learn about things, but when it comes to this, I don't want to read about it. I just want it all to go away. My goal is just to forget about it and move on."

Concluding this first session, I told her that to understand her anxious thoughts more clearly, she needed to learn more about rape and the common feelings victims feel after being raped. This would help her feel less alone. I stressed that what she's experiencing is a normal reaction to what happened to her and that talking about it with me would help her feel better and then be more able to feel relaxed and less anxious.

She came into the next session ready to tell me what had happened that night. I explained to her that we could do it at her own pace; she could take breaks if necessary. I reminded her that this should be challenging but not overwhelming. Certainly, I didn't want her to be retraumatized by becoming flooded with uncomfortable feelings. She was confident that she could tell me, since she had told several of her friends already. She also said, "I already told my doctor and have been tested for sexually transmitted diseases, which, thank God, were all negative."

Then she began to describe what had happened. "It was a Friday night, in the second week of February. I had stayed up half the night before, studying for a test, and I was tired. My roommate, Stacey, told me about this frat party. I was tired and didn't really feel like going out, but she convinced me that it could be fun. I told her I probably would want to leave early, and she was fine with that. Stacey and I had become good friends, and she's a lot of fun to go out with, but I can't help but think I should have listened to my gut and not gone. If I didn't go to that stupid party, none of this would've happened to me. I keep thinking of that. Anyway, we went to the party. I had a few beers. I know how to drink. I drank in high school, got trashed a few times, and don't like that feeling."

I told her she was doing great and asked her to continue. "I don't drink a lot; everybody here knows that about me. I didn't even smoke weed that night. I knew that would put me right to sleep, because I was so tired to begin with. So, we had been there for a few hours, the music and so many people made it very loud. I was ready to go back to the dorm and went to find Stacey, because we'd agreed to walk back together. We felt safer that way. Ironic, isn't it? We thought it was dangerous to walk alone at night, and I get raped at a big party, with lots of people around. It makes no sense. So I was walking around looking for her, and I heard my name called."

At this point Monica slowed down. "This is where it all went bad. It was Don. He's a junior, pre-med. We'd hung out a little in the fall. I hadn't seen or heard from him in months. I figured I'd talk to him for a few minutes. He said something like he wanted to catch up with me. I went into this room with him and quickly realized he was drunk. Really drunk. He smelled like hard liquor, weed, and sweat, all combined. I remember thinking I was too tired to listen to him slur his words and talk nonsense, I just wanted to go back to my dorm, to sleep. But I didn't want to be rude. How stupid is that? Why was I worrying about being rude? I should have just left right then. I quickly told him I was tired and heading back to my dorm.

"He said, 'Oh no, you're not.'

"I thought he was kidding, and I said, 'Oh yes, I am. Stacey's waiting downstairs for me.'

"At that point he grabbed me hard and pulled me down. I remember telling him to stop, to leave me alone; I still couldn't believe what he was doing. I told him he was hurting me and tried to get away. Then, I will never forget this, he said, 'Shut up, bitch.'

"I started to struggle, and he put his hands around my neck like he was going to strangle me. Then I was really scared. That's when time seemed to slow down. I felt like I was going to die. I never felt that before."

Tears started to roll down Monica's face. She was shaking, and her face and neck were beet red. I suggested she might want to take a break. She said, "No, I'm fine. I know it's over. I really thought I could die. He's a big guy, a football player. I don't know why I didn't scream. Or bite him or punch him. Why didn't I fight more? If I fought more, maybe this wouldn't have happened. I got so scared, I froze. I remember him being so big, on top of me, hurting me and out of control. And then, it was over, just like that. He got up, and this is weird, he mumbled something about it being good, and stumbled out of the room, leaving me there. I got up and felt . . . nothing, numb, like I was in a daze.

"I guess I was just walking around, and Stacey came up to me. She knew immediately something was wrong. She asked if I was okay. I told her I just needed to get out of there. We left and started walking back to the dorm. Right away, she asked me about my neck. She said it was all red. She kept asking me what was wrong. I didn't want to tell her. I didn't know what to say, I felt so ashamed. How could I have let this happen to me? Finally, I blurted out, 'I was just raped.'

"I remember the words coming out of my mouth with no emotion. I felt nothing, nothing except dirty. I felt filthy dirty. I just wanted to take a shower and wash all this off me. Stacey was shocked and so upset, she started to cry. I told her I was fine. I remember she said something about how I should report it. I told her no way. I was not going to report it. I have seen what happens to girls who report these things. It gets ugly. At that point I just wanted to get clean and forget it ever happened.

"As soon as we got to the dorm, I headed straight for the shower and kept washing and washing. I wanted to scrub every inch of my body. I washed until I was too exhausted to continue and had to stop. I still felt dirty. Finally I came back to the room, and Stacey was still up. She asked me who it was. I didn't want to tell her, but then she said, 'Was it Don?' I was surprised and asked her how she knew. She said she heard rumors that he was known to be a creep like this when he was drunk. She said, 'I never believed the stories. He's such a nice guy and so smart, pre-med. He's always talking about going to Harvard where his dad went.' I made her promise not to tell anyone. It was all so confusing. I felt so ashamed. That night, Stacey cried, but I didn't cry. I still felt nothing, numb."

Monica looked at me at this point and asked, "You're not going to tell anyone, are you? Don't make me tell anyone. I don't want to report this to anyone at school. I can't go through that. I know I can't."

I reassured her about confidentiality and that reporting it or not was in her control. Monica started crying. I told her it was good for her to cry, and I asked her to let herself feel what Stacey felt for her that night—so sad that something like this had happened to her.

In the next session, we were ready to take a closer look at her anxious thoughts:

- It was my fault this happened.
- I should've fought harder.
- I could've stopped him.
- I should've screamed and caused a scene.
- I was a complete coward.
- If I hadn't talked to him, this never would have happened. I knew he was wasted; I shouldn't have talked to him.
- If I hadn't gone to this party, it wouldn't have happened. I shouldn't have gone.
- I shouldn't have gone upstairs in that house; I should have kept close to Stacey.
- Maybe it was what I was wearing. I threw out the jeans and sweater I wore that night.

- This could have been prevented. It's my fault this happened.
- I can't let anyone find out about this. They'll think it was my fault and that I'm an idiot. Why did this happen to me? There must be a reason this happened to me and not all the other girls at that party.
- Don isn't a bad person. Everyone thinks he's great. He's on the football team. He's smart. How could he be a rapist? No one would believe he did this to me.
- Now I'm afraid of men. I guess I think any guy could just rape me. I'm scared this will happen again.

Next we worked on challenging those thoughts with facts. I explained to Monica that one in five college girls is sexually assaulted while in college. She was hardly alone. It is an epidemic on campuses across the country. She was shocked to hear that. I told her this was not her fault, but when bad things happen to good people, they tend to blame themselves. Rape victims almost always first blame themselves. I emphasized that she did nothing to cause this to happen, and she couldn't have stopped it. She did what her instincts told her to do, and she was probably right. If she had fought him more, he could have escalated his violence. She was afraid for her life, but she survived his attack, even though she had thought he was going to kill her. He's the criminal who raped her.

As I said these words, tears came streaming down her face. She said, "I never thought of it like that. I don't know why. He's hurt me so much by doing this to me; my whole life has changed since that night. I hate him."

From this point on, we started to see a transformation. Changing how she thought was changing her feelings from numb to sad and even angry. She was starting to challenge her thoughts. We were making progress.

I asked Monica to list her anxious behaviors:

- I get anxious going to parties, especially large parties. I panic.
- I feel like my libido is gone. I avoid guys completely, even the nice ones. I'm afraid of them.
- Oh, the smell of hard liquor and weed, that combination, I can't stand it. It literally makes me sick, and I have to get away. Let's face it, I live on a college campus—that smell is everywhere. But I stay away from it as much as I can.
- I hate walking near where it happened, that frat house.

- I feel ashamed when I talk about it. Like it's my fault.
- I love my parents, and I know they're upset about me and want to know what's wrong, but I can't tell them. I feel too ashamed. I just want to block it all out. I feel like they will think differently about me.

After listing these behaviors, it was time to rate them.

Step 2: Rate the Anxious Thoughts and Behavior

Although Monica felt a high level of anxiety related to the incident, I told her we needed to view the relative numbers before we started to deal with the specific issues.

Her list:

- Going to a small party with friends **3**
- Going to a large party **6**
- Doing anything sexual, including masturbation **7**
- Talking about the details of what happened and not feeling ashamed **8**

- Reading or watching anything about rape or PTSD **3**
- Smelling hard liquor or marijuana **5**
- Telling parents **7**
- Going to frat house **7**
- Walking by frat house and looking at it **4**

This gave us a framework for the next step.

Step 3: Agree on Challenges to Work On

After Monica agreed to write out her anxious, irrational thoughts about being raped, she then needed to write the realistic thoughts. This is called *cognitive restructuring*, helping her change the way she thinks about this trauma. She decided to write it in her phone, so she could read it anytime she found herself feeling bad about herself because of being raped. She wrote: "I was raped. Rape is a crime, and it was not my fault. I'm angry he did this to me. I'm not alone. Too many students are raped, and he probably did this to other students. I shouldn't feel ashamed. I did nothing wrong. I did the best I could. I'm not dirty because of this. All men are not rapists. It's okay to have feelings that are all mixed up. I will feel better." She agreed to read this every day.

This was the cognitive part of the therapy, changing the way she thinks.

She also agreed to do graduated exposures around the things she was avoiding, starting with spending time having fun with her high school friends, who were also home for the summer. She also agreed to read more about rape and learn about how her experience is very typical of victims of rape. She had resisted this because she wanted to avoid anything about rape; she just wanted to forget about it. But she was starting to understand that trying not to think about it only made her anxiety worse. Learning more about rape could only help her change the negative way she was thinking about herself.

It was time to move forward.

Step 4: Initiate and Teach Strategies to Practice

We discussed various relaxation strategies that she could work on. She agreed to learn meditation and practice it twice a day. She also agreed to take a yoga class and practice stretching with deep breathing. Being trauma-tized often creates an intense physical reaction that can become associated with anxiety, and combining physical relaxation with cognitive restructur-ing and exposure therapy can be useful in the recovery from trauma.

Monica has felt both numb and flooded with intense feelings. These strategies could help her modulate her feelings and reduce her anxiety. She went back to working as a lifeguard but was worried about having a panic attack at work. It's very common to get anxious after having a panic attack—panicking about panicking. We reviewed what she could do if she had a panic attack. She chose to make a plan for herself that included self-talk (it's just anxiety, it will pass, I'm okay), distraction (go in the pool or take a break and go to the bathroom), and focusing on "ground-ing herself" (letting all her senses tune in to where she is, so she's in the here and now and not focused on her anxious feelings). She learned to acknowledge her feelings as they moved through her. We practiced this in the office.

Step 5: Note and Chart Progress Made

Monica decided to keep her progress chart in her phone. When she went to chart her progress, she agreed to also read what she had written to challenge her anxious thoughts. She would also keep track of how often she did the following and rate how hard it felt:

- Spending time with guy friends
- Going to parties
- Reading about rape and PTSD

Step 6: Offer Incentives to Motivate

Sometimes, this is the most critical step. Given Monica's age and her strong motivation to feel better, at first glance this step may not seem necessary. In discussing this with Monica, however, we talked about how hard the work was and how she needed to move forward, not backward. She also needed to acknowledge her strength and power as she regained control over her feelings and worked to recover.

She felt ashamed of what happened, so she needed to develop more feelings of pride in her accomplishment as a trauma survivor. She decided to think of ways she could treat herself as she moved along in her goals. She made a list of things she could reward herself with:

- Getting a manicure and pedicure
- Getting a massage
- Getting a frozen yogurt
- Watching a marathon session of the latest TV show she wants to catch up on
- Buying herself a new outfit

Step 7: Reinforce Progress and Increase Challenges

Monica worked hard and was feeling better. She was enjoying yoga and meditation, and she'd been spending more time with friends; she had even gone to two small parties.

We discussed increasing the goals. Even though it was the middle of her summer break, she needed to go back to school for a long weekend to meet with one of her professors, so we discussed doing exposures on campus. She agreed to go to the frat house where it had happened, even just walking by it at first, until that felt okay, and then going inside if she could.

We also discussed her parents, who were still not aware of what had happened. I disclosed to Monica that they had called me. They were concerned about her, and still very worried and confused. They wondered if she should go back to school in September. Monica said again that she felt too ashamed to tell them. We discussed how she would feel about telling them if she had been mugged on campus and her wallet had been stolen. She immediately said that would be no problem. I explained how she would never blame herself for any other crime that could have been committed, so why should she be to blame for this?

I suggested that it was a good goal for her to tell her parents, to overcome her shame.

She then said, "Could you tell them?" We discussed them coming in for a session, and I would tell them first, and then she could join the session and we could talk about it together. This way, I could help her parents understand the depth of her shame and provide more information about PTSD. She agreed, and the joint session was positive. Her parents initially had a very strong reaction of anger toward this boy and her college. They needed to process their feelings and realize that their focus had to be on supporting their daughter. They were relieved to finally know what was causing their daughter such distress. They also agreed to learn more about campus rape and PTSD.

Next Steps

When September approached, Monica was ready to go back to school, and her parents supported that decision. She sees a therapist on campus to continue the work we started. She joined a rape support group, and this is helping her blame herself less and realize she's not alone. It's also helping with her sense of shame. Telling her parents and getting their support has also helped her feel stronger and not ashamed.

Monica was right: her father's immediate reaction was wanting to kill the boy, and her mother was ready to sue the school. They were able to calm down, however, and learn more about how to help their daughter get through this. As they learned more about rape on campus, they realized that this could have happened at any school. Knowing what was bothering her all this time helped them offer her more understanding and support.

DSM-5 Guidelines

Post-Traumatic Stress Disorder

The *DSM-5* identifies the diagnostic criteria necessary for a diagnosis. The assumption is that many readers will have children who meet some but not all the criteria.

Note: The following criteria apply to adults, adolescents, and children older than 6 years. For children 6 years and younger, see corresponding criteria below.

A. Exposure to actual or threatened death, serious injury, or sexual violence in one (or more) of the following ways:

1. Directly experiencing the traumatic event(s).

2. Witnessing, in person, the event(s) as it occurred to others.

3. Learning that the traumatic event(s) occurred to a close family member or close friend. In cases of actual or threatened death of a family member or friend, the event(s) must have been violent or accidental.

4. Experiencing repeated or extreme exposure to aversive details of the traumatic event(s) (e.g., first responders collecting human remains; police officers repeatedly exposed to details of child abuse).

Note: Criterion A4 does not apply to exposure through electronic media, television, movies, or pictures, unless this exposure is work related.

B. Presence of one (or more) of the following intrusion symptoms associated with the traumatic event(s), beginning after the traumatic event(s) occurred:

1. Recurrent, involuntary, and intrusive distressing memories of the traumatic event(s).

   Note: In children older than 6 years, repetitive play may occur in which themes or aspects of the traumatic event(s) are expressed.

2. Recurrent distressing dreams in which the content and/or effect of the dream are related to the traumatic event(s).

   Note: In children, there may be frightening dreams without recognizable content.

3. Dissociative reactions (e.g., flashbacks) in which the individual feels or acts as if the traumatic event(s) were recurring. (Such reactions may occur on a continuum, with the most extreme expression being a complete loss of awareness of present surroundings.)

   Note: In children, trauma-specific reenactment may occur in play.

4. Intense or prolonged psychological distress at exposure to internal or external cues that symbolize or resemble an aspect of the traumatic event(s).

5. Marked physiological reactions to internal or external cues that symbolize or resemble an aspect of the traumatic event(s).

C. Persistent avoidance of stimuli associated with the traumatic event(s), beginning after the traumatic event(s) occurred, as evidenced by one or both of the following:

1. Avoidance of or efforts to avoid distressing memories, thoughts, or feelings about or closely associated with the traumatic event(s).

2. Avoidance of or efforts to avoid external reminders (people, places, conversations, activities, objects, situations) that arouse distressing memories, thoughts, or feelings about or closely associated with the traumatic event(s).

D. Negative alterations in cognitions and mood associated with the traumatic event(s), beginning or worsening after the traumatic event(s) occurred, as evidenced by one or both of the following:

1. Inability to remember an important aspect of the traumatic event(s) (typically due to dissociative amnesia and not to other factors such as head injury, alcohol, or drugs).

2. Persistent and exaggerated negative beliefs or expectations about oneself, others, or the world (e.g., "I am bad," "No one can be trusted," "The world is completely dangerous," "My whole nervous system is permanently ruined").

3. Persistent, distorted cognitions about the cause or consequences of the traumatic event(s) that led the individual to blame himself/herself or others.

4. Persistent negative emotional state (e.g., fear, horror, anger, guilt, or shame).

5. Markedly diminished interest or participation in significant activities.

6. Feelings of detachment or estrangement from others.

7. Persistent inability to experience positive emotions (e.g., inability to experience happiness, satisfaction, or loving feelings).

E. Marked alterations in arousal and reactivity associated with the traumatic event(s), beginning or worsening after the traumatic event(s) occurred, as evidenced by one or both of the following:

1. Irritable behavior and angry outbursts (with little or no provocation) typically expressed as verbal or physical aggression toward people or objects.

2. Reckless or self-destructive behavior.

3. Hypervigilance.

4. Exaggerated startle response.

5. Problems with concentration.

6. Sleep disturbance (e.g., difficulty falling or staying asleep or restless sleep).

F. Duration of the disturbance (Criteria B, C, D, and E) is more than 1 month.

G. The disturbance causes clinically significant distress or impairment in social, occupational, or other important areas of functioning.

H. The disturbance is not attributable to the physiological effects of a substance (e.g., medication, alcohol, or another medical condition).

Specify whether:

With dissociative symptoms: The individual's symptoms meet the criteria for post-traumatic stress disorder, and in addition, in response to the stressor, the individual experiences persistent or recurrent symptoms of either of the following:

1. **Depersonalization**: Persistent or recurrent experiences of feeling detached from, and as if one were an outside observer of, one's mental process or body (e.g., feeling as though one were in a dream; feeling a sense of unreality of self or body or of time moving slowly).

2. **Derealization**: Persistent or recurrent experiences of unreality of surroundings (e.g., the world around the individual is experienced as unreal, dreamlike, distant, or distorted).

Note: To use this subtype, the dissociative symptoms must not be attributable to the physiological effects of a substance (e.g., blackouts, behavior during alcohol intoxication) or another medical condition (e.g., complex partial seizures).

Specify if:

With delayed expression: If the full diagnostic criteria are not met until at least 6 months after the event (although the onset and expression of some symptoms may be immediate).

Post-Traumatic Stress Disorder for Children 6 Years and Younger

A. In children 6 years and younger, exposure to actual or threatened death, serious injury, or sexual violence in one (or more) of the following ways:

1. Directly experiencing the traumatic event(s).

2. Witnessing, in person, the event(s) as it occurred to others, especially primary caregivers.

Note: Witnessing does not include events that are witnessed only in electronic media, television, movies, or pictures.

3. Learning that the traumatic event(s) occurred to a parent or caregiving figure.

B. Presence of one (or more) of the following intrusion symptoms associated with the traumatic event(s), beginning after the traumatic event(s) occurred:

1. Recurrent, involuntary, and intrusive distressing memories of the traumatic event(s).

   Note: Spontaneous and intrusive memories may not necessarily appear distressing and may be expressed as play reenactment.

2. Recurrent distressing dreams in which the content and/or effect of the dream are related to the traumatic event(s).

3. Dissociative reactions (e.g., flashbacks) in which the child feels or acts as if the traumatic event(s) were recurring (such reactions may occur on a continuum, with the most extreme expression being a complete loss of awareness of present surroundings). Such trauma-specific reenactment may occur in play.

4. Intense or prolonged psychological distress at exposure to internal or external cues that symbolize or resemble an aspect of the traumatic event(s).

5. Marked physiological reactions to internal or external cues that symbolize or resemble an aspect of the traumatic event(s).

C. One (or more) of the following symptoms, representing either persistent avoidance of stimuli associated with the traumatic event(s) or negative alterations in cognitions and mood associated with the traumatic event(s), must be present, beginning after the event(s) or worsening after the event(s):

Persistent Avoidance of Stimuli

1. Avoidance of or efforts to avoid activities, places, or physical reminders that arouse recollections of the traumatic event(s).

2. Avoidance of or efforts to avoid people, conversations, or interpersonal situations that arouse recollections of the traumatic event(s).

Negative Alterations in Cognitions

3. Substantially increased frequency of negative emotional states (e.g., fear, guilt, sadness, shame, confusion).

4. Markedly diminished interest or participation in significant activities, including constriction of play.

5. Socially withdrawn behavior.

6. Persistent reduction in expression of positive emotions.

D. Alterations in arousal and reactivity associated with the traumatic event(s), beginning or worsening after the traumatic event(s) occurred, as evidenced by one or more of the following:

1. Irritable behavior and angry outbursts (with little or no provocation) typically expressed as verbal or physical aggression toward people or objects (including extreme temper tantrums).

2. Hypervigilance.

3. Exaggerated startle response.

4. Problems with concentration.

5. Sleep disturbance (e.g., difficulty falling or staying asleep or restless sleep).

E. Duration of the disturbance is more than 1 month.

F. The disturbance causes clinically significant distress or impairment in relationships with parents, siblings, peers, or other caregivers or with school behavior.

G. The disturbance is not attributable to the physiological effects of a substance (e.g., medication, alcohol, or another medical condition).

Specify whether:

With dissociative symptoms: The individual's symptoms meet the criteria for posttraumatic stress disorder, and the individual experiences persistent or recurrent symptoms of either of the following:

1. **Depersonalization:** Persistent or recurrent experiences of feeling detached from, and as if one were an outside observer of, one's mental process or body (e.g., feeling as though one were in a dream; feeling a sense of unreality of self or body or of time moving slowly).

2. **Derealization:** Persistent or recurrent experiences of unreality of surroundings (e.g., the world around the individual is experienced as unreal, dreamlike, distant, or distorted).

Note: To use this subtype, the dissociative symptoms must not be attributable to the physiological effects of a substance (e.g., blackouts, behavior during alcohol intoxication) or another medical condition (e.g., complex partial seizures).

With delayed expression: If the full diagnostic criteria are not met until at least 6 months after the event (although the onset and expression of some symptoms may be immediate).

American Psychiatric Association. "Posttraumatic Stress Disorder." In *Diagnostic and Statistical Manual of Mental Disorders.* 5th ed. Washington, DC: American Psychiatric Association, 2013.

Chapter 9

And There's More

Hair Pulling, Skin Picking, Tics, Picky Eating, and the Like

Disorders or habits like hair pulling and skin picking are often associated with anxiety and are frustrating for kids and parents. Helping children with these problems involves *habit reversal*, not exposure treatment, so our seven steps don't fit the way they do for the other disorders. Though the strategies differ somewhat, the treatment is still cognitive behavioral, which helps kids change the way they think and behave so that they can gain control.

Hair Pulling

Parents are often horrified and confused when they first notice their child pulling out her hair. Seeing their beautiful child with no eyelashes or eyebrows, or with bald spots on her head, can be shocking. Parents naturally respond with panic and concern about what could be causing such self-destructive behavior. It seems like there must be something terribly wrong if a child is pulling out her hair.

Parents have questions and admonitions: "Why are you doing this to yourself?" "You need to stop pulling." "Just stop doing this!"

Unfortunately, there are no easy answers. Kids don't know why they pull; they just do it. They don't want to pull and usually want desperately to stop pulling, but they can't. They feel ashamed and upset about being so out of control. They don't understand why they do it and often feel judged and misunderstood by others, especially their parents.

Kids who pull usually don't want to talk about it and even deny doing it. But parents seeing hair loss want to do something about it. The more parents want to stop the pulling, the more kids feel criticized and ashamed. This leads everyone to feel helpless and worried about the effect of the hair pulling.

Trichotillomania (trich) is the name of the condition where people pull out their hair. Most commonly, kids with this condition pull out their eyelashes, eyebrows, or head hair. Less commonly, they may pull other body hair, including pubic hair, leg hair, or arm hair.

Having a child who pulls hair is often a painful experience for parents. Mothers, in particular, are often deeply disturbed by this behavior. Hair and appearance often have more meaning and importance for women than for men, and mothers are often worried about their child being teased or bullied because of the hair loss.

Both girls and boys can have trich. It may be more common among girls, or it may be that more girls than boys seek help with it.

Parents often feel embarrassed and judged as hair loss becomes more noticeable. Among psychiatric disorders, this one usually involves the most mentally healthy kids, yet it is also the most visible to others. Parents often feel others are judging them. "What are you doing to make your child pull her hair?" Parents often blame themselves and try to figure out what they are doing wrong.

Zoey and Gary's Story

Zoey and Gary came seeking help with their 15-year-old daughter, Olivia.

"Olivia is a beautiful girl," Zoey said. "An excellent student. She gets great grades. She's an athlete—she plays hockey. She's never had any problems. About a year ago, I started noticing she looked different. Her eyebrows looked like they were getting smaller and smaller, until one morning, I looked at her, and they were totally gone. I mean gone. She had no eyebrows at all. I probably didn't react the right way. I yelled at her and said something like 'What have you done to yourself? What were you thinking to pull all your eyebrows out? Don't you ever do that again. It looks awful.'

"It was not my best parenting moment, but I was so shocked and upset. I had never seen anything like this before. Of course, Olivia burst into tears and ran out of the room. I felt terrible and tried to calm down. I told her

I was sorry for getting so upset, but I needed to know why she did this to herself. At first, she denied even doing it, then said it was an accident, then finally, after lots of tears and hugs, she admitted that she couldn't stop pulling, and she doesn't know why. Well, that really confused me. I admit, I really don't get this. It's so hard for me. I keep thinking, why would my beautiful daughter want to do this to herself?"

She composed herself and continued. "So, I knew we needed help and got her into a therapist right away. I called my insurance company, and they gave me names of therapists. I was desperate and called over fifteen. Most never got back to me. Some said they had a long waiting list. I finally got someone who took my insurance and had an appointment after school. So we met. She was very nice but admitted she didn't have much experience with this. I just wanted help for Olivia, and the therapist said she thought she could help her, and they started meeting weekly. Soon she wanted her on Prozac. I didn't want to put my child on drugs, but the therapist said it would help, so I agreed.

"Yet Olivia still had no eyebrows, and I was willing to do anything to help her. She took the Prozac, and she seemed more easygoing and relaxed. Her grades improved. She seemed happier. But still no eyebrows. When I asked her about the therapy, she said they just talked about things."

Gary then interrupted. "The reason we're here is she is now pulling her eyelashes. Maybe there's something bothering her so much she feels she needs to pull her hair out? What are we missing? This problem is getting worse even though we are doing everything we think we should do. Her therapist has no answers for us. She is very nice, but our daughter is still on medicine and now pulling not only her eyebrows but her eyelashes. This is not working. Last week, Olivia was crying. She thinks she will never have eyebrows or eyelashes. Is this true? Will they ever grow back?"

Gary didn't wait for a response. "It's bad enough she has no eyebrows, but the poor kid puts this dark powdery makeup on where her eyebrows should be. It looks awful. Sometimes I think she would look better with no eyebrows than with that fake black stuff. She's still beautiful and such a wonderful kid. I wish this didn't have to be such a big deal."

"You don't understand," Zoey cut in. "She likes boys. She wants to go to the prom. But there are school pictures, and I wonder what kids are saying about her. She may be getting teased, for all we know. That makeup does make her look very odd, but I think she would be worse if she had nothing there. Now she's pulling out her eyelashes. Eye makeup doesn't work if there are no eyelashes. Mascara can't work if there's nothing there."

Zoey looked defeated. "All this therapy and medicine, and she's worse. We don't know how to get her to stop pulling. I feel like we've tried everything and still no eyebrows."

Gary became more reflective. "It's hurting my relationship with my daughter. If I see a little improvement, I get excited, and then when it's all wiped out, I can't help it, I get so disappointed and angry. I try not to show it, but I just don't get it. Why can't she just stop pulling out her hair? We fight about it a lot, and she now just refuses to talk about it. I want to help her. I worry so much about this, but I don't know how to help her."

It was clear that we had to hear from Olivia.

Olivia's Story

I chatted with Olivia one-on-one a bit, and then she started to open up: "I began pulling my eyebrows about a year and a half ago. At first it was just a little here and there. Then one night I pulled a lot out. I didn't realize how much until I looked in the mirror. Oh my god, I was shocked. There were big gaps in my eyebrows. I felt so mad at myself. How could I have done this? And I felt embarrassed, afraid everyone was going to see what I'd done. I tried to cover it up with a little makeup, but it still showed the gaps. I prayed no one would notice, but as soon as I saw my mother, she freaked. She started yelling at me as if I did this on purpose."

She seemed distraught. "Who would want to do this? I hate it! I want to stop, but I can't. Since then, it seems the more I pull, the more I want to pull. I get urges to pull. Sometimes I look in the mirror and feel I just have to pull the hair out. Other times I could be studying or on the computer or watching TV, relaxing, and my hands go up there, and I pull without even really thinking about it. Then the damage is done, and I feel awful."

I encouraged her to continue.

"I think my mom calmed down about it a bit after she read about trichotillomania. It's such a weird name. I think she knows I don't want to do this, but I don't think she really gets it. She's always staring at my face and looking at my eyebrows. I feel we can't even have a conversation without her asking me about it or just staring. I know what she's looking at, to see if I've been pulling or if anything is growing back. It feels like that's all she thinks about now. And she always wants to talk about it. I hate that. Sometimes I wasn't even thinking about it, and she has to bring it up, and then I start thinking about it. I told her to stop it, but she can't. I know I get angry at her, and I'm not really angry at my mom. I'm angry about this whole thing. I'm angry that I pull."

"I found this powder online," she continued. "It's dark but it goes on and stays on, sort of like eyebrows. I know it doesn't look natural, but it's the best I could find. It's such an ordeal. I have to get up an hour earlier for school. I have to put it on, and sometimes it takes a long time to get it right. Then I worry all the time. I think kids are staring at my eyebrows. I try to look away from people so they won't see my face. I also worry constantly that it will get smeared, and I sometimes have to go to the bathroom at school to check that it's okay. And at hockey, I have to be so careful with the helmet not to mess up my eyebrows. I think about all this constantly. I used to be outgoing and popular. Now I feel just shy. I don't want anyone to notice me and my eyebrows. I'm constantly thinking kids are saying things about it."

She sighed deeply. "I don't know how it happened, but one night I had a lot of homework, and I had no more eyebrows to pull, so I started pulling my eyelashes. The next morning when I looked in the mirror, I was horrified. Most of my lashes were gone. I knew my mother was going to be so upset. I tried to avoid her, but she noticed. The look on her face . . . Sometimes I think she thinks I must be really crazy to be doing this. I know she was trying. She didn't yell at me, but she looked shocked, and she had tears in her eyes. She asked me about it, and I acted like I didn't know what she was talking about and quickly left for school. I hate when she asks me about this.

"I try so hard not to pull. I use squeeze balls and fidget toys, and I keep a journal about my feelings. I don't know why I do it. I hate myself after I pull. I feel like such a freak."

She said she had been to another therapist. "She kept asking what my week was like and what was making me upset. So awkward. She was nice, but I'm concerned about my hair pulling and nothing else. I started to think it was all hopeless.

"I'm afraid they won't ever grow back, and this is the way I'll always be. That really scares me. Everyone thinks it should be easy to just stop. Nobody understands how hard this is; even I don't understand why it's so hard. And I hate taking medication. It doesn't work, and if anything, the pulling is worse."

It was time to start looking for solutions, and we agreed to meet together, Olivia and her parents. Zoey, Gary, and Olivia were clearly feeling pretty hopeless. Olivia's eyebrows looked fake. Though I could tell much effort went into making them look right, under the makeup, I could tell there really weren't many hairs. Most of her eyelashes were also gone.

So we started by discussing the disorder. I explained that there is not much research on trich, due to a lack of funding and interest. Even though trich causes so much distress, it is often not viewed as a critical psychiatric problem compared to others. Add to that the shame associated with it, and finding subjects to study can be difficult. Those who are studied may not be representative of all the people who have trich.

Still, I have learned a lot about this disorder from clinical experience treating hundreds of hair pullers, and the kids I have seen who pull their hair have had several characteristics in common:

- They don't want to pull their hair. They want to stop.
- Unlike other disorders I treat, trich is not caused by anxiety. Although anxiety can be a trigger, so can boredom or being highly focused on something.
- Kids who pull often have family members who either pull their hair or pick at their skin, which lends support for a genetic component.
- Trich often comes with an obsession with hair, a hyperfocus on how hair feels and looks. Often, these kids are fidgety, their hands eager to touch and fiddle with something. For people with trich, in some ways it feels good to pull hair, since it's self-soothing. But it can quickly become a compulsive habit that feels out of control.
- Trich is not a symptom of an underlying serious psychiatric problem, but it can cause anxiety, depression, and low self-esteem. It is a burden for kids, and it carries social consequences because everybody can see it, yet it can be hard to understand.

- Kids often feel a great deal of shame about pulling and will often deny it to parents and others. Kids who never lie about anything will lie about pulling.
- It's not surprising that pulling can have a negative effect on parent-child relationships. Parents, often mothers, can feel upset about the pulling and may be desperate to stop it. They're aware of the negative social consequences pulling can have on their child. They see their child so out of control with this behavior that they want to take control and stop the pulling. Unfortunately, they can't.
- Willpower alone is usually not enough to stop the pulling, because it can be such a strong compulsive habit.
- It is very important to assess if the child is eating the hair. Although rare, some children have trichotillomania along with pica, meaning they eat the hair they pull out. These children often find hair in other places in addition to their head. For example, children with pica may eat other people's hair, pet hair, or hairs found on a brush. They are obsessed with hair and feel great satisfaction eating it. This can be very dangerous because the hair can form a ball in the stomach, called a bezoar, or a mass that would have to be removed surgically.
- Sometimes kids pull other people's hair or their pet's hair. They love their pets but can't resist pulling the hair.

The good news is, the longer a child goes without any hair pulling, the weaker the urge to pull becomes until the habit is reversed. The brain becomes retrained against pulling, and in my experience, it is extremely rare for the hair not to grow back. So even though stopping the pulling can be difficult initially, it does get easier over time.

I explained that Zoey and Gary had to stop thinking something they were doing wrong had caused this, and Olivia also had to stop blaming herself. Together they needed to work on helping Olivia stop pulling. In my experience, the most effective way to stop pulling is to make it so the child can't easily pull. This is difficult since the urge to pull is so strong. Imagine going on a diet and sitting in front of chocolate cake with a fork in your hand, or imagine trying to quit smoking with a cigarette hanging out of your mouth and a lighter in your hand. That's how hard it is to stop pulling when you have trichotillomania. Hair is always there, waiting to be pulled.

Using barriers, so the child can't feel the hair and get the grip needed to pull it, is a powerful strategy. Kids usually feel the hair before pulling it. So preventing this touching and making it hard to grip the hair to pull it can help prevent the pulling. This often entails wearing something on the fingers that takes away the ability to pull, usually Band-Aids or tape, and often gloves at night. Wearing hats, headbands, or other barriers can also be useful.

To implement this, the first step is to identify when the pulling occurs. Does the child pull throughout the day and at night, or only at certain times? Where does pulling happen? At home? In school? In bed? When on electronics? When anxious? When bored? In the car? Doing homework? In the bathroom? In front of the mirror? With tweezers? This information becomes helpful in deciding which strategies to use and when.

Olivia knew that she pulled at school, in boring classes. She also pulled in front of the TV, doing homework, when she was on her phone or the computer, and basically during her down time. Recently she had pulled some of her eyelashes in front of a mirror. Sometimes she pulled in the car, especially on long drives. She also pulled when reading. Obviously, she never pulled when playing hockey.

Kids usually pull when they are alone or feel alone. So not spending time alone is a strategy. If pulling is in front of a mirror, covering the mirror is another strategy. If tweezers are used, get rid of the tweezers. Then we look at which fingers are used to pull, usually the thumb and one or two other fingers. Covering those fingertips with Band-Aids so that kids can't grip the hair makes it impossible to pull. In addition, having the fingers covered increases awareness, because when the hand goes up to feel the hair, the Band-Aid is in the way. Wearing gloves at night can help kids who pull before going to sleep or if they wake up at night. Gloves are also helpful for morning pullers. Some pulling is so automatic and impulsive, it's almost like scratching an itch. The awareness is there a little bit, but the pulling is experienced as a thoughtless, impulsive action. Other pulling is very obsessive, with a hyperfocus on the hair and a feeling that certain hairs must be pulled. Most kids experience both impulsive and obsessive pulling. Remember that it's a self-soothing, relaxing behavior. Think of it like thumb sucking, which babies do when they're relaxed as well as when they're anxious.

As with other disorders, Olivia had to learn to "talk back" to her urge to pull. Saying no and using willpower, in addition to the strategies discussed so far, are important. She didn't automatically know what fingers she used to pull, so she put her fingers up to her eyebrows as if she were going to pull. She used two fingers on both hands. Those are the fingers that needed to be covered.

She then agreed to wear Band-Aids on her four fingers, covering the tips so that she couldn't feel the hair and couldn't pull the hair. She agreed to wear Band-Aids during the day and gloves at night. She would keep extra Band-Aids with her at school in case they fell off.

Avoiding isolation was a huge step. Her parents had never seen her pull because she always did it when she was alone or felt alone. Like most teenagers, she spent a lot of time in her room doing schoolwork and on her computer. This had to change, at least temporarily, to help her avoid pulling out her hair. So Olivia agreed to do her homework in the kitchen and not in her room for now and to try to stay out of her room as much as possible. In addition, we decided to cover the mirror in her room so it wouldn't tempt her.

Zoey and Gary agreed to remind her to wear the Band-Aids but not be the "Band-Aid Police." Olivia had to do the work herself. Nagging her about the Band-Aids will only cause friction among them. On the other hand, she was a busy girl, and she might forget, so reminding her and having lots of Band-Aids around the house could be very supportive.

I cautioned all three of them that if these strategies were used only some of the time, they would not work. There would be no progress. The behavior has to stop totally to reverse the habit, because every time Olivia pulled, she stirred up the urges all over again. Simply put, the more she pulled, the more she wanted to pull; the less she pulled, the less she wanted to pull. So to change this behavior, the practice had to completely stop.

Easier said than done. For instance, keeping fingers covered all the time can be very annoying. But it works to extinguish the behavior gradually. Over a few months, the hair usually grows back, and the desire to pull lessens. Gradually, the strategies can be decreased as the results are apparent, which increases motivation.

Incentives can also help motivate. Olivia was interested in earning money, so we discussed a system where she could earn something for every day she used these strategies. Consecutive days of implementing the strategies would get her the most money. Not pulling for an extended period would reverse this habit. Tying the incentive to the use of the Band-Aids and gloves was much better than tying it to the pulling. Kids who never lie about anything else will sometimes deny pulling because of the shame they feel. Some will say they didn't know when it happened and lie about how it happened. Arguments then can start with parents saying, "I know you pulled!" and the child saying, "I didn't pull!" Parents should not get sucked into a struggle about this; it's an argument that can't be won. Denial is a symptom of the shame. Focus on supporting the use of the strategies and measuring them, and the results should follow.

Olivia worked hard using the strategies, and she did very well. Her eyebrows and eyelashes grew back. She and her parents talked to her psychiatrist, and they all agreed to taper her off Prozac. Olivia thought it was making her tired, and no one thought it was helping with the pulling. We discussed the fact that she might become more anxious after stopping the Prozac, because it might have been alleviating her anxiety without her realizing it. Sometimes kids come off medication and then realize it was helping; other times they feel no different and are glad not to take a pill every day. Olivia was firm. She wanted to stop taking the medication.

When she stopped pulling, she became acutely aware of the burden she had endured. It had affected her socially, creating more anxiety and isolation. It had also hurt her self-esteem.

She freely expressed her relief: "I thought I was the only one who did this freaky thing. I felt like no one could understand this. I didn't understand it. I can't believe how great it feels not to have to worry about the makeup and about people looking at me all the time."

Olivia spent a lot of time every morning making sure her makeup covered the hair loss, and this had caused her to feel depressed. "It was hard not to feel hopeless about this. I kept trying to stop pulling but couldn't."

As mentioned, this behavior had certainly affected her relationship with her family, especially with her mother. "I always felt like she was looking at my eyebrows and eyelashes and judging me. Always."

Yet Olivia turned things around and did very well for many months.

Finally, she was able to suspend the strategies. After a year, however, she had a relapse and starting pulling again, which was very discouraging. Why had she slipped? She doesn't know, saying it "just happened," and she felt all the urges come back again. Fortunately, she went back to using the Band-Aids, and the pulling stopped again.

Some kids never slip; others have relapses and need to reactivate the strategies.

Olivia talked about her frustration with this. "In some ways, my mom still doesn't get it; she still thinks I do this on purpose, like I want to pull my hair. She doesn't understand how it feels. I told her, 'You know when you've had a long day, and you're exhausted, and you just feel so good putting your head down on your pillow at night? That's how it feels for me when I am pulling.'"

Children with trichotillomania, like Olivia, often say, "No one understands how hard this is." And this is why communication and education are so important.

Skin Picking

Skin picking (excoriation) is a disorder that is a lot like hair pulling, and some children do both. But with skin picking, the obsession is noticing any little imperfection, bump, or scab on the skin and feeling the need to pick at it. Kids who look like they have terrible acne may actually have minor acne, but because they feel the need to keep picking at it, it looks far worse and doesn't heal. Similarly, kids with mosquito bites may pick at the bites so much that they don't have a chance to heal.

Children with skin picking disorder can pick at their fingers, scalp, ears, face, legs, arms, feet—any place on their skin. And of course, there are kids who compulsively pick at their nose, as if their nose has to be perfectly clean inside.

A major problem with skin picking is the risk of infection. In these days of super bugs that are resistant to antibiotics, infections are not something to take lightly. When a child picks, putting antibiotic cream on the area and seeking medical attention if there's even a question of it being infected is important.

Like hair pulling, skin picking often runs in the family, and the strategies used are similar: barriers to make it difficult to pick, such as long-sleeve shirts and pants, Band-Aids on the picking fingers and sometimes on the area picked; keeping the skin clean; and having things to fidget with to prevent picking.

Among the scores of children I have treated for skin picking is the experience of Liam.

Nevan and Pete's Story

Nevan and Pete saw me about their 7-year-old son. "Liam has always been a nail biter and picked at his fingers, but lately it's gotten worse," Nevan told me. "He's been picking his nose, which I know is such a terrible habit. In the last couple of months, he started having nose bleeds, which he never had before. So we took him to the pediatrician. He admitted to the doctor that he's been picking his nose, and this is causing the nose bleeds.

"We realized then, this is serious. Nothing we say or do seems to make a difference. We tell him to stop, that he's going to get teased, that it's dirty, that he can get an infection if he keeps picking. Sometimes I don't even think he's aware he's doing it. If we punish him, it doesn't work. It's like he can't stop himself. We found bloody tissues in the bathroom the other night, and I'm sure it was from his picking."

Pete added, "He also picks at his feet at night, and if he gets a mosquito bite, forget it. He can't seem to leave it alone. When he was younger, he used to chew his clothes, but that's stopped. I've caught him picking at his head; at one point hair was missing, because he was picking so much. And one more spot, I know this is weird, but right inside his ear, he picks at sometimes, and that can lead to a scab. I know it's just a matter of time before kids start to make fun of him or he gets an infection. We don't know how to get him to stop."

I explained that we could implement strategies, and we decided to all meet together.

Liam's Story

Liam was a little fidgety in his chair as we started, but he was honest. "I know I pick. I can't help it. I feel like when I have a scab, I just have to pick it until it's gone. Any bump I feel, I need to pick at it. Lately it's been my nose. I feel like there's something in there, and I have to pick and pick until I get everything out. Then a couple of weeks ago, all this blood came out, and it scared me. I thought something was really wrong. Now it's happened a few times. I can't stop picking, and I know it's gross, but I feel like I have to do it. Sometimes I don't even realize I'm doing it, and my mom and dad will yell at me to stop. They get angry at me and sometimes grab my hand to get me to stop. I try to stop when they tell me to, but then it starts up again. It feels like they're always nagging at me to stop. In school, sometimes I feel like I just have to pick my nose, so I do it so nobody sees me. I sneak it so the kids don't see me do it."

As with hair pulling, we needed to initiate strategies to help Liam stop picking. Since the dynamics of picking and pulling are very similar, so are the strategies to reverse the habits. A Band-Aid on the picking finger forms a barrier and is particularly effective for nose picking. Plus it increases awareness, which is important because kids who pick often don't realize they're doing it.

Other strategies include a Band-Aid on skin that was picked at, long-sleeve shirts and pants if the picking is on the arms and legs, and a tight-fitting shirt if the picking is on the back or chest. Some kids pick their feet, but this is usually at night, and socks can be a barrier. Many kids pick their head, and a hat or a headband that covers the picking spot serves as a barrier.

Naturally, children who pick have to resist the urge so that the urges gradually lessen. They particularly need to understand that taking care of the open wounds from picking is crucial because infections can be dangerous.

Liam agreed to wear a Band-Aid on his picking fingers, wear socks at night, and try hard to stop his picking. He agreed to wear a baseball cap to help with his head picking. He also agreed to let his parents be aware of any spots he's been picking at, so they can monitor for infections.

For incentives, we discussed earning points every day for using the strategies, with big bonus points for successful consecutive days. As the points accumulated, Liam got closer to the prize of going to a baseball game with his dad.

I emphasized that not picking for many days in a row was what would reverse the habit.

Liam, like Olivia, worked really hard to reverse the habit and did a good job, with less and less picking. After a couple of months, he didn't need the strategies anymore. But if he slips, he knows he has to go back to wearing the Band-Aids until the urge passes.

Like most conditions, skin picking and hair pulling can be mild, moderate, or severe, and more strategies and closer monitoring are needed when the problem is severe.

Tics

Tics are involuntary movements or vocalizations that are associated with Tourette syndrome and transient tic disorder. Some kids have what look like classic tics, but the tics are more anxiety-driven, obsessive compulsive movements. Many kids have both: tics that are involuntary or thoughtless as well as other movements they feel they "have to do." These latter tics are more obsessive and in a sense voluntary. Understanding which kind of tics a child experiences is important because both the CBT technique and the appropriate medications are different for tics than for OCD.

Anxiety-driven, obsessive movements often look like classic tics. These can include eye rolling, head shaking, mouth movements, breathing rituals, sniffing, and vocalizations. How do you tell the difference? I have learned to ask the children and listen to the parents. Parents often have a sense of how much control their children have over these movements. And asking the children what makes them do these things often provides a clue to how voluntary the movements are.

True tics are like hiccups: they just happen without the person thinking about it. More obsessive movements happen for a reason, although the reason is irrational. The CBT treatment for tics is called habit reversal training and does not involve exposure response prevention (ERP), which is most effective with anxiety-driven movements. (See chapter 6 for a description of ERP.)

Kids with tics are often very accepting of them. It can be more difficult for parents who are watching their child's tics. For parents, often the best approach is to accept the tics, knowing that the child will most likely outgrow them.

Sometimes tics are severe and can cause the child distress or discomfort. Fortunately, habit reversal training has been found to be an effective treatment. This training involves increasing awareness and developing a "competing movement" that the child can apply to fight tics. Practicing this technique generally helps reduce tics; medication can sometimes help as well.

Sally, 7 years old, had generalized anxiety. She had a fear of choking that developed into a fear of not getting enough air. She would take frequent short quick breaths that seemed like tics. Her mother insisted that this habit was not a tic, that it was based on her fear: "She will be rapidly breathing periodically, which seems automatic and thoughtless. For example, when we are having a conversation, or when she is relaxed and playing. The rapid breathing started with a fear, but she has been gasping so often, it has become a habit."

We worked on Sally "talking back to the worries." Her fears were worse when she had a cold, because she then worried more about her breathing. She made progress with this approach but was also put on antianxiety medication by another doctor. This combination caused the "breathing tic" to disappear, as did her fear of not getting enough air. Her mother was right: It was an anxiety-based movement and not a tic.

A teenage boy I worked with had head-shaking and hand-wiping movements and vocalizations. He had been diagnosed with Tourette syndrome. He was taking medication to help reduce his tics. As I met with him, however, it became clear that these were obsessive compulsive movements that looked like tics. He explained, "When I get a 'bad' thought, I have to cancel it out by shaking my head. When I see kids I don't like—you know, the kids who do drugs and don't do well in school—when I walk by them or even think of their names, I have to shake my body. I know it sounds weird, but it feels like if I don't do this, I could turn into them, or be like them, so I have to shake, sometimes just my head, sometimes my whole body. Then if I touch something they have touched, I have to wipe my hands on something, you know, wipe it off."

He also mumbled under his breath sometimes. When asked about that, he said, "When I get a bad thought I have to say my name quickly three times to cancel out the thoughts."

His treatment consisted of exposure response prevention because these "tics" were really OCD rituals. He stopped his tic medication because he didn't have Tourette syndrome.

I worked with this young man to help him not do the movements while looking at the kids who triggered him to do the movements. Then we worked on him intentionally having a "bad thought" (which for him was either sexual or violent) and not doing the vocalizations. The exposure to the kids and to the thoughts took the power out of them and made it easier for him to stop doing his movements. One by one, he was able to stop all his movements and vocalizations.

As noted above, sometimes treatment can be complicated because kids can have both tics and anxiety-driven movements. A boy I worked with had eye tics, including blinking and eye rolling. When asked about it, he explained that the blinking just happens. "I don't even know I'm doing it. But the other thing, with my eyes, that's different. If I see something in the corner of my eye, I feel I have to roll my eye back and forth. It's kinda like needing to even it out."

One eye movement, the blinking, is a tic; the other is an obsessive compulsive movement. I never would have known that if I hadn't asked him about it, because they both looked like classic eye tics. The treatment for the eye rolling was exposure response prevention. He worked on intentionally seeing something in the corner of his eye and not doing the eye rolling. He was able to work on that successfully, and the movement went away.

He still has the eye-blinking tic, but that doesn't bother him.

Picky Eating

Many kids restrict what foods they will eat, but when this behavior is extreme, it may be anxiety based. When children have no physical reasons for eating difficulties, yet they limit their food choices dramatically, anxiety is likely at the root of the problem. If we think of anxious kids as wanting to stay in their comfort zone and not wanting to try new things, or take risks, it makes sense that this can be applied to food. Parents often become alarmed because the food selections can be so limited.

An example of this is 8-year-old Jackson, who has generalized anxiety. His diet consists primarily of pasta with butter, but it has to be Ronni pasta shells. He will eat pizza, from one pizza restaurant, with no cheese. Jackson also eats chicken nuggets and fries, but only from McDonald's. In addition, he eats raw carrot sticks and grapes. He used to eat cheese, but not anymore. Recently, he has started eating sugar puff cereal. That's his entire diet, and he refuses to try any other foods except, like most kids with this problem, sweets—he will gladly eat candy, cookies, and cake.

What helped Jackson expand his palate was graduated exposure with incentives. This included eating some nonpreferred food before he was able to eat his preferred food. He was involved in the choices of food, but he had to eat the nonpreferred food repeatedly until he became more used to it and was able to incorporate it into his diet.

Of course, parents can play a large role in this problem. Some parents are extremely tolerant of picky eating and may make different meals for each child. Other parents are more concerned and able to be more firm in their approach to eating. With an anxious child, the sooner we work on this, the better. Eating a variety of healthy foods is learned behavior that starts very early in life. Avoidance of new foods, just like avoidance of new experiences, should not be permitted in an anxious child.

Stomach Problems, Constipation, and Headaches

Another anxiety-related behavior is the problem of constipation, a common problem with anxious children. Young children can be afraid of having a bowel movement and may withhold it until they are "backed up." Often they need to take a stool softener daily, to make it easier for them. Once they are constipated, it can become a vicious cycle, because having a bowel movement then becomes painful, causes avoidance, and results in further constipation.

Using a stool softener and having sitting times on the toilet is the best approach. Of course, parents have to monitor bowel movements so that constipation doesn't develop into a chronic problem. I also encourage them to work closely with their pediatrician.

We all know that tension can cause headaches, and among anxious children, headaches can be a real concern. Relaxing, staying hydrated, and eating a balanced diet can help keep headaches under control. As with all anxiety-related physical problems, reducing the anxiety lessens the problem. When needed, pain medication can also be used. It's important to keep the headaches from interfering with a child's functioning. Kids have to learn to ignore the pain and keep active.

The same with stomach pains. Kids have to recognize that these pains are "the worries" and not a sign that they are sick. They need to push themselves to continue their activities; often the distraction helps the pain go away. In addition, by "pushing through their anxiety," kids find out that the anxiety decreases, and with that, the pain decreases. Physical problems caused by anxiety should not be used as a reason to avoid anxiety-producing situations.

More Reasons for Hope

Although the above conditions aren't classic anxiety disorders and don't easily lend themselves to the seven steps, they can be extremely frustrating. The good news is that cognitive behavioral techniques can solve these issues and help children and their parents move on.

Chapter 10

Easier Said Than Done

When More Help Is Needed

Anxiety disorders can be mild, moderate, or severe. When applying cognitive behavioral therapy (CBT) strategies at home is not enough, professional guidance is often needed. But be forewarned: the mental health system for children can feel like a maze that is difficult to navigate. There are social workers, mental health counselors, school counselors, psychologists, nurse practitioners, and psychiatrists. If that's not confusing enough, there are different kinds of therapies, from play therapy to talk therapy, family therapy to biofeedback, psychoanalytical therapy to mindfulness therapy, cognitive behavioral therapy (CBT) to dialectical behavior therapy (DBT).

My considered preference is CBT because it is evidence based, meaning that much research has been done proving its effectiveness, especially for children with anxiety disorders.

Psychiatrists are medical doctors who have a medical degree (MD) and specialize in treating psychological disorders with medication. Some child psychiatrists provide medication and therapy; some focus only on prescribing the right medication for children. Child psychiatrists are very skilled in understanding psychiatric medications and choosing among many different choices for individual children and adolescents. Most therapists have relationships with psychiatrists they trust. Therapists can guide you if they feel medication should be added to your child's treatment, though medications should be the last treatment option in most cases, not the first. If your child is severely ill or at risk of serious harm to self or others, including talking about doing harm, you should seek immediate medical care for your child.

Finding a Therapist

Unfortunately, there are many therapists who say they do CBT with kids after they have taken a weekend workshop in it, and the truth is that their training is limited. Therefore, you need to meet with any potential therapist for your child and feel comfortable with that person. I recommend meeting first without your child, so you can more freely discuss your child's problems and ask questions about the therapist's approach.

For instance:

- What is your training?
- Are you licensed?
- How much experience do you have doing CBT with children?
- How much do you involve the parents in this process?
- How will we be able to judge if it is working?
- What is the cost, and do you take my insurance?
- How often will you meet with my child?
- Do you have after-school and/or weekend hours?
- Now that you know some of my child's difficulties, what is your approach?

Social workers and mental health therapists usually have one to two years of schooling after their BA or BS. Psychologists have at least four years of graduate schooling, plus an internship, dissertation, and postdoctoral study. A social worker with extensive clinical experience and training in CBT, however, could be a better fit for a particular child or problem than a psychologist who specialized in research and has far less clinical training. As in any field, there are good people who know what they're doing, and there are other good people, with less training and experience, who are not as competent. You want someone who is skilled and experienced in CBT and who will involve you in understanding how the process works.

You also want to be able to see measurable progress. Although there are plenty of well-meaning professionals your child can chat with, you want to ensure that the right treatment is being provided to reduce your child's anxiety.

Recommendations from friends and from your child's pediatrician can be good sources for finding a therapist. You probably know people whose children have been in therapy, and these personal recommendations can be useful. Schools also can be a resource for referrals to a therapist, if you feel comfortable sharing this need with your child's guidance counselor.

When you meet with the therapist, trust your feelings. Do you feel comfortable that this is a good match? Will the therapist do an assessment and give you a diagnosis? Many parents seek therapy for their child because they want help and because they want to know what's wrong. A diagnosis is a starting point in understanding how to help your child.

Also keep in mind, once you engage with a therapist, you are not married to that person. If you don't feel it's working, or are not feeling comfortable, it's fine to find another therapist who is a better match. Never worry about a therapist's feelings when it comes to this issue. Finding the right match for your child is most important in making the therapy work.

Deciding on Medication

When a child has an infection or other physical medical problem, a responsible parent will seek and administer appropriate medication. No responsible parent will hastily medicate their child to treat anxiety, however. For most parents, it's a very difficult decision to make. I think medication should be considered, under certain circumstances, but not as a first line of treatment. When anxiety is severe, it can be too hard for children to apply the CBT strategies and do the necessary work because they are so flooded with overwhelming feelings. Severe anxiety can be crippling to a child and very painful, and for these children, medication plus therapy may be needed.

When should an evaluation for antianxiety medications be considered? Consider the following three examples:

1. When the anxiety is so severe that it's interfering with the health of the child

An example is a teenage girl I worked with who had a severe phobia of choking that caused her to stop eating. She was rapidly losing weight, and although we were making progress getting her to drink and eat bits of soft foods, it wasn't enough. It was so hard for her to challenge this fear and eat. So medication was added, and she made significant, rapid progress. The medication made it possible for her to realize how irrational her fear was. Gaining that insight helped her eat more and enabled us to continue the therapy.

Another example is a little girl with severe separation anxiety. She had been doing CBT, but her anxiety was pervasive. The anxiety started triggering headaches and exhausting her. She said, "Mommy, it's just so hard, and I'm only 11 years old." Medication made a big difference in reducing her anxiety and her headaches.

2. When the anxiety is so severe that it's interfering with the child's functioning, including the ability to respond to CBT

The "exposure" for these children with severe anxiety is simply to get through the day. They can't function because they are paralyzed by irrational anxiety. Severe anxiety may have psychotic features. Gaining insight and applying the cognitive strategies of challenging anxious thoughts may be impossible. Medication added to therapy can help the child be better able to apply the CBT.

A good illustration of this is children who have school phobia, with significant trouble attending school. These situations are often complicated and demand coordination with family and school, but medication to help the child feel less anxious can make the difference needed to get the child to school.

3. When kids are so anxious, they are often angry, with panic attacks and explosive behavior that interferes with family life

When the anxiety seems pervasive and is not responding enough to CBT, adding medication can make a big difference.

For instance, I worked with a 12-year-old who was very anxious and angry and took it out on her family, especially her mother. The medication decreased her anxiety, and because she was feeling more comfortable and less anxious, her anger lessened. Adding medication made a big difference for her and her family. Her father said, "I have my daughter back."

Are kids overmedicated? Many are, since medication can be seen as a quick fix. Insurance companies, when approving therapy sessions, often routinely ask if a medication evaluation was done, and if not, why not? Frankly, covering the cost of medication can be cheaper than covering the cost for therapy. But giving children medication for anxiety without therapy gives children the wrong message. Pills can't take the place of working to manage anxiety. This is a very important point: children are working and learning useful skills, and medication can help them apply these skills. My concern about medication without therapy is that children don't learn about themselves and how to control their feelings; rather, they put their faith in a pill instead. Not a great message to grow up with.

Medications also may come with side effects. Most kids are easy to medicate, and a low dose of a medication can make a big difference, sometimes with no side effects. Yet other kids have major side effects, so finding the right medication or combination of medications can be a challenge. Unfortunately, no one knows who will be easy, and who will be difficult, to medicate. And yes, these medications are powerful: they work on the brain. Therefore, children starting on a medication for anxiety need to be carefully monitored for side effects. When side effects occur, one medication is usually discontinued and replaced by another.

Unlike some other medications, where the choices and dosing are standard, antianxiety medications vary considerably from child to child. A small child may need a high dose of a medication to get a positive response, and a big teenager may need a low dose of the exact same medication. Two children with identical anxiety symptoms may have totally different reactions to the medications aimed at alleviating those symptoms. Prescribing these medications is more of an art than a science, so it's important to work with a doctor who is very experienced and knowledgeable about these medications.

Some pediatricians are comfortable prescribing medications for anxiety; others are not. If it appears to be a "simple" solution, and the pediatrician's initial medication works, that's great. But if it becomes more complicated, most pediatricians will refer to a child psychiatrist or nurse practitioner who specializes in medications for anxious kids. This is their expertise. They don't prescribe for infections and fevers; they prescribe only for psychiatric illnesses. They are the specialists who know these medications, in contrast to the pediatrician, who is a generalist. Overall, while a generalist may be fine in some circumstances, sometimes a specialist is needed.

The most common medications prescribed for children with anxiety disorders are selective serotonin reuptake inhibitors (SSRI). Believed to increase the level of the neurotransmitter serotonin, they are taken daily and may take several weeks before the effects are felt. Children usually start with a very low dose, and several weeks later, if no response, the dose is increased as needed. This interval continues until the dose is making a difference in reducing the anxiety. Many kids are on these medications for only nine months to a year, though some are on them longer. The younger the child, the more conservative I am about the use of medications. I also prefer to attempt to get kids off medications when they have an extended time of being symptom-free. I never assume children have to stay on medications for the rest of their lives.

A common side effect of the SSRIs can be sexual dysfunction—reduced arousal and difficulty having an orgasm—for both women and men. This information is not frequently shared with teenagers, because we like to think they don't have sex. However, it's an important side effect to discuss with them. I'm sure many kids who have been on these drugs through puberty have had a diminished sex drive but didn't realize it. Very little is known about how that diminished sex drive affects their development and feelings about themselves.

The other class of medications that is sometimes used for anxiety is benzodiazepines. They enhance the effect of the neurotransmitter gamma-aminobutyric acid (GABA), resulting in a sedative, sleep-inducing, anticonvulsant and muscle-relaxing effect. They can be short or long acting, and they do not take long to take effect, unlike the SSRIs. The anxiety-reducing effect is felt right away. Short-term use of these medications, or using them "as needed," is most common. Long-term use is not generally advised due to their addictive qualities. These drugs can be abused, unlike the SSRIs, because they have immediate antianxiety effects.

In addition, melatonin, which is a hormone sold over the counter (without a prescription) in health food stores and pharmacies, in the vitamin section, is often used to help kids sleep. If your child has difficulty falling asleep and gets more anxious before sleep, melatonin can be a useful sleep aid. It is natural and does not require a prescription. Check with your child's doctor about the appropriate dose. *Always discuss this and all medications with your child's pediatrician.*

School Involvement

When is it necessary to get help from your child's school?

It's important to involve your child's school when the anxiety shows itself at school and when school performance is affected. You want the school to understand your child, and there may be supports the school can offer. If the anxiety is only evident when your child is at home, and there are no symptoms at school, the school doesn't have to be involved.

I have worked with many anxious children who are very disruptive at home but are model students at school. Alice, an 8-year-old with OCD, is a good example of this. She couldn't wear underwear, had night rituals that sometimes brought her mother to tears, experienced anxiety-driven tantrums at home, and was so rigid in her thinking that any change in plans caused a meltdown. When her mother went to her teacher conference, the teacher said that she wished all her students were like Alice, who was a role model for others. Needless to say, her mother almost fell off her chair. Even though that was surprising to her mother, there was no need to involve the school, because she was fine there. Sometimes the structure, consistency, and predictability of school is containing for anxious children, in a way that home life can't be.

Jacob, a 6-year-old with selective mutism, is the opposite. He's fine at home, happy, a normal kid; all his anxiety is school focused. At school he's silent and withdrawn. His school has to be directly involved and give him a lot of supports to help him talk more and be less anxious.

School Bullying

Many anxious children have a lot of school-based social anxiety that can severely affect their school performance. Kids spend a great deal of time in school, interacting with their peers. These interactions are not always positive, and when toxic, they can create intense anxiety. Issues of bullying are unfortunately all too common. Bullying can take the form of a child being targeted and harassed or excluded in hurtful ways. Victims of bullying often feel helpless and overwhelmed because they have to face a hostile school environment every day. Bullies can be sneaky, with so much of their behavior happening off the teacher's radar. This dynamic can create intense anxiety for a child.

The issue of cyberbullying remains an ongoing problem among kids through the role of social media. Kids may write mean things they would never say to another child face to face. The written word is often very public, read by large groups of kids who get involved rapidly in the group chat. The intensity of this interaction is amazing because anything written is read and often responded to quickly by many kids. Within minutes, a child can feel violated by a crowd of kids and feel overwhelmed and unable to respond.

I have worked with girls, often in middle school, in situations where fifteen girls are online chatting, saying very mean things about one particular girl. Sometimes it takes the form of online battles among groups of girls, almost like schoolyard fighting, only far more intense. Unlike the spoken word, the written word lasts forever, for anyone to see. Not having face-to-face contact during these fights elevates the cruelty. Understandably, these exchanges can cause severe anxiety. Words are written and read, but the writing doesn't show the faces of sadness and fear these kids feel; it doesn't reveal the sound of the crying among these girls. Words can be very cold, and without face-to-face communication, so much is missed. These increasingly common experiences can be overwhelming for children and the cause not only of panic attacks, but of suicidal feelings.

Schools need to be actively involved in promoting a less hostile environment for kids, and parents should alert the administration when these things are happening. Kids need to be held accountable for bullying behavior, and there needs to be a zero-tolerance policy. Kids also need to be taught that whatever they write is public—that there is no privacy.

School Stress

Schools sometimes also play a role in increasing anxiety among kids. The pressure to excel, the excessive homework load, and "teaching to the test" all can contribute to overwhelming anxiety. Middle school kids start worrying about getting into the "right college." High school kids often can't possibly get the amount of sleep they need for their health because of the homework load. Many of them fall asleep at school, or wish they could. Schools and communities have to look at how the culture is causing kids to be far more anxious than they should be, and they need to work to promote a healthier environment for kids. With more progress in this area, I believe we would see fewer children not only on antianxiety medications, but also on stimulants to stay focused and alert.

504 Plans and IEPs for Anxious Children

Anxiety is a medical illness, and anxious children who need accommodations can request a 504 Plan. This is a legal document that guarantees your child certain accommodations due to a medical illness.

Many parents are also familiar with IEPs (Independent Educational Plans), which are for children who have difficulty accessing the curriculum due to learning disabilities or more severe social and emotional problems. An IEP may be appropriate if a child needs intensive support to learn, including placement in a more therapeutic school setting. A 504 Plan is more common for children who have anxiety disorders and provides accommodations to help them manage their anxiety in school.

Common accommodations that anxious kids may require include:

- Extra time for tests
- Extended deadlines for homework
- Ability to take breaks when needed
- Ability to meet regularly with the school counselor
- Frequent communication between parents and teacher concerning anxiety
- Ability to meet with the teacher before school starts in the fall
- Ability to have friends in the same class
- Ability to be excused from class participation as needed
- Reduced homework load
- Ability to eat outside the cafeteria
- Ability to use the nurse's bathroom
- Ability to have a counselor-led social group, often called "lunch bunch"

The hope is that kids will need less of the above as they work on reducing their anxiety. These supports can be crucial, however, to help children feel less anxious at school. School counselors can be a huge support when anxiety situations result at school, because they know the peers and the teachers and are right there to help. Many kids who have social anxiety or school anxiety can benefit from a counselor who is on site and able to help, in addition to an outside therapist.

When to Get a Neuropsychological Evaluation

When children appear to be struggling at school and showing a lot of anxiety, it's easy to attribute the school difficulties to the anxiety. But kids can be complicated. If there is an underlying undiagnosed learning disability or problems with attention and focus, an already anxious child becomes far more anxious. Imagine an anxious child, sitting in a classroom, and not understanding what the teacher is teaching, or an anxious child spacing out and having no idea what's going on in the classroom. These situations could trigger panic in an already anxious child.

Too often the focus of all problems is on the child's anxiety. But the anxiety could be a normal reaction to a difficult school situation. Having a comprehensive neuropsychological evaluation can tease out what's anxiety and what might be something else going on with your child. Understanding your child's needs can help guide treatment decisions and decide what supports your child may need at school. As noted earlier, your child may need supports in the form of an IEP. The neuropsychological evaluation can help determine if that's what's needed, and if so, how to get it for your child.

These evaluations should be done by a licensed neuropsychologist, trained and experienced in working with children. They should include an IQ test; achievement tests; tests of attention, organization, memory, and processing speed; psychological assessments; and other tests, depending on the questions needing answers. As a parent, you should expect to receive a comprehensive report outlining the tests conducted and the results, and providing a summary and recommendations for your child. Testing results can help you understand your child's cognitive and emotional functioning as well as how best to support your child.

Many parents seek independent neuropsychologists, who usually provide a far more comprehensive evaluation, and as a result, they may make different conclusions and recommendations. Parents have a right to bring this information to their child's school and expect their child's educational needs to be met.

Parent as Advocate: Working with Your Child's School

It can feel very frustrating to see your child suffering with anxiety, clearly needing more school support and not getting it. Parents can hire advocates who know the laws and your rights in relation to your child's school-based needs. It's not something everyone wants to do, but sometimes hiring an advocate can be a useful way to get what your child needs from the school system. In addition, attorneys may be useful in advocating for your child.

When to Get More Medical Tests

When a child with anxiety presents with headaches or stomachaches, anxiety may be the cause of these pains. It's important to involve a pediatrician, however, especially if children experience these problems when they're not anxious. I always feel more comfortable ruling out a medical cause for physical symptoms before assuming they're anxiety based.

A good example is an 11-year-old boy who had OCD and lots of anxiety. He also complained randomly of stomach pain, but his complaints didn't always come when he was anxious; in fact, he sometimes complained when he was having fun with friends. It was easy to assume it was his anxiety causing his pain, since anxiety often causes stomach discomfort. His parents pursued this with his pediatrician, and I recommended that they follow up further. And sure enough, tests revealed that this boy had celiac disease. With a change in his diet, the stomach pain disappeared.

On the other hand, I have also worked with kids whose physical pain was an expression of their anxiety and who underwent too many medical tests to find a physical cause. Tests that come back normal are a sign that anxiety is the cause of the pain. This can become a vicious cycle. Anxiety causes the pain, and the pain causes anxiety, which causes more hyperfocus on the pain and even more anxiety. There are always more tests that can be done, and knowing where to draw the line on medical tests is important.

Sometimes the expression of pain really is caused by the anxiety, or becomes a way to avoid anxious situations. Saying, "I'm sick," is for many kids easier and more effective than saying, "I'm worried and scared." And parents often respond differently, with more patience and support, to sick kids than to anxious kids. As parents, if we think our children are truly in pain, we don't want to push them. Many anxious kids know this and complain about pain to avoid anxiety-producing situations. Sorting this out as a parent is not always easy. A child who uses sickness as an avoidance strategy is a very anxious child who can look comfortable and relaxed when avoiding situations and challenges.

Parents have to become aware that their child is "faking it" out of the desperate need to avoid challenging situations, which can include social activities, extracurricular activities, and in the worst cases, attending school. Anxiety can cause children to become very "manipulative" due to the intense need to avoid feeling anxious.

Alternative Approaches

Tools that promote relaxation can be useful for children as well as adults. Physical exercise can reduce anxiety and improve mood. So having your child involved in regular aerobic exercise can be as powerful as medication for anxiety. In addition, kids today spend so much time in front of screens; they are often not getting the exercise they need. Being away from a screen and being involved in other activities is important, not just for a child's physical health, but for a child's mental health as well.

Making sure your child is getting enough sleep is also very important. With too little sleep, kids may become more anxious. So many kids are sleep deprived, especially teenagers. Without enough sleep, children are at greater risk for anxiety, mood, and attentional disorders. Kids need their sleep, and with computer games and social media often done in isolation—without parents knowing if the child is sleeping—sleep is often sacrificed.

Overuse of screens can be a huge problem for anxious kids. It allows them to avoid healthier activities. Sleep, exercise, and social activities need to take priority over the use of screens. Parents need to set limits and follow through with those limits so anxious kids can't hide for hours every day behind screens. And "virtual friends" are not the same as face-to-face, real-life friends. Kids need to be with other kids away from screens.

Depending on the child, meditation and yoga can also offer relief from anxiety symptoms. In addition, biofeedback is a structured way of teaching children how to relax their bodies; depending on the child, biofeedback can be useful.

When Parents Need Support

Parenting an anxious child can be challenging for many reasons. For one, these children can be demanding of time and energy. When the anxiety symptoms are severe or include more explosive behaviors, the whole family is affected. Since anxiety is contagious, the atmosphere in the family of an anxious child can become intense and stressed.

Parents of anxious children often feel overwhelmed and in need of support. For some parents, this experience causes them to seek therapy and even medication for themselves. They may benefit from guidance to keep their anxiety under control. Sometimes parents have conflicts with each other about how to parent their anxious child. Disagreeing about when to push and when to be more protective of the child is common. Knowing how hard to push, and how much to protect, can be confusing. When one parent is more firm and another more lenient, parents who don't fight about anything else may argue about their anxious child. When your child feels out of control, it's easy to blame each other. Many couples consider therapy to help resolve conflicts about parenting. It strengthens the ability to support each other and can be beneficial, not only to the parents, but to the whole family.

There are support groups for almost everything but few support groups for parents of anxious children. Why? There's a great stigma about any kind of mental illness, including one as common as anxiety. As mentioned before, many anxious kids are high functioning, so they often have a hard time integrating their sense of being so "normal" with having an anxiety disorder. They may not want anyone to know they have anxiety, because they feel ashamed.

Many of my teenage patients suffering with severe irrational fears are also successful students, fine athletes, and popular kids. They often say, "None of my friends would ever believe I'm sitting here in a therapist's office. Everyone thinks it's the weird kids who need this help. I'm not one of the weird kids."

I understand how these kids feel and why they want to keep it all very private. Yet another part of me hopes that more anxious kids will speak up about their struggles, because that's what will help break down the stigma. It will also demonstrate to others how many "normal" kids suffer from anxiety disorders and affirm that it's not something to feel ashamed about.

Parents are also aware of the stigma about mental illness, and often want to protect their child from any negative consequences that might follow if others know about their child's anxiety. They don't want their child to be harshly judged, and they don't want to be judged as bad parents. When a child has a mental health problem, many people still believe that the parents must be doing something wrong.

One of the parents I work with noted that parents of autistic children certainly have their own challenges, but they are not blamed the way parents of children with psychiatric problems are blamed. Autism is understood to be biologically based and not caused by bad parenting. The same acceptance isn't offered to parents of children with psychiatric problems, even though these problems are also biologically based. As a result, parents of anxious children often suffer in silence, not wanting others to blame them for their child's problems and not wanting others to know what they're going through.

The notion that all children are born the same, and some children simply end up with anxiety or other problems because of bad parenting, is incorrect. The idea that kids who are calm and relaxed are that way because of superior parenting is also incorrect. Clearly, kids are born with different wiring. The proof of this is how often, in the same family with the same parents, one child can be calm and anxiety-free, and the other can be the polar opposite. One child makes parenting look like a breeze, while the other is far more challenging and demanding.

A 10-year-old patient with anxiety and explosive behavior was disruptive in his church group. Parents complained, and he was asked to leave. His mom was naturally very upset, especially because she had a long relationship with this church, and her son liked going to the classes. Yet she understood, she said, "I used to be one of those mothers. I hate to say it, but back then, I would've complained. Before I went through this with my son, I had no clue."

The isolation that parents feel, the sense that no one really "gets it," can be profound. The stigma of so many other things in our society has been discarded, but the stigma of having a child with any kind of mental illness lives on.

This stigma can be broken only if we break it together, through educating others and sharing with friends and family what it's really like to parent an anxious child. Speak up when people give you well-meaning but annoying advice, like "Why don't you just tell her to relax?" "Ah, if only I'd thought of that." Explain that if it were that easy, there'd be no problem. People need to be educated about anxiety. The more parents talk openly about their challenges with anxiety, the more support they will find, because this is an epidemic that affects so many families.

Parents of anxious children could be a more effective resource for each other. Navigating the mental health system alone is a challenge. What if parents shared information about their helpful therapists and talked about strategies they've found effective with their children? Lending support, breaking down the myths, and feeling less alone as your family is turned upside-down by anxiety could be of great benefit. To do this, parents have to confront the stigma about having an anxious child.

What could this look like? Monthly meetings led by parents on a rotating basis, with community speakers and time allotted so parents can share stories and suggestions. This sounds easy, but when you're exhausted with an anxious child and everything else, it's not so easy. I believe that community mental health centers and schools could offer more of this kind of support, in coordination with parents. These meetings could also help the wider community examine ways to decrease children's anxiety on a broader scale.

In short, the epidemic of anxious children demands that kids learn how to manage their anxiety, that parents learn how to help them, and that communities learn what they can do to reduce anxiety among their youth. We all have to share in the responsibility for this problem affecting our kids.

Acknowledgments

I offer sincere thanks to the following individuals. Without their contributions and support, this book would not have been written.

I am grateful to Gary Woonteiler and Woonteiler Ink for editing and writing support, Dr. Jerome Rogoff for ongoing support, Margaret Sharkey for cheering me on, Lisa Tener for her amazing voice giving form to this book, Regina Brooks for believing in this project, and Jackie Wehmueller, who brought this book to press.

And my thanks also go, as always, to my patients—my greatest teachers—who have allowed me the privilege of getting to know them, laughing with them, and helping them overcome anxiety.

Notes

1. Jane E. Costello, Helen L. Egger, and Adrian Angold, "The Developmental Etiology of Anxiety Disorders: Phenomenology, Prevalence, and Comorbidity," in *Phobic and Anxiety Disorders in Children and Adolescents: A Clinician's Guide to Effective Psychosocial and Pharmacological Interventions*, ed. Thomas Ollendick and John March, 61–92 (New York: Oxford University Press, 2011); Kathleen Merikangas, Jian-ping He, Marcy Burstein, Sonja A. Swanson, and Shelli Avenevoli, "Lifetime Prevalence of Mental Disorders in US Adolescents: Results from the National Comorbidity Survey Replication—Adolescent Supplement (NCS-A)," *Journal of the American Academy of Child and Adolescent Psychiatry* 49, no. 10 (October 1, 2010): 980–89; H. Egger Bittner, A. Erkanli, Jane Costello, and D. Foley, "What Do Childhood Anxiety Disorders Predict?" *Journal of Child Psychology and Psychiatry* 48, no. 12 (October 2007): 1174–83.

2. E. Costello, S. Mustillo, A. Erkanli, G. Keeler, and A. Angold, "Prevalence and Development of Psychiatric Disorders in Childhood and Adolescence," *Archives of General Psychiatry* 60, no. 8 (August 2003): 837–44; Julia D. Buckner and Norman B. Schmidt, "Marijuana Effect Expectancies: Relations to Social Anxiety and Marijuana Use Problems," *Addictive Behaviors* 33, no. 11 (November 2008): 1477–83; P. C. Kendall, S. Safford, E. Flannery-Schroeder, and A. Webb, "Child Anxiety Treatment: Outcomes in Adolescence and Impact on Substance Use and Depression at 7.4-Year Follow-Up," *Journal of Consulting and Clinical Psychology* 72, no. 2 (April 2004): 276–87; L. J. Woodward and D.M. Fergusson, "Life Course Outcomes of Young People with Anxiety Disorders in Adolescence," *Journal of the American Academy of Child and Adolescent Psychiatry* 40, no. 9 (September 2001): 1086–93.

3. Kathryn A. Kerns, Shannon Siener, and Laura E. Brumariu, "Mother-Child Relationships, Family Context, and Child Characteristics as Predictors of Anxiety Symptoms in Middle Childhood," *Development and Psychopathology* 23, no. 2 (May 2011): 593–604.

4. Kathryn Degnan, Alisa Almas, and Nathan Fox, "Temperament and the Environment in the Etiology of Childhood Anxiety," *Journal of Child Psychology and Psychiatry* 51, no. 4 (April 2010): 497–517.

5. Allison M. Waters, Melanie J. Zimmer-Gembeck, and Lara J. Farrell, "The Rela-
    tionships of Child and Parent Factors with Children Anxiety Symptoms: Parental
    Anxious Rearing as a Mediator," *Journal of Anxiety Disorders* 26, no. 7 (October
    2012): 737–45.
6. Merel Kindt, "Malleability of Fear Memory: A Behavioral Neuroscience Perspec-
    tive on the Etiology and Treatment of Anxiety Disorders," *Behavior Research and
    Therapy* 62 (September 2014): 24–36; Feng Lui, Chunyan Zhu, Yifeng Guo, Wenbin
    Li, and Meilling Wang, "Disrupted Cortical Hubs in Functional Brain Networks in
    Social Anxiety Disorder," *Clinical Neurophysiology* (November 27, 2014); Jeffrey
    Strawn, John Wegman, Keli Dominick, Max Swartz, and Anna Patinor, "Cortical
    Surface Anatomy in Pediatric Patients with Generalized Anxiety Disorder," *Journal
    of Anxiety Disorders* 28, no. 7 (October 2014): 717–23.
7. Shaozheng Qin, Christina Young, Tian Duan, Tianwen Chen, and Kaustubh
    Supekar, "Amygdala Subregional Structure and Intrinsic Functional Connectiv-
    ity Predicts Individual Differences in Anxiety during Early Childhood," *Biological
    Psychiatry* 75, no. 11 (June 2014): 892–900.
8. Desmond J. Oathes, Brian Patenaude, Alan F. Schatzberg, and Amit Etkin, "Neu-
    robiological Signatures of Anxiety and Depression in Resting-State Functional
    Magnetic Resonance Imaging," *Biological Psychiatry* 77, no. 4 (2015): 385–93.
9. Marta Andreatta, Evelyn Glotzbach-Schoon, Andreas Muhlberger, Stefan Schulz,
    and Julian Wiemer, "Initial and Sustained Brain Responses to Contextual Condi-
    tioned Anxiety in Humans," *Cortex* 63 (February 2015): 352–63; Jonathan Isper,
    Leesha Singh, and Dan Stein, "Meta-Analysis of Functional Brain Imaging in Spe-
    cific Phobia," *Psychiatry and Clinical Neurosciences* 67, no. 5 (May 2013): 311–22;
    Melisa Carrasco, Christina Hong, Jenna Nienhuis, Shannon Harbin, and Kate
    Fitzgerald, "Increased Error Related Brain Activity in Youth with Obsessive Com-
    pulsive Disorder and Other Anxiety Disorders," *Neuroscience Letters* 541 (Febru-
    ary 2013): 214–18.
10. Julia Zito, Daniel Safer, Susan dosReis, James Gardner, and Myde Boles, "Trends
    in the Prescribing of Psychotropic Medications to Preschoolers," *Journal of the
    American Medical Association* 283, no. 8 (February 2000): 1025–30; Thomas
    Delate, Alan Gelenberg, Valene Simmons, and Brenda Motheral, "Trends in the
    Use of Antidepressants in a National Sample of Commercially Insured Pediatric
    Patients, 1998–2002," *Psychiatric Services* 55 (2004): 387–91.
11. Wendy Silverman, A. Pina, and Chockalivgam Viswesvaran, "Evidence-based Psy-
    chosocial Treatments for Phobic and Anxiety Disorders in Children and Adoles-
    cents," *Journal of Clinical Child and Adolescent Psychology* 37, no. 1 (2008): 105–30;
    D. Chambless and S. Hollon, "Defining Empirically Supported Therapies," *Journal
    of Consulting and Clinical Psychology* 66, no. 1 (February 1998): 7–18; S. Hollon
    and A. Beck, "Cognitive and Cognitive Behavioral Therapies," in *Bergin and Gar-
    field's Handbook of Psychotherapy and Behavioral Change*, 6th ed., ed. M. J. Lam-
    bert, 393–442 (New York: Wiley, 2013); T. Ollendick and N. King, "Evidence-based
    Treatments for Children and Adolescents: Issues and Commentary," in *Child and*

Adolescent Therapy: Cognitive Behavioral Procedures, 4th ed., ed. P. C. Kendall, 499–520 (New York: Guilford Press, 2011).

12. Dina Hirshfeld-Becker, Jamie Micco, Heather Mazursky, L. Bruett, and A. Henin, "Applying Cognitive-Behavioral Therapy for Anxiety to the Younger Child," *Child and Adolescent Clinics of North America* 20, no. 2 (April 2011): 349–68.

13. Paula Barrett, Amanda Duffy, Mark Dadds, and Ronald Rapee, "Cognitive Behavioral Treatment of Anxiety Disorders in Children: Long Term Follow Up," *Journal of Consulting and Clinical Psychology* 69, no. 1 (February 2001): 135–41; Courtney Benjamin, Julie Harrison, Cara Settipani, Douglas Brodman, and Philip Kendall, "Anxiety and Related Outcomes in Young Adults 7–19 Years after Receiving Treatment for Child Anxiety," *Journal of Consulting and Clinical Psychology* 81, no. 5 (2013): 865–76; P. C. Kendall et al., "Child Anxiety Treatment"; Laura Seligman and Thomas Ollendick, "Cognitive Behavioral Treatment for Anxiety Disorders in Youth," *Child and Adolescent Psychiatric Clinics of North America* 20, no. 2 (April 2012): 217–38.

14. K. Brendel and B. Maynard, "Child-Parent Interventions for Childhood Anxiety," *Research on Social Work Practice* 24, no. 3 (2014): 287–95; Jennifer Podell and Phillip Kendall, "Mothers and Fathers in Family Cognitive Behavioral Therapy for Anxious Youth," *Journal of Child and Family Studies* 20, no. 2 (2011): 182–95; John Piacentini, Lyndey Bergman, Susanna Chang, Audra Langley, and Tara Peris, "Controlled Comparison of Family Cognitive Behavioral Therapy and Psychoeducation: Relaxation Training for Child Obsessive Compulsive Disorder," *Journal of the Academy of Child and Adolescent Psychiatry* 50, no. 11 (2011): 1149–61; Barbara Esbiorn, Michael Somhovd, Sara Nielsen, Nicole Normann, and Ingrid Leth, "Parental Changes after Involvement in Their Anxious Child's Cognitive Behavioral Treatment," *Journal of Anxiety Disorders* 28, no. 7 (October 2014): 664–70; Allison Smith, Ellen Flannery-Schroeder, Kathleen Gorman, and Nathan Cook, "Parent Cognitive Behavioral Intervention for the Treatment of Childhood Anxiety Disorders: A Pilot Study," *Behavior Research and Therapy* 61 (October 2014): 156–61; Kirsten Thirlwall, Peter Cooper, Jessica Karalus, Merryn Voysey, and Lucy Willetts, "Treatment of Child Anxiety Disorders via Guided Parent-Delivered Cognitive-Behavioral Therapy: Randomised Controlled Trial," *British Journal of Psychiatry* 203, no. 6 (December 2013): 436–44.

15. Patricia Porto, Leticia Oliveira, Jair Mari, Elaine Volchan, and Ivan Figueira, "Does Cognitive Behavioral Therapy Change the Brain? A Systematic Review of Neuroimaging in Anxiety Disorders," *Journal of Neuropsychiatry and Clinical Neurosciences* 21, no. 2 (2009): 114–25; Vincent Paquette, Johanne Levesque, Boualem Mensour, Jean-Maxime Leroux, and Gilles Beaudoin, "'Change the Mind and You Change the Brain': Effects of Cognitive-Behavioral Therapy on the Neural Correlates of Spider Phobia," *Neuroimage* 18, no. 2 (February 2003): 401–9; Andrea Reinecke, Kai Thilo, Nicola Filippini, Alison Croft, and Catherine Harmer, "Predicting Rapid Response to Cognitive-Behavioral Treatment for Panic Disorder: The Role of Hippocampus, Insula, and Dorsolateral Prefrontal Cortex," *Behavior*

Research and Therapy 62 (November 2014): 120–28; Ulrike Leuken, Benjamin Straube, Carten Konrad, Hans Wittchen, and Andreas Strohle, "Neural Substrates of Treatment Response to Cognitive-Behavioral Therapy in Panic Disorder with Agoraphobia," *American Journal of Psychiatry* 170, no. 11 (November 2013): 1345–55; Phillipe Golden, Mifal Ziv, Hooria Jazaieri, Justin Weeks, and Richard Heimberg, "Impact of Cognitive-Behavioral Therapy for Social Anxiety Disorder on the Neural Bases of Emotional Reactivity to and Regulation of Social Evaluation," *Behavior Research and Therapy* 62 (November 2014): 97–106; V. Miskovic, D. Moscovitch, D. Santesso, R. McCabe, and M. Antony, "Changes in EEG Cross-Frequency Coupling during Cognitive Behavioral Therapy for Social Anxiety Disorder," *Psychological Science* 22, no. 4 (April 2011): 507–16; J. Strawn, A. Wehry, M. DelBello, M. Rynn, and S. Strakowski, "Establishing the Neurobiological Basis of Treatment in Children and Adolescents with Generalized Anxiety Disorder," *Depression and Anxiety* 29, no. 4 (April 2012): 328–39.

16. Eli Lebowitz, Lyndsey Scharfstein, and Johanna Jones, "Comparing Family Accommodation in Pediatric Obsessive-Compulsive Disorder, Anxiety Disorders, and Nonanxious Children," *Depression and Anxiety* 31, no. 12 (December 2014): 1018–25; Johanna Thompson-Hollands, Caroline Kerns, Donna Pincus, and Jonathan Comer, "Parental Accommodation of Child Anxiety and Related Symptoms: Range, Impact, and Correlates," *Journal of Anxiety Disorders* 28, no. 8 (December 2014): 765–73; C. Wei and P. Kendall, "Child Perceived Parenting Behavior: Childhood Anxiety and Related Symptoms," *Child and Family Behavior Therapy* 36, no. 1 (January 2014): 1–18.

17. Hirshfeld-Becker et al., "Applying Cognitive-Behavioral Therapy."

18. Martina Gere, Marianne Villabo, Sven Torgersen, and Phillip Kendall, "Overprotective Parenting and Child Anxiety: The Role of Co-occurring Child Behavior Problems," *Journal of Anxiety Disorders* 26, no. 6 (August 2012): 642–49.

19. J. Silk, L. Sheeber, P. Tan, C. Ladouceur, and E. Forbes, "You Can Do It!' The Role of Parental Encouragement of Bravery in Child Anxiety Treatment," *Journal of Anxiety Disorders* 27, no. 5 (June 2013): 439–46.

Index

abuse of benzodiazepines, 225

accommodation, educational, 228–29

accommodation, parental: avoidance and, 10–11; problems with, 13–14; separation anxiety, 92, 111; specific phobias, 164–66

ADHD (attention deficit hyperactivity disorder): *DSM-5* diagnostic criteria for, 63–65; GAD and, 60–61

advocates for working with school system, 230

agreeing on challenges to work on, 22–23; GAD, 43–44, 55–56; OCD, 129–31, 139–40; PTSD, 178–79, 191–92; selective mutism, 72–73; separation anxiety, 99–100, 113; social anxiety, 84–85; specific phobias, 157–58, 169

alcohol and drug addictions: abuse of benzodiazepines, 225; anxiety and, 5; faith in pills and, 224; GAD and, 50–52; social anxiety and, 82

amygdala, 6

anger: of child, over anxiety problems, 40, 96, 223; oppositional behavior and anxiety, 84; of parent, at child's anxiety, 10, 92; as resistance and denial, 79–80; at therapist, 97

anterior cingulate cortex, 6

anxiety disorders, 4–5; ADHD and, 60–61; biological underpinnings of, 5–8, 11; irrationality of anxiety, 90; prevalence of, 1; resistance and, 79–80, 172–73; social isolation and, 31, 82; tantrums and, 8, 36, 92. *See also* physical symptoms; talking back to anxiety; targeting anxious thoughts and behaviors; *specific disorders*

Asperger syndrome and bug phobia, 161–66

attention deficit hyperactivity disorder (ADHD): *DSM-5* diagnostic criteria for, 63–65; GAD and, 60–61

autism spectrum disorders: communication difficulties and, 77; selective mutism and, 67

avoidance: as common reaction, 19; complaints of pain and, 231; as defense against anxiety, 13, 20, 34; enabling of, 172; parental accommodation and, 10–11; social anxiety and, 81; targeting, 83

bathroom at school, using, 76

behavioral part of CBT, 13

behaviors: normalizing, 31, 41, 71, 85, 192; oppositional, and anxiety, 84, 96. *See also* rating anxious behaviors; targeting anxious thoughts and behaviors; targeting behaviors

benzodiazepines, 225

biological underpinnings of anxiety, 5–8

brain: experience as changing, 13; "fear circuitry" of, 5–7; plasticity of, 9–10

bugs, fear of, 161–66

bullying, 226–27

calendar format for charting progress, 26–27, 28–29

calm-down list: fear of vomiting, 24; GAD, 45–46; separation anxiety, 114–15

campus, rape on, 183–85, 190, 195

case studies, 2; fear of vomiting, 17–20; GAD, 35–40, 49–53; hair pulling, 203–12; OCD, 122–25, 135–37; PTSD,

The Pact

The Pact

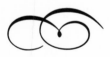

HILARY NORMAN

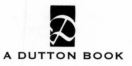

A DUTTON BOOK

DUTTON
Published by the Penguin Group
Penguin Books USA Inc., 375 Hudson Street, New York, New York 10014, U.S.A.
Penguin Books Ltd, 27 Wrights Lane, London W8 5TZ, England
Penguin Books Australia Ltd, Ringwood, Victoria, Australia
Penguin Books Canada Ltd, 10 Alcorn Avenue, Toronto, Ontario, Canada M4V 3B2
Penguin Books (N.Z.) Ltd, 182–190 Wairau Road, Auckland 10, New Zealand

Penguin Books Ltd, Registered Offices:
Harmondsworth, Middlesex, England

First published by Dutton, an imprint of Dutton Signet, a division of Penguin Books USA Inc.

First Printing, June, 1997
1   3   5   7   9   10   8   6   4   2

 REGISTERED TRADEMARK—MARCA REGISTRADA

LIBRARY OF CONGRESS CATALOGING-IN-PUBLICATION DATA:
Norman, Hilary.
The pact / Hilary Norman.
p.   cm.
ISBN 0-525-94256-4 (acid-free paper)
I. Title.
PR6064.0473P33   1997
823'.914—dc21   96-50131
                                      CIP

Printed in the United States of America
Set in Bembo
Designed by Jesse Cohen

PUBLISHER'S NOTE

This is a work of fiction. Names, characters, places, and incidents either are the product of the author's imagination or are used fictitiously, and any resemblance to actual persons, living or dead, events, or locales is entirely coincidental.

For my mother, Herta Norman,
still my first reader and critic.

ACKNOWLEDGMENTS

Grateful thanks are due, as always, to many people, old and new friends, and as usual, I list them in alphabetical order:

Staff at The American School, London; the concierge at the Hotel Amigo in Brussels for answering my many strange and unusual questions; Dorothy and David W. Balfour, for going out of their way (literally) to help me, yet again; Howard M. Barmad; Carolyn Caughey; my cat, Charlotte, for helping me understand Cleo; the public relations department of Eurostar; Sara Fisher; Jim Gilles of the *Newport Daily News*; John Hawkins; Jonathan Kern, my husband, for many things (including knowing when I'm a no-go area); Audrey LaFehr; special, sincere gratitude to Mr. Nicholas Parkhouse, D.M, M.Ch, F.R.C.S., for his expertise, valuable time, and kindness; Mr. Robert Purdy at St. Mary's Church in Newport, Rhode Island; Helen Rose, my sister, who always helps, and Neal Rose, who seriously helped this time; Lynne Sacks for her British advertising know-how; Dr. Jonathan Tarlow, who always guides me through the medical mire, but who really came through in a major way for this one; Michael Thomas; Norman Waterman for his U.S. advertising knowledge and experience; and the staff of the Westminster and Wiener Libraries for their guidance.

Greek mythology tells us that when Pandora, overcome by curiosity, opened the box that she had been forbidden to open, she released from it all the evils and ills that would beset man, leaving only hope within.

PROLOGUE

BRUSSELS: JULY 26, 1995

Olivia Segal sat, with Cleo, her little tortoiseshell cat, on her lap, on the faded Kashan silk prayer rug and looked up at the clock.

Seven minutes past five in the afternoon in Brussels. Seven past eleven in the morning in New York.

She picked up her little black Ericsson phone, ready finally to make her last-resort call. The Belgian police had been courteous and kind enough, she supposed, but she knew they hadn't really believed her story, knew they thought she was crazy, and she had tried and failed again to reach Jamie, and now there was no one left to try but Annie.

Jamie and Annie. Her two dearest friends in the world. Olivia wished, more than anything, that she could have spared them both this—she had tried so hard to handle it alone. But now she was too afraid. She had never considered herself a coward—Annie was always telling her how tough she was—but at that moment, with her left arm broken and the mass of still-darkening bruises flowering over her rib cage and legs, Olivia, all alone in her beautiful but suddenly vulnerable home—about to use a cellular telephone in case her land line had been bugged, for God's sake—was more than afraid. She was terrified. And not just for herself. For all she knew, Jamie—darling, blissfully unaware Jamie—might already be in danger. And from the moment Olivia took Annie into her confidence, from the instant she shared the long-hidden, dark, *monstrous* secrets of the box she had opened, Pandora-like, Annie, too, might be equally at risk.

Olivia considered, for at least the hundredth time, leaving it all alone, trying to push the ugly truths to the back of her mind. Maybe if she stopped now, kept silent now, they might leave her alone, let her try to forget. Let her live. But Olivia knew that was no longer really a possibility. For one thing, her conscience would not allow her to forget; she owed it to the ghosts, to the long-dead victims, to let the truth be told. To give justice a fighting chance.

And besides, she knew they would not let her live.

It was eight minutes past five.

Olivia made the call.

Annie Aldrich Thomas put down the phone, still sitting on the edge of the king-size bed, and stared around at the lovely room she was sharing with her husband, Edward, at the St. Regis Hotel. It all looked so normal, just as it had a few minutes earlier, before Olivia's call. Yet nothing, Annie knew, was really the same, not for her. Not anymore.

She stood up and walked mechanically into the bathroom, got into the shower, and tried to gather her wild, racing thoughts. For one thing, she was due to meet Edward for lunch at twelve-thirty, and now she would have to call and leave word, make an excuse, and she knew that Edward wouldn't mind too much, but Annie hated lying to him, had told too many lies in her own troubled past. Though this time she had no alternative, because it was Olivia who was in trouble and there were things that Olivia needed Annie to do for her. And Annie knew that Olivia would never have made that call if she hadn't been desperate, because even though eight years had passed since her own problems, Olivia and Jamie both still had a tendency to protect Annie from bad things.

They didn't come any worse than this.

She got out of the shower and started drying her hair. In the twenty-something years she had known Olivia, Annie could not remember her ever being really frightened of anything. Calm Olivia. Clever, independent Olivia. The coolest, the most self-sufficient, the boldest of them all. But just now, on the telephone, Annie had recognized actual terror in her friend's voice.

"I wanted to keep it from you," Olivia had said, breathless and low. "But I can't seem to find Jamie, and there *is* no one else I can trust, and I can't go on alone."

"It's all right," Annie had said gently. "You don't have to."

So Olivia had told her. And now nothing, Annie realized with a sick, awful chill, would ever be the same again.

In his suite at his family's twenty-five-room Ocean Drive "cottage" in Newport, Rhode Island, Jamie Arias was sitting in a comfortable old armchair beneath a Vuillard original of which he had always been fond, rereading a dog-eared edition of *War and Peace* and putting off going downstairs to join the others. He had come for his cousin Michael's fifty-second birthday celebration, but Jamie planned on spending no more time at the Arias compound than he had to because it was hard these days—as the others all realized—for him to be around Peter, his older brother, for too long.

Jamie did not intend to allow Michael's birthday to be ruined by family sniping. He had nothing but respect for his cousin, always had, for Michael Arias had been the head of their family for almost twenty years now, since Jamie and Peter's father had died, and Michael had returned that respect by leaving Jamie to get on with his own life. Yet still, respect aside, they had little in common except blood, and Jamie would be frankly relieved when it was time to get away from the too large, art-and-antique–laden Newport house, glad to get back to his own place in Boston, back to work at the agency. His own life— modest beside the Arias wealth—but his own.

Sitting now in the comfort of his room, immersed yet again in Tolstoy, Jamie was quite unaware that Olivia had been trying to reach him. Had no idea that she was in danger. If he had known that, he would have been out of Newport and on the first flight to Brussels, family celebrations or not. No matter what.

Annie and Olivia in trouble—especially Olivia, if he allowed himself to be honest—came first with Jamie. Before family. Before everything. They had for the last nineteen years.

The small black phone on the floor beside her, still wishing she could have reached Jamie but comforted nevertheless by the sound of Annie's reassuring voice, Olivia remained painfully huddled on the rug on the parquet floor of her Brussels living room. Staying away from the windows, wishing for the very first time that she had chosen a less intimate high-rise instead of her characterful, ground-floor apartment, Olivia was aware that some of the trembling and just a little of the sick, clenched feeling in her stomach had eased.

She had known since leaving London that all she had to do was make two calls and Annie and Jamie would drop everything and come to her. It was one of the unwritten rules of their pact, made so many years before when they had all sworn to be there for each other, no matter how far apart they were living—no matter how heavily committed they might be, to family or to work, to *anything*.

She and Jamie had been there for Annie eight years ago during her troubles, and three years after that she and Annie had been there for Jamie when he had needed them. Being there for each other was what they were all about, and now that Annie knew what was going on, she was sure to follow Olivia's instructions, and then she would find Jamie, and they would come to her.

The real question, the truly frightening question, was, would they get there in time?

OLIVIA'S BOX

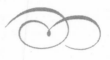

he story had lain inside the thick cardboard box, sealed shut with shiny
brown tape and locked into the black, airless vault beneath Leadenhall
Street in the City of London, for almost twenty years. Its author had
been a young man named Anton Rothenburg; its guardian for all those
years, one Paul Walter Osterman of Philadelphia. A seeker after justice,
Osterman had carried the weight of the Family Rothenburg's tale of
evil for a quarter of a century until, close to death, he had passed the
burden to another man who—understanding the enormity of what
Osterman had given him—had, in turn, placed it for safekeeping inside
the vault.

> I never knew Anton Rothenburg [Osterman had written] nor
> his parents or his two sisters. Their tale was passed on to me by a
> total stranger, a man taken into confidence by seventeen-year-old
> Anton when they were both nearing their lowest ebb. It was a tale
> I never asked or wished to hear, but once the horror had burned
> its scars into my mind, into my soul, I knew they could never be
> eradicated.
>
> The story changed me—I can't say exactly why. I'd heard
> many other tales, of course, worse tales, of that nightmare period,
> and was always appalled by them, but the feelings of sorrow and
> rage had always moved on after a time, had shifted sufficiently—as
> such things must—to enable me to go on with my own life. Yet
> when I learned what had happened to that particular family in

Nazi Germany, I became so profoundly affected that my own everyday existence seemed to fade into insignificance and never returned into its formerly sharp, clear-cut focus.

I did not know Emanuel Rothenburg, Anton's father, yet I suppose that he reminded me, in some ways, of my own father. He, too, was born in the town of Baden-Baden—though unlike Emanuel Rothenburg he came to live, peacefully, and to die, in the United States. My father, too, loved fine art. I remember, at an early age, watching him standing for the longest time before a beautiful painting in the Philadelphia Museum of Art, remember the look on his face, the passion in his eyes, as he gazed at it. I think maybe I understand just a little of the depth of emotion that a wonderful piece of art can stir in a human soul. My father died many years ago, of natural causes, with his wife and son at his deathbed, loving him, bringing him comfort. Emanuel Rothenburg died when a bullet pierced his brain. After he had already lost much of what had been precious to him.

Once I had heard and read the story of the Rothenburgs, I knew that I was changed forever. Once I'd learned about that tale of evil deeds, I felt that I had been somehow charged with trying to avenge their memory.

I have failed to do that, and now my own time is almost up. Yet the torch still burns fiercely in my mind, and hope still surges. And so I'm doing the only thing I still can.

Passing on the torch.

THE PACT

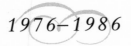

1976–1986

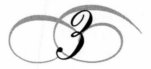

They stood together, about halfway up Dukesfield Fell, twenty or so rugged miles southwest of Newcastle-upon-Tyne and ten miles south of Hadrian's Wall, where it had happened a decade earlier to that very day. It was a little after noon on July 4, 1986, and they had climbed a long way to reach the spot, yet Olivia, Jamie, and Annie all felt chilled to the bone. They said it was the wind, blowing from the east off the North Sea, cold enough, they said, to rip the warmth from the hottest day, but they all knew that the chill came from within, from remembering.

"Maybe this was a mistake," Olivia said.

She looked at Annie's white face and felt a sharp pang of guilt because she had organized the day, had pushed and harried and prodded them, the way she always did when she believed in something, *wanted* something to happen, and now Annie looked as if she might pass out and Jamie just looked so sad, so bleak. And it could all have been so much easier, they could all have met up in London and had lunch someplace civilized—the Connaught maybe, eating roast beef and drinking something red and wonderful—and they'd have been warm and ten years past the grief, instead of standing on this lovely, terrible hill and seeing it all again in their minds—and when would she ever *learn*?

"I don't think it was a mistake," Annie said softly, kindly.

"Nor do I," Jamie echoed on her other side.

Olivia felt gratitude and love pass through her, felt a little of the ice inside her melt away along with the guilt. She never felt guilty for long; it was not in her nature, she supposed. "I guess maybe we did have to come," she said. "No other place we could really be today."

They linked arms, stood still and silent for a while, eyes closed, letting themselves rerun the old images in their minds. They had not been allowed to see the wreckage firsthand back in '76, but the pictures on television had been graphic enough. The debris had been strewn over a considerable distance, but the main part of the cabin had lain here, beneath their feet. With the bodies.

"Anyone want to say anything?" Olivia asked after a while.

"I don't think so," Jamie answered.

"I think we've said it all," Annie said. "They know what we think."

No one spoke for a time. The wind blew harder, nipped at their ears, tore at the roots of their hair, drove the gentle, summery scents of grass and soil and wildflowers into their faces, brought back again the ugly discordance of that dreadful remembered time when fire and death had scorched savage scars into the hillside.

"Shall we?" Jamie said at last.

"I'm ready," Annie said.

They both looked at Olivia.

"Livvy?" Annie said.

Olivia nodded. "Yes."

They walked away slowly, arms still linked until the narrowness of the path forced them to separate, and then they reached the road and the hired car waiting to take them back to Riverdale Hall, a country house hotel near Hexham where Olivia had booked rooms. Restored by hot showers, changes of clothes, one shot of malt whisky apiece—even for Annie, who seldom drank wine and never touched spirits—and a fine lunch of fresh-caught wild salmon, the three friends felt themselves coming slowly back to the present, felt the memories slipping and sliding away again, for the original rawness had long since gone, the jagged edges smoothed over by time and life.

"Ten years," Olivia said later, after lunch, as they walked near the river. "Who would have thought it possible ten years ago that we could ever be happy again? Ever be normal again."

"Yet here we are," Jamie said. "Annie a mother of three—me an old married man—"

"Even if it is to Carrie," Olivia said wryly.

"Livvy, don't," Annie scolded.

"We both know what Olivia thinks of Carrie," Jamie said lightly. "And you too, Annie, even if you are too nice a person to say it out loud."

"Meaning I'm not a nice person?" Olivia inquired.

"You're a very honest person," Jamie said, and smiled.

"I know." Olivia kicked at a clod of earth. The sun had broken through the clouds, and it was warm now, the wind just a gentle breeze; Dukesfield Fell seemed a million miles away. "I guess I'll never be as nice as either of you two, which is probably why I'll stay an old maid."

"You enjoy sex too much to qualify as an old maid," Jamie said.

"So now I'm not nice *and* a slut. And I'm pushy, too."

"True," Jamie said. "But we love you anyway."

"What you are," Annie said reflectively, "is a natural leader."

"No, I'm not."

"Sure you are," Annie said.

"You're our motivating force," Jamie agreed. "You keep us together, no matter how many thousands of miles we drift apart." He stopped walking and looked around. "This'd be a good spot for some photos."

The bringing of cameras to each of their reunions was one of their rituals, the updating of the records they had all kept of one another for so long. Whenever and wherever they came together, it always seemed to them as if nothing had changed; they *felt* the same, their friendship was the same. Only the photographs, pored over later, would record that petite, golden-haired, blue-eyed, exquisitely turned out Annie had grown perhaps a little too thin; or that sleek, elegant, worldly-looking Jamie's dark eyes had new care lines around them or that his almost black hair had one or two silvery threads; or that within the frame of Olivia's dark brown, bouncing mass of hair, her mobile, expressive, strong face with its not quite perfect nose, its slightly Slavic cheekbones and striking green eyes, a little of the youthfulness—of the carefree, sometimes careless, spark that had always been her trademark—had been rubbed away by passing years.

"When you say I'm your leader," Olivia said later, photographs snapped, "what you really mean is that I bully you."

"True," Jamie said.

"I prod you, I nag at you, I drive you both nuts until we find a way of getting back together again."

"Every time," Annie said.

"And we love you for it," Jamie added warmly.

"It's why we're here today," Annie said. "You're why we're here."

"That's not true," Olivia said. "We're here because of what today is."

"Not entirely." Jamie shook his head. "Perhaps not at all. If it hadn't been for you, Annie and I would probably have let the day go by—oh, we'd have called each other, and I guess we'd have raised a glass or two to them, but we wouldn't have climbed up to Dukesfield Fell. And, more importantly, we would have been apart." He paused. "Mostly because we'd have chosen not to face up to it. We're not as brave as you are, Olivia."

She flushed. "That's nonsense."

"It isn't, Livvy," Annie argued. "I'm a dreadful coward."

"You've had three babies," Olivia reminded her.

"Having babies is the easy part of life," Annie said.

"You and Jamie have both had the courage to make commitments."

"You've had the strength to stay alone," Jamie told her.

"I'm not alone," Olivia said softly. "I have you two."

Other people, outsiders—like Edward Thomas, who had married Annie in 1981, and, a few years later, Caroline Beaumont, who had become Jamie's wife—tended to assume at first that the pact among the three friends had been sealed during their school days. It was a natural enough assumption for them to reach, for it seemed the kind of passionate covenant usually entered into by emotional adolescents and, after all, Olivia, Jamie, and Annie had attended that enclave of the United States in Britain: the American School in London's leafy St. John's Wood, a coeducational day school committed to helping young Americans away from their homeland ease into and grow in their new environment.

It was certainly true that Jamie, Annie, and Olivia had developed a fairly close friendship at the school and that their parents, too, were acquainted with one another, but there had been nothing overly intense about the friendship back then. They had shared classes and outings and gossip; Olivia and Jamie had played basketball and watched Annie play violin in the chamber orchestra; they had gone out on field trips together and had liked one another very well, but they'd all had other friendships, too. Thanks to their good fortune, none of them had ever felt like insecure foreigners tossed into an alien or hostile environment. Like many of their contemporaries, Olivia, Jamie, and Annie all hailed from secure family backgrounds, their lives, either temporarily or permanently, being lived in England instead of back home in the United States. Annie's father, Franklin Aldrich, was a partner in an old and trusted international law practice and, at that time, heading the London office, and their English home was a splendid mews house near Belgrave Square immaculately organized by Grace Aldrich, Annie's mother. Jamie's father, Carlos Arias—a widower of distinguished Spanish descent left with two sons of his own and the care of the son of his late brother and sister-in-law—headed the venerable Arias shipping empire from their Pall Mall offices and ruled, with gentle command, their sumptuous Regents Park apartment. And Olivia's mother, Emily Segal, was a cardiac consultant at Great Ormond Street's Hospital for Sick Children, while her father, Arthur Segal, worked from their house near Kenwood in Hampstead collecting art and antiques and raising funds for numerous charities that encompassed Simon Wiesenthal's Nazi-hunting center in Vienna and other Jewish charities, as well as UNICEF and whichever current, needy appeal captured his sympathetic eye.

At eighteen, just graduated from high school, Olivia Segal, Jamie Arias, and Annie Aldrich had been secure, confident, successful, and contented young people. With the exception of Jamie's mother's sudden death from cancer nine years earlier, nothing grievous had ever befallen any of them.

Until the Fourth of July that year, 1976.

Years later, they all remembered where they were and what they had been doing immediately before they heard the news. That was, of course, what people always said about President Kennedy's assassination, but Olivia, Jamie, and Annie had been just five years old at that time and had, therefore, no true memories of their own, just the awareness, passed through to them later, of a vast, daunting, adult, collective grief. What happened to them on Independence Day of 1976 was so entirely personal, so infinitely and intimately shattering, that their memories of that day were etched, and would be forever, like deep, sharp, painful carvings, upon each of their minds.

They had all just arrived at David Orbach's party in Dulwich. The Orbachs had a big house amid several acres of gardens with a swimming pool and tennis courts, and their Fourth of July parties were famous both for their lavishness and for the shenanigans reported by all those fortunate enough to attend them. Jamie had gone the previous year and had come back to school to tell Annie—whose parents had not let her go—that contrary to popular myth no one had swum nude, but any number had dived into the pool with their clothes still on; and he'd told Olivia—who hadn't been able to go either because her parents wanted her at their own party at home—that he'd seen not a single sign of a real-live orgy, though he'd seldom seen so much unabashed necking in an arena where parents were present.

This year they were all going, partly because they were eighteen, but mostly because all their parents were flying up to Scotland for an Independence Day celebration in aid of one of Olivia's father's charities. That, of course, meant there would be no arguments about what they decided to wear, no curfew that night, and no repercussions next morning if they showed up long after breakfast and with hangovers.

"What are you wearing?" Olivia asked Annie on the phone at five o'clock that afternoon.

"A dress my mother bought me in New York last month."

"What's it like?"

"White crepe, with a halter neck."

"Long?"

"Yes." Annie sounded suddenly uncertain. "Is that all right, do you think?"

"It sounds gorgeous. You always look lovely," Olivia said, meaning it.

"What about you?" Annie asked.

"I've been shopping. You'll hate it," Olivia added with relish.

"Why should I hate it?"

"I waited for Mom and Dad to leave," Olivia said, "and then I went right over to this little boutique off Heath Street—I'd already asked them to hold everything for me."

"What did you buy?" Annie was intrigued. Olivia Segal came from a family not quite, but almost as conventional as her own, yet Annie thought Olivia the most exciting person she knew.

"I've gone punk—well, kind of punk, anyway."

"You haven't."

"Would you believe black bermudas and a black silk camisole?"

"You're kidding." Annie was half aghast, half impressed.

"And I found this really wild studded belt *and* a pair of those wrap-around sunglasses we saw in *Vogue*. And a dog chain necklace." Olivia stopped short of telling Annie that she'd had scarlet streaks sprayed into her dark hair.

"It sounds—lovely." Annie hesitated.

"But?"

"Isn't it black-tie tonight?"

"I forgot to buy a tie."

"I didn't mean that, Livvy."

"I know you didn't, Annie." Olivia liked teasing Annie.

"What if they don't let you in?"

"They will. Jamie said that some people were dressed pretty wildly last year."

"Still, a *dog* chain—" Annie was lost for words.

"David Orbach has a German shepherd," Olivia said confidently. "I can always take it off and pretend it was a present for him."

The party was due to begin at eight-thirty, and Annie had told Olivia that she and Jamie had arranged to get a lift with Jenny Lee Barnsworth, another student from the American School, and there was plenty of room in Jenny's car if Olivia wanted to join them; but Olivia had already made plans to go with Bill Murray, who lived in Highgate, much closer to the Segals than either the Aldriches or the Ariases, and she and Bill were probably going to have a drink somewhere en route to Dulwich, and no, she and Bill were not an item, but he was an okay guy, and it was a long drive, so she might as well enjoy it.

By the time Olivia and Bill got to the party, the driveway and the street were jammed with cars, and Bill, a gentleman, let Olivia out at the house while he went off to hunt for a parking space. Her gift for David Orbach in her right hand, her small black bag swinging from her left shoulder, Olivia headed jauntily across the big gravel drive toward the brilliantly lit house.

She saw Jamie almost immediately, standing in the entrance hall, saw that his face was ashen and that he seemed to have been weeping, and that David Orbach, close by, was looking at her strangely.

"What's wrong?" Her voice caught in her throat. "Jamie, what's happened?"

He looked so strange, so perfectly, immaculately dressed in his tuxedo and black tie—Jamie was always such a lovely mix of slenderness and strength—yet at the same time he looked somehow, Olivia thought with a sudden and terrible fear, destroyed.

"Our parents," he said in a whisper.

"What about them?" Olivia found she still had David Orbach's gift in her hand, and she pushed it at David and reached out to seize Jamie's left arm. "What's happened, Jamie?"

He shook his head.

"Jamie, what? *Tell* me."

Behind her, Bill Murray came through the door, laughing at first, then going very quiet as someone hushed him, drew him away, pulled him and another pair of late arrivals out of the entrance hall and into the first of the music-filled rooms.

"They're dead," Jamie said tonelessly, his dark eyes beseeching Olivia's, as if he hoped that she might put him straight, tell him that he was wrong, that he was crazy.

For a long moment, Olivia said nothing.

"What did you say?" she asked, very quietly, at last.

"All killed," he said.

Someone put a hand on Olivia's arm and she jumped as if they'd burned her.

"It's true, my dear." Mrs. Orbach, David's mother, stood beside her. "I'm so very sorry." Magnificent in black Chanel, she looked compassionate and afraid and deeply uncomfortable all at the same time, and Olivia realized in a flash of instinct that, as shocked and sympathetic as their hostess clearly was, she wanted, more than anything, to get her and Jamie out of her entrance hall—if possible out of the house and away from her party.

"Your friend's waiting upstairs," Mrs. Orbach said gently.

"Friend?" Olivia felt confused, disorientated, almost dizzy.

"She means Annie," Jamie told her.

"Why?" Olivia stared up at him. "What's happened to Annie?"

"It's all of them," Jamie said. "On the way to Scotland."

And finally Olivia understood.

"The helicopter," she said.

Annie was in a bedroom on the first floor, away from the noise. She was sitting on the floor, on a white rug, all curled up, partly camouflaged by her white crepe dress. She, too, had been crying, but now her eyes were dry and she looked shocked, almost absent. A moth, drawn by the light through the open window, fluttered close to her blond hair, but she made no move to brush it away.

Olivia and Jamie came into the room. Jamie got down on the floor beside Annie, put one arm around her, and Olivia, her legs suddenly weak, sat on the edge of the big bed.

There was a cheval mirror facing her from across the room. She saw her reflection, saw the black bermudas and the silk camisole that had seemed so daring and sexy, saw the crazy, idiotic wraparound sunglasses pushed up into her scarlet-streaked hair, saw the bizarre dog chain around her neck—and abruptly that seemed so offensive, so revolting, that she tried to pull it off, but it was too tightly fastened and she was hurting herself, didn't know that she was making small, choking, whimpering sounds until Jamie's hands were on hers, stopping her from dragging at the thing around her neck.

"Let me," he told her gently. "Let me, Olivia."

She let him, watched the chain hang loose from his hands, watched him lay it on the bedspread. She stared at him.

"Are they really all dead?" She sounded incredulous, like a child.

"Yes," he said.

Annie still sat curled up on the floor, saying nothing. The moth

was resting on the skirt of her dress now. Jamie took Olivia's hand and
drew her off the bed and down onto the rug, and they were all three in
a row, him in the middle.

"It happened this afternoon," he said very softly. "Somewhere near
Newcastle."

"How?" Olivia asked.

"They crashed. That's all we know." Jamie paused. "There's a man
downstairs, waiting. My cousin, Michael, sent him. To take us all
home." He paused again. "We wanted to wait for you."

"I'm sorry," Olivia said. "I was late, wasn't I?"

"It doesn't matter," Jamie said. "There's no hurry."

"No," Olivia said. "I guess there isn't."

The wheels of death ground into motion. They were none of them
young children, to be protected from reality or shielded from harsh for-
malities. Postmortems were conducted, funerals were arranged, inquests were held in conjunction with the main accident inquiry which
found, in due course, that the helicopter had crashed because of a
mechanical failure. No human error, no suspicious circumstances, no
violent storm. Just some hunks of steel and electrical circuits failing to
keep the machine in the air. Olivia, Annie, and Jamie flew to their
respective family homes in the United States for the funerals, fumbled
their way numbly through the interments and various rites—the Segals'
Jewish service in New York, the Aldriches' Protestant burial in San
Francisco, and the Ariases' Roman Catholic mass in Rhode Island—
and then returned to Britain for what seemed, to each of them, the
most harrowing, the most inescapably tangible part of the ritual, the
clearing up of their parents' homes.

There was plenty of help available for the packing up and removal
of the large objects, but as with all deaths there were wardrobes to be
gone through, and dressing tables and cabinets and desk drawers. In
Jamie's case, there was his older brother, Peter, to help, and Michael,
their cousin—the son of Carlos Arias's late brother, Juan Luis—came
through for them magnificently well. Michael was, as he pointed out to
Jamie, almost twice his age, and as the new head of the Arias family it
was his duty to take over the dismal tasks involved with closing down
the Pall Mall office and Regents Park house and transferring their

belongings to the main family residence in Newport and the New York offices, from where Michael intended to rule. Annie, still seeming less able to cope than the others, began the process of trying to sift through Franklin's and Grace's personal files by herself but all too swiftly crumbled and gave up, asking Richard Tyson, her father's London-based partner, if he would mind having all the papers in the mews house—unsorted for the moment, perhaps forever—packed up and laid to rest in the archives of her father's London office.

Olivia tackled her own task head-on, the only way she could, the only way she wanted to. In her mother's case it was, in a sense, straightforward. Grief and loss, both accentuated by the sight and touch and smell of Emily's belongings. But Emily Segal had been orderly and not overburdened by sentiment, a thousand miles away from the average Jewish mother. Arthur, on the other hand, had been both disorderly and an unabashed nostalgia collector. Immersed as he had been in so many diverse fields, with his art collection and his numerous charities—which would from now on be administered by the Arthur Segal Foundation—proud as any archetypal Jewish husband and papa of his beloved wife and only daughter, fervent as he had been to hold on to his past and to as many shreds of his heritage as possible—Arthur's wardrobes and drawers and filing cabinets, once opened, seemed almost to seethe with scrapbooks and photograph albums and diaries and other keepsakes.

And the correspondence! Once released from the cabinets and boxes that had until now held them in check, a veritable mountain of her father's letters confronted Olivia. Much of it was commonplace, dull business communications that could now, without question, be consigned to black rubbish bags, and old postcards from friends, including three from Max Wildenbruch, the art dealer, on holidays in Tuscany and France, but hidden among all these were other things of infinite value. The skullcap Arthur had worn for his bar mitzvah, neatly labeled by his mother. Every birthday card Olivia had ever sent her father. Ancient school reports: Arthur's own, describing a boy to whom friendship had clearly always mattered more than studies; Emily's, the kind to make any parent glow with pride; and Olivia's, every single comment from first grade upward, good or bad or someplace between, preserved. And love letters, simple but intensely moving, that Olivia read unashamedly and wept over, then carefully folded again, keeping to each original crease, feeling she had drawn a little closer to Arthur and Emily with every word.

On the third day of her delvings and sortings, Olivia found in her father's study an old battered pigskin briefcase he had continued using from time to time in preference to the more handsome black calf attaché case that Emily had bought him from Asprey for his birthday two years before. Like just about every single container in the house used by Arthur, it seemed to contain papers, but it was locked and Olivia could find no key. She looked for a while at the tiny gold lock and thought it would be an easy matter to force it open, but the idea of breaking into something her father had locked seemed somehow offensive to her. *Which makes no real sense at all,* she thought, *when I've just spent the last few days reading his private mail.*

Olivia wondered abruptly, guiltily, why people assumed that death made them privy to everything about those who had died. She had told herself that her own invasion of her parents' privacy was a means of bringing them closer again, of drawing them back, temporarily, from the void. She thought, on reflection, that she had truly felt that, and it was done now, anyway, their intimate words had bled into her mind, were part of her now, and there was no going back and no point in feeling guilty. Jewish though she was, Olivia had never been big on guilt.

She fetched a small, sharp, black-handled knife from the kitchen, returned to Arthur's study, and worked at the lock until the pigskin case was open. It was enjoyable work, had a rather satisfying edge of petty villainy to it, and she wondered idly if that, perhaps, was one of the attractions of burglary, the small battle to pick the door lock or quietly break the window, all the while anticipating the opportunity of trespass into another person's private world.

More letters. One from Coutts, the bankers. Two from a firm of insurance brokers. An invitation, on thick white card, to a dinner at the Israeli embassy, the date already past; another, to the opening of an exhibition at the Hamilton Gallery. And a strange, brief note from Jamie's father, dated June 4, one month before the helicopter crash, handwritten with a fountain pen and curiously worded in a hurried, uncomfortable, almost telegraphic style.

Dear Arthur,

Deeply shocked and dismayed to learn that your suspicions are not, after all, unfounded.

We must meet soon.

Carlos Arias

Olivia told Annie about the note on the telephone later that evening.

"It sounds important. Do you suppose it is?"

"You mean should you ask Jamie about it?" Annie was calm tonight, partly, perhaps, because she'd taken one of the tranquilizers a cousin had given her before the funeral, but then again she thought that she had been feeling a little better, a little easier, ever since Richard Tyson had agreed to house all the Aldrich papers in their office archives.

"Should I?"

Annie paused. "I wouldn't."

"Why not?"

"Because it could mean anything at all, and there's nothing Jamie can do about it now, and it might just worry him."

"You're right," Olivia said. "I guess."

"But you're not sure," Annie said.

"Not quite," Olivia admitted. "There I was, prying into my own parents' private affairs, and suddenly there was Jamie's dad, and I'm not sure I have the right to keep it from him."

"Keep what, Livvy? It's just a note. It's nothing."

"It doesn't sound like nothing."

"Not when it was written, maybe," Annie said softly. "But it is nothing now."

Olivia had said nothing to Jamie, and the note was long forgotten by the time the three friends next saw each other at the communal, non-denominational memorial service held at the end of August at All Souls Church in London, a thanksgiving for the lives of all those who had died in the helicopter crash: the pilot, an Edinburgh man named John Wilkes; Carlos Arias; Arthur and Emily Segal; and Franklin and Grace Aldrich.

There were colleagues, business partners, cousins, uncles, and aunts, but both Olivia and Annie were only children, and the only close blood relatives present were Peter and Michael Arias.

"I've never seen them before, have you?" Olivia said to Annie as they were preparing to file out after the service.

Annie shook her head. "They're both very handsome, aren't they?"

Olivia studied the two men as they stood at either side of Jamie. "Michael's very distinguished, isn't he, in a piercing kind of way?"

"Peter's even better looking than Jamie," Annie whispered, a moment of foolish gossip infinitely welcome after the sorrow of the service. "A bit like Alan Alda, don't you think?"

"He's too smooth," Olivia said. "Look, they're both putting their sunglasses on while they're still inside." She quelled a sudden, inappropriate urge to laugh. "They look like Spanish Mafia."

"Yes, they do." Annie gave her black cloche hat a little pat in a gesture of tidiness inherited, unconsciously, from Grace Aldrich. "Jamie doesn't, though, does he?"

Olivia shook her head. "Jamie's more elegant. More like Carlos." She'd thought, for a while now, that she might be attracted to Jamie Arias, but he was such a warm, easygoing, friendly guy, was that way with just about everyone he came into contact with, that it was impossible to tell if he felt the same way about her. Now, she supposed, with all the brightness and normality gone, and with all of them going their separate ways, she would never find out.

They walked a little farther toward the exit, were spoken to by a number of people, had their hands shaken and their cheeks kissed, and Jamie came and walked out with them into Portland Place, into the shock of sunlight and traffic and the rest of the world going about its business.

"I felt so sorry for Mrs. Wilkes," Jamie said suddenly.

"Who?" Olivia asked stupidly, confused.

"The pilot's wife," Annie said.

"Oh, yes. Of course."

"She looked so sad," Jamie said, "and so guilty."

"No one's blamed him, have they?" Annie asked.

"Not at all," Olivia said. "Mechanical failure. Not his fault."

"But still," Annie said. "Poor lady."

Olivia glanced at her, realized how extremely white her face was, remembered how she had been that night at the Orbach party, how utterly silent and remote.

"Annie, are you okay?" she asked softly.

"Not really." Annie's voice was flat. "Are you?"

"No," Olivia said. "I guess not."

"How can we be?" Jamie said.

Olivia hesitated for a moment.

"Are you both free the day after tomorrow?"

"I am," Jamie said. "I don't leave till next Monday."

"Annie?"

"I have nothing special," Annie said.

"I think we should go up there," Olivia said.

"Up where?" Jamie asked, though he thought he knew.

"To where it happened." Olivia paused. "Just us. I want to be there. I want to say good-bye." She paused again. "I think it might do us all some good."

"I don't know," Annie said slowly, "if I could bear it."

"It would be a fair climb," Olivia said.

"We'd need boots and hiking gear," Jamie added. "It's quite a way up."

"You don't have to come, Annie," Olivia said. "It's just an idea."

"Can I think about it, please?" Annie asked.

They all traveled north two days later, having extricated themselves from well-meaning relatives and acquaintances. They took an Intercity train to Newcastle, rented a car, picked up a local road map, drove as far as they were able, and then hiked the rest of the way up to Dukesfield Fell. Both Jamie and Olivia kept a watchful eye on Annie, conscious that of the three of them she was emotionally the most obviously fragile, but she seemed perfectly in control today, as prepared for whatever awaited them as they were.

There was very little, and yet there was everything. Of the wreckage and debris, not the tiniest scrap remained; if blood had been scattered, it had been washed away, either by officialdom or by nature. But the crater made by the body of the helicopter falling from the sky was there, roped off for safety, and there, too, was the wounded earth, scorched and gouged and ripped.

It was August, the height of summer and a clear day, yet up there it seemed to Olivia and Jamie and Annie that no birds sang, that it was cold and bleak as November, and their losses weighed down on them more heavily there, were suddenly rendered far more real than they had been. For when they had seen the pictures on their television screens, and when they had listened at the inquests and sat at the memorial service—even when they had stood at the gravesides and watched the coffins lowered into the ground—the harsh, unrelenting truth of their parents' deaths had never quite come home to them. But here was where they had fallen, here was where the life had been crushed out of them, where the fire had half consumed their bodies before the Northumbrian rain had put out the flames.

"I'd like to go down soon," Annie said after a while.

"All right," Olivia said.

"I can go by myself, if you and Jamie want to stay."

"No, you can't," Jamie said quickly. "We have to stick together. I'm ready to leave, too." He looked at Olivia. "How about you?"

"I wouldn't mind another minute or two. You two go ahead."

"Just a little way," Jamie said. "Will you be okay?"

"Of course," she said.

Olivia waited until they were some distance away, and then she sat down on the ground. She was glad they had come with her, but now she was glad to have been left alone. It had felt too much like the memorial service with them beside her, that sense of having to stand still and behave well for the sake of others, when what she really wanted to do was to get down on the ground, get as close as possible to where her mother and father had died, and say good-bye to them properly.

She put her hands, palms down, on the cool earth, and shut her eyes. She thought about her parents: about Emily Segal, doctor, wife, mother, and individual; about Arthur Segal, philanthropist, husband, father, collector of memories and beautiful things. They had always been such busy people, their lives had been so full, yet they had always found time for each other and for their daughter, had given her so much, all that she'd needed and more, all the love, comfort, sound advice, and friendship. It was cruel, Olivia supposed, that they had died so young, when they still had so much to do, so much to give, and yet, she realized suddenly, there at the place where they had died, at least they had had little time to be afraid, and at least they had gone together.

They stayed at an old hotel in the village of Blanchland in the Derwent Valley that night, in no rush to return to London, for they would all be leaving England for the foreseeable future within the week. Jamie and Olivia had both always planned to leave before September in any event, though Annie had intended to remain with her family awhile longer. Now there was no longer any alternative. The process of closing down their London homes was almost complete and their lives, as they had formerly known them, were at an end. Jamie was to go to Harvard University, where he would be within about sixty miles of the magnificent, art-filled Arias family estate in Newport; Olivia was to go to Paris to study French at the Sorbonne; and Annie, at a complete loss, was going home to lick her wounds at the Aldrich house in San Francisco. This, they suddenly realized with an unexpectedly acute sense of fresh loss, would be their last chance to be together for a long time.

They had dinner in the restaurant, drank a lot of wine—even Annie had a glass—and adjourned to Olivia's bedroom, the biggest, where Olivia and Jamie drank some cognac too, to which they were unaccustomed, and began to talk, honestly and openly, about their feelings and their fears. Nothing, they had all become aware, would ever be the same again. Their frames of reference had been irrevocably distorted; the bedrock on which their personalities had been formed was all broken up; the very people who would, they all knew, have done anything in the world for love of them, had disappeared.

"We had a fight," Annie said suddenly from her chair.

"Who?" Olivia asked, startled.

"My father and I."

Annie's chin came up, abruptly, and they saw that her blue eyes were filled with anguished tears, and Olivia realized then that Annie was the only one of them who had, until then, said hardly anything at all about her personal feelings.

"The last time I saw my father," she said, "we had a terrible fight."

Neither Jamie, on the bed, nor Olivia, sitting on the floor, said anything, both sensing that this was not a moment to interrupt her, that Annie needed time.

"It started about the party," she went on. "Just a silly argument, really. He didn't want me to go, but I told him I was eighteen and he couldn't stop me, and he gave way and I was so glad, because Daddy and I never fought, or hardly ever, but then he started making all kinds of rules, about what I should wear and how I should get there and when and how I should get home."

"All fathers do that," Olivia said, putting down her cognac glass on the carpet.

"I know," Annie said. "I knew it then, too—and I'd never really minded before, and I don't know what was wrong with me that day, but it just seemed to get to me, and I couldn't seem to stop arguing with him. Even when he said things that I knew made perfect sense, I argued."

"I expect he understood," Jamie said.

"No," Annie said, and the tears were really flowing now. "He didn't understand at all. I saw it in his face. He looked so hurt, and I knew I'd hurt him, but I just told myself it was my fault for always having given in to him about everything—for having always been such a good little girl—and it would do us both good if I made a stand once in a while."

They waited for her to go on.

"And you didn't get a chance to make up with him," Olivia said at last.

Annie shook her head. "My mother came home from the hairdresser's, and she heard what we'd been arguing about, and she smoothed things over a little because she could see it was all a storm in a teacup, nothing we wouldn't both get over."

"She was right," Jamie said. "You would have."

"But we didn't," Annie whispered. "He still looked so hurt, and I just left the room, and my mother asked him to go and help her with their packing, and when it was time for them to leave for Scotland I was in the bath—and I could have gotten out and gone to kiss him good-bye, but I didn't. My mother stuck her head around the door and blew me a kiss and told me to enjoy myself, and that was that."

Olivia looked up at Jamie, then back over at Annie.

"And you've been tormenting yourself about that all these weeks."

"Yes." Annie took the handkerchief Jamie reached across to offer her, and wiped her eyes. "Of course."

"Then you're a bit of a goose, Annie Aldrich. I guarantee your dad forgave you—probably forgot all about it—before they even got into the helicopter." Olivia paused. "He knew you loved him, didn't he?"

"I guess so."

"You know so."

"Olivia's right," Jamie said. "Your dad would hate to think you were making yourself crazy—that's the kind of fight all kids have with their fathers."

"I know," Annie said.

"Your lips say that," Olivia said gently, "but your eyes don't look so sure."

Annie bit back the tears that were threatening again. "I'm just so sad, you know?"

"We all are," Jamie said. "I guess we'll all be sad for a long time."

"At least," Olivia said, "we have each other."

"Not for much longer," Annie said miserably. "You'll be in Paris; Jamie'll be at Harvard. I'll be thousands of miles from you both."

"That's just distance." Olivia got up from the floor, bent to pick up her glass, and poured a little more cognac for herself and Jamie. "We can write letters and phone and visit each other. We're none of us short of funds—we can get on a plane pretty much whenever we want to."

"It's not the same as being in the same city, though," Jamie said. "I know I'm going to miss you both like hell."

"It's strange, in a way." Olivia joined him on the bed, glass in hand. "We were friends in school, but we weren't all that close, yet now I feel this really strong bond with both of you."

"It's not so surprising," Jamie said, "given the circumstances."

"Grief, you mean," Annie said.

Olivia shook her head. "It's more than grief, Annie. I think it's that we all realize that no one else in the whole world will ever be able to comprehend better than us what we've been through—the way the crash has changed our lives—has already started to change us."

"I know what you mean," Jamie agreed. "This afternoon, standing up on Dukesfield Fell, there was such a strong connection between us—I felt it, I mean I *really* felt it, tangibly. I knew—or I thought I knew—what you were both thinking—I don't mean I was reading your minds, but—" He shrugged, unable to express exactly what he wanted to say.

"I think I understand, too," Annie said quietly. "Though I'd be lying if I said I'd felt it up on that place—I was too wrapped up in my own misery. I don't think I was paying much attention to either of you."

"We were all pretty wrapped up," Olivia said. "That was why I wanted to stay behind on my own for a few moments." She paused. "But I still knew that you were both there for me, and it helped a lot."

They all fell silent for a time.

"Do you think we will all write regularly?" Jamie asked. "I mean, when we all get hooked up in our new lives—I'm not saying we won't intend to write, or that we won't want to, but—"

"But you're just being a realist," Annie said.

"It doesn't matter if we write letters or not," Olivia said. "What matters is just that we keep in touch somehow. Knowing me, I'll pick up the phone more often than a pen, or I might send tapes—"

"Good idea," Jamie said.

"And Livvy's right about paying visits once in a while," Annie said.

Olivia took one more sip, then put down her glass. "But none of those things," she said slowly, thoughtfully, "are what really matters when the chips are down."

"What do you mean?" Annie asked.

"I mean that what really counts is what we're going to need the most." She paused. "And that's being there for each other. When things get rough—*really* rough, I mean—for any one of us. Which they will, sometime. By the law of averages."

"So what are you saying?" Jamie asked her.

Olivia stood up. The mix of cognac and wine was buzzing in her veins, yet her mind felt curiously clear and resolute. "I'm saying that we all take a vow—make a pact, I guess—to always be there for each other when we're needed."

Annie, still in her chair, took a breath. "Yes," she said. "I'd like to do that very much."

"Jamie?" Olivia looked down at him.

"Sure." He smiled at her. "You want to do this properly? Swear to stay in touch—swear to do all we can for each other?"

"No." Olivia shook her head. "Not just 'all we can.' People always say that—it's like having a get-out clause all neat and ready in case we have something better on. I'm talking about a real pact, a solemn promise that if any of us gets in any kind of a serious jam and needs help, then the other two will drop everything and be there to see them through."

Annie stood up. "Like family, you mean."

"Just like family," Jamie said, getting up, too. "The way our parents would have been there for us if we really needed them."

"In loco parentis." Annie smiled. "My father would have liked the sound of that."

"They all would," Olivia said softly. She felt a new warmth that had little to do with liquor coursing through her, a renewed strength and sense of hope.

"We need our glasses," Jamie said. "One more toast to our pact."

They found them, came to stand close together, and raised them.

"To always being there," Jamie said.

"No matter what," Annie added.

"Come hell or high water," Olivia said, and drained her glass.

For the next ten years, as they grew and worked and lived their separate lives, the friends exchanged letters and phone calls and got together mostly for the odd vacation. They reunited, too, for Annie's wedding, in London in 1981, to a banker named Edward Thomas, and the following year Annie and Jamie went to New York, where Olivia was living, to celebrate her engagement; five months later, they returned to commiserate with her on her split from her fiancé—only to find that she felt she'd had the luckiest of escapes and needed no commiseration. In 1985—by which time Jamie and Olivia had attended the christenings of Sophie, William, and Liza, Annie and Edward's children—they were all together again in Boston for Jamie's marriage to Caroline Beaumont, a rising star in the advertising world. And on the Fourth of July, 1986, they all climbed Dukesfield Fell again to commemorate the tenth anniversary of the helicopter disaster.

None of those reunions—not even the last, they all agreed—came under the category of "being there" for one another; they were simply moments of importance, of substance in their lives, snapshots in time when good friends wanted to be together. They had been lucky in those ten years, had had no real need to call for help.

But those times would come. They had all gone on with their lives determinedly, courageously, and successfully, yet those grievous losses, that massive body blow to normality, could not be sustained without some damage. They were all strong in their own ways, yet like the rest of the human race they all had their Achilles' heels, too, and it was, perhaps, to be expected that the violent, untimely deaths of their parents would exacerbate those weaknesses.

In Annie's case, it was her fear of admitting that she was not always able to cope perfectly with everything life threw at her. With Jamie, it was his need to live up to the memory of the father he had lost. And for Olivia, it was, more than anything, her compulsive passion for truth.

Three times in the next decade, still stirred by the distant but unfailingly dark backwash of the helicopter crash, those vulnerabilities would threaten each of them, and on each occasion, the strength of their pact of friendship would be tested to the limit.

The first call for help would come from Annie.

OLIVIA'S BOX

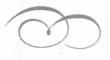

My name is Anton Rothenburg. By the second half of the
nineteen twenties, when I was still just a young child, my family
had lived in our large gray stone mansion on the outskirts of
Baden-Baden for two generations. We—my father, Emanuel
Rothenburg, my mother, Hedi, and my two younger sisters, Lili
and Trude—were, I now realize, an archetypically successful, contented, comparatively wealthy and assimilated German Jewish
family. Our religious practices were liberal; we went to synagogue
on the high holy days, on Jarhzeits—the anniversaries of the
deaths of our grandparents—and when we were invited to wed-
dings or bar mitzvahs. My parents had a wide circle of acquaintances in which they were respected and popular, and my sisters
and I had good friends and were happy inside and outside school.
Mama loved throwing parties, played bridge and canasta twice a
week, and went shopping on Sophienstrasse, and, at least twice
each month, in either Stuttgart or Frankfurt. Papa cherished us all
and went about his business of dealing in fine art with a joy that
he readily transmitted to us, often telling us how conscious he was
of his great good fortune in having some of life's loveliest and
often precious creations pass through his hands, and, above all,
in being in a position, from time to time, to add to his personal
collection of late-nineteenth-century Symbolist paintings. As a
small boy, of course, I understood and appreciated little of these
things—I only came to understanding later, when, from the time

of my own bar mitzvah, my father began to share confidences with me, to talk to me almost as if I were a man. But in those early years, before the troubles began to touch us, all I really knew, all I really understood, was that we were happy.

By the beginning of the thirties, the Rothenburg Symbolist Collection had become moderately well known in Baden-Württemberg and beyond, and our mansion was something of a lovingly protected treasure trove that encompassed works by Bonnard, Gauguin, Emile Bernard, Vuillard, Redon, Munch, Hodler, and more. Well before January of 1933, when I was almost twelve and when Adolf Hitler became Chancellor, my sisters and I became used to hearing our parents discussing whether or not they should be making plans to move us and the collection from Germany to America.

"There's no great rush," Papa would tell our mother regularly when she raised the question. "No need to panic. We can make our arrangements carefully, take our time."

The stranger had come to call for the first time almost a year earlier, in the second week of February 1932. I still remember that day quite clearly. It was a Sunday, after lunch, and we were all in the salon, with Mama playing Chopin at the piano, when Maria, our housekeeper, brought in his visiting card. The card announced him as Georg Brauner, but Papa said later that he thought it might not be his real name. The man spoke fluent German, but with a foreign accent that Papa said he was unable to place. Not that either his name or his accent especially mattered to my father.

Georg Brauner said that he had come to help.

"What makes you think that I am in need of help, Herr Brauner?" Emanuel was forty-two years old, with light brown hair that had lately begun to gray and recede a little, and a waistline that was not as slim as it had once been. He was an easygoing, placid man, and until recently he had also been gregarious and outgoing, the kind of man who enjoyed welcoming strangers into his lovely home, but the times were growing increasingly troubled, and these days Emanuel tended toward caution. That February afternoon, sitting opposite the elegant, composed, dark-haired stranger—whom he estimated to be at least ten, or maybe even fifteen years younger than himself—in the tranquil, familiar and secure setting of his own library, surrounded by fine leather editions of Goethe, Dumas, Scott, and the like, Emanuel felt curiously and uncharacteristically uncomfortable.

"I'm aware, Herr Rothenburg, that you wish to leave Germany." Brauner, having come directly to the point, did not wait for Emanuel either to confirm or to deny what he had said. "I'm also aware—as you must be—that it's likely to prove extremely difficult, perhaps even impossible, for you to take your collection with you to the United States."

Emanuel sat perfectly still. He was unsure which aspect of Georg Brauner's statement had upset him most: the man's presumptuousness or the sudden, discomfiting knowledge that a stranger knew his private business. He regarded his cigar box on the rosewood-and-leather table, his urge to light a cigar only controlled by the awareness that he would have to offer Brauner one out of common courtesy, and Emanuel wanted Georg Brauner out of his library, out of his house, far more than he wanted the cigar.

"I can't imagine," Emanuel said slowly, "where you have obtained your information, Herr Brauner, but I have to tell you that it is inaccurate."

"Which part of it?" Brauner asked.

"I beg your pardon?"

"Which part of my information is inaccurate, Herr Rothenburg? That you plan to leave Germany for the United States, or that you will encounter problems if you try to remove your paintings?"

"As I said," Emanuel replied, irritated but still picking his words carefully, "I cannot imagine how or where you could have learned anything about my plans, but I can assure you that it is all entirely inaccurate." He paused. "Now, if there's nothing else—" He prepared to stand up.

"Please, Herr Rothenburg—" The younger man's voice was softer now and clearly conciliatory. "I can see I have annoyed you."

"Not at all," Emanuel said. "I'm simply a busy man who doesn't want to waste your time any more than my own."

"Just a few moments more," Brauner went on, "and I assure you that neither of us will be wasting his time."

He wore a beautifully cut, dark gray three-piece suit, a lighter gray silk tie, and immaculate black shoes. As Emanuel watched him reaching into an inside pocket for a slim gold cigarette case, which he opened and offered to his host before taking a lighter, also gold, from his right outside pocket, Emanuel thought that there was something suave and altogether too smooth about Brauner that might perhaps, in another man, have spelled confidence trickster; and yet it was patently clear to Emanuel that neither the expensive suit nor any of the accessories were a sham. The outer skin matched up to the inner man; something about Georg Brauner, in spite of his youth and his instantly dislikable slickness and sharpness, spelled old European money, inherited elegance, and innate sophistication. All of which warned Emanuel that he might be sensible to swallow his irritation, at least for the few moments more that Brauner had asked for.

"Very well."

Brauner, legs crossed and relaxed, leaned forward, his manner suddenly conspiratorial. "I really can help you, Herr Rothenburg. I have a great deal of cash at my disposal, but more relevantly to you, I have a most useful network of contacts both inside and outside Germany."

Emanuel made a small, slightly dismissive gesture with his hands but said nothing.

"Your personal collection is a great tribute to you," Brauner went on. "I, too, am a lover and something of a collector of art—though I don't, of course, have either your experience or expertise—but you have my utmost admiration for what you have achieved."

"Thank you." Emanuel waited for more.

Brauner gave a small nod. "To business, then." He paused. "I believe that I can assist you in moving your entire collection to America." He noted the fresh flicker of annoyance in the other man's eyes and went on swiftly. "Please don't trouble to tell me again that I'm wrong. Even if I am—even if this whole conversation is purely hypothetical—it surely can't do any harm just to let me finish what I have to say."

Emanuel sighed. "If you insist."

"As I said, I can help. Believe me, I can."

"Why?" Emanuel asked.

"Why would I help?" Brauner smiled. "What's in it for me, you mean?" There was no response. "Payment in kind," he said, and again he paused. "A Bonnard for a Hodler, perhaps, theoretically—and, of course, hypothetically—a Munch for a Redon. All negotiable, naturally."

"Naturally," Emanuel said, almost amused for the first time.

"That's it." Brauner gave a little shrug. "All very simple, on the surface. Much more complicated beneath, of course."

"Of course." Emanuel's voice was tinged with soft irony.

"So." Brauner leaned back again. "What's your first reaction to my proposition?"

"First and last," Emanuel said, and the irony and amusement were both gone. "I thank you, Herr Brauner, most sincerely, but the fact remains that I do not need your help."

"Because you have your own contacts in the United States?" Brauner's question was gentle. "Fellow art lovers and friends?" He paused. "Your colleague, Max Wildenbruch, in Manhattan, for example."

For the second time, Emanuel felt a frisson of unease. "I'm sure you'll understand if I don't choose to discuss my personal acquaintances with you," he said stiffly.

"Of course," Brauner said. "After all, you don't know too much about me."

"I know nothing about you, sir."

Again, Brauner smiled. "Except one thing. That I am in a position to help you. And that I am willing to help you. At a price."

"And I say to you again, and for the last time, that I don't need your help." Emanuel rose from his chair and waited while the other man, left with no real alternative, stood up, too. He put out his right hand. "Thank you for coming, Herr Brauner. I'm sorry it's been a wasted journey."

Brauner shook his hand. "Not wasted at all."

They walked out of the library along a corridor into the high-ceilinged, wood-paneled entrance hall. The Rothenburgs' two Great Danes, lying on either side of one of Hedi's favorite Hodlers, stirred and wagged their tails but did not get up.

"I shall be staying at Brenner's Park," Brauner said at the front door, "if you change your mind."

"Will you be in town long?" Emanuel was still cordial.

"A few days," Brauner said.

"I hope you enjoy them." Emanuel opened the door. A blast of cold winter air blew in from the driveway.

"I shall," Brauner said. "Though I'd prefer it if the casino were open. I hear there'll be roulette again next year." He paused one last time. "Are you a gambler, Herr Rothenburg?"

"Occasionally, on my travels. I'm not a true gambler."

"A pity," Brauner said. "Had you been, I might have suggested a wager on how long it would take you to change your mind about my offer."

Emanuel almost admired the man's persistence.

"And I would have advised you not to waste your money," he said.

Georg Brauner did not return to our house for fifteen months, but once inside Papa's library for the second time, he became morbidly insistent upon reminding my father of the many injustices being heaped upon the Jews in our country. Papa hardly needed reminding that the Gestapo had, for almost a month, had powers to arrest, interrogate, and intern without due process of law; or that Jewish artists were being excluded from exhibitions; or that books by Jewish writers were being burned; or that Jews were not only being discriminated against but humiliated and, in a growing number of cases, murdered. When he pointed out that Brauner had told him nothing he had not already known, Brauner asked him why, in that case, when so many of his people were leaving, and if he had such wonderful contacts abroad, were we still in Baden-Baden?

Because, in our case, my father replied, honestly—as he had so often told our mother—there was no urgency. No attempt was being made to halt the mass emigration, which was, after all, the Nazis' main aim: to rid Germany of what Brauner called "his people." Papa said that he had never achieved anything fine in his life by being hurried, and he did not plan to start now.

"So," said Brauner, "you still believe you don't need my help."

Papa looked him straight in the eye.

"I know that I don't," he said.

My father meant what he had told Brauner. Ours was not an ordinary position; we were, he firmly believed, less vulnerable—at least for the time being—than many German Jews because of Papa's status in the local community and because of our family's wealth. My father had often told us that money itself meant little and that love, good health, and contentment were of infinitely greater importance. Yet as the rumors and increasingly hard evidence of growing brutality and shocking discrimination around the country began to bite more regularly into my parents' peace of mind, Papa said that he had begun to appreciate the true value of his riches. His money and his respected position were, after all, enabling us to continue our lives in an almost unaltered manner. Even if there were difficulties for some local Jews in the shopping streets of Baden-Baden or Stuttgart or Frankfurt, Mama could always send Maria, our housekeeper, or Rudi, the chauffeur, to do the shopping and avoid unpleasantness or embarrassment. At the earliest hint of anti-Semitism at our school, Papa had arranged special tutoring for Lili, Trude, and myself at home, and I, for one, was happy about that plan, since my best friend and neighbor Leo Landau's father, Samuel, who agreed with Papa, had arranged for Leo to share lessons with us. Our tutor, Professor Eichinger, was younger and less stuffy than many of the teachers at school had been, but while our lessons were certainly less formal and more enjoyable, he kept discipline and made sure that we worked harder than we might otherwise have done. And as for Papa himself, as he pointed out, he still dealt, as he always had, with artists, and the vast majority of artists were, by nature and design, liberal human beings, above and beyond the baseness of racism and thuggery. In other words, we were luckier than most.

Still, my father was neither foolish nor complacent. Month after month was passing with no sign of any improvement in the general situation. Any lingering hopes he might have been harboring that our family could simply continue to ride out the storm and remain in our lovely home were crumbling. But worse than that, it was becoming increasingly clear to Papa that if he wanted to remove us to America before things grew any uglier, then he might, after all, have to consider losing perhaps the greatest part of the Rothenburg Symbolist Collection. Lately, I heard him say to Mama, the country seemed to be overflowing with so-called dealers claiming to be prepared to "take care of" Jewish-owned artworks, but Papa said he had no faith in the promises of double-dealing opportunists. At least Georg Brauner, he remembered wryly, had been frank enough, even at the outset, about his plans to gain from helping them, and at least Brauner had claimed—even on his second visit—that he would be able to spirit at least 50 percent of the collection over the Atlantic.

"Perhaps," Papa confided in Mama, "I was wrong not to have listened to him."

"I don't think so," Mama reassured him gently. "I think you were right not to trust him."

"Maybe." Papa sighed. "But right or not, if he were to return again now, I can tell you I might almost be glad to do business with him."

Brauner did come back on the afternoon of September 30, 1935, fifteen days after the passing of the Nuremberg Laws. Fifteen days for Emanuel to have fully absorbed the new laws that meant that Jews were no longer eligible as German citizens, that marriage and physical relations between Germans and Jews were forbidden, that any remaining hope of normalization was gone. Fifteen days for Emanuel to finally extract his head from his rich native soil and to try to complete the travel arrangements for himself and his family irrespective of the losses he now knew their departure would entail.

Brauner looked fit and suntanned.

"You look well," Emanuel told him cordially.

Hedi and the children were all at home, the two young girls and fourteen-year-old Anton and Leo Landau being tutored in the library, and so Emanuel had brought Brauner into their salon, the family's favorite room, cozier and less intimidating than the large lounge in which they had so often, in happier times, entertained many of the top families in Baden-Baden. This room contained the wireless and gramo-phone, a well-stocked bar, the baby grand piano that Hedi and Anton liked to play, the most comfortable, well-used furniture in the house, and three paintings, a de Chavannes, a Denis and, in pride of place, a Bonnard.

"I've had a good holiday this year," Brauner replied.

Emanuel had used the moments in which Hedi had organized coffee for them to compose himself, to try to quiet the almost violent surge of relief that had overcome him when he had learned that Brauner was at the front door. To show eagerness would be not only undignified but counterproductive, he warned himself as his guest settled himself into an armchair facing him. He wanted Brauner to be in no doubt of his own change of heart; he wanted him to know that there was business to be done between them, but he wanted, also, des-perately, to try to maintain control over the bargaining.

"Am I correct in thinking," Brauner asked, "that you are, at last, beginning to come to terms with reality?"

"You mean am I planning to leave Germany?" Emanuel knew they were beyond game playing, was conscious that this might be his last chance with Brauner.

"That is what I mean."

"When we last met," Emanuel said at last, "you made an offer of help."

"The last time," Brauner said, "and the first, too."

"For which I was grateful," Emanuel said. "But which I rejected."

"I can't say I noticed the gratitude," Brauner said.

"In which case, I apologize."

"No need."

"That's kind." Emanuel felt a knot of sickness in his stomach but forced himself to continue. "I realize now, with hindsight, that I was perhaps too hasty in my response."

"Really?" Brauner picked up his cup and saucer and drank some coffee.

"I need to know"—Emanuel saw there was no point delaying, that it was better to get it over and done with—"I need to know, Herr Brauner, if your offer of assistance is still available."

Brauner set down his cup and saucer. "It is," he said.

"Then perhaps"—Emanuel prided himself that his relief did not show—"we could discuss some business in a little more detail." He paused. "The terms you originally mentioned were, as you yourself said, purely hypothetical. Not realistic."

"Not at all realistic," Brauner agreed. "I believe I suggested something to the effect of a Bonnard for a Hodler, and a Munch for a Redon."

"Exactly." Emanuel smiled. "Perhaps you might be ready to make a more workable suggestion."

"With pleasure," Brauner said.

"Some more coffee?" Emanuel asked.

"No, thank you." Brauner paused. "The price for my help, given the worsening of your situation, has, of course, grown higher. Considerably higher."

"How much higher?" The knot in Emanuel's stomach grew tighter, though he had tried to prepare himself for this moment, had realized that old money and influence notwithstanding, Georg Brauner—whoever he really was—was still, of course, not much better than most of the other opportunists he had lately encountered.

"You agree that there is little time to waste," Brauner said.

"I do."

"You understand, also, that though I am a far freer agent than you, able to travel where I wish and with any of my possessions I see fit to take, a private arrangement to remove items belonging to you could still be risky for me."

"Yes," Emanuel said, "I understand."

"Good." Brauner paused. "Can we see the works right away?"

"We can."

"And do you agree that, subject to our agreeing upon the terms, I may also select and extract certain items right away?"

Emanuel's stomach fluttered again. "Subject to agreement, yes."

"Very well. Let's begin." Brauner looked directly, piercingly, at him. "You are in possession of two Gauguins; am I correct?"

"You are."

"And a number of sketches by Munch."

"Correct."

"I shall take both the Gauguins and all the sketches, and in return, I shall see to it that one of the paintings in this room—the Denis, I think—begins its journey to New York within one week."

Emanuel stood up. His face was very pale. "It's out of the question."

"Which part?"

"All of it. You know it's impossible."

"On the contrary," Brauner said pleasantly, looking up at him, "it's perfectly possible. And it's the kind of bargain I intend for the whole collection."

"But it's ludicrous—derisory. It's no bargain at all." Outraged, Emanuel struggled to find the words. "It's like comparing the Kurhaus and the casino with this house—it's quite out of proportion."

"Of course it is." Brauner shrugged. "Nevertheless, that is my offer."

"Then with respect, sir, I cannot deal with you."

"Are you quite certain of that?" Brauner was perfectly calm and mild.

"Absolutely certain. You could surely not have expected me to agree?" Emanuel stood up, rage beginning to boil inside him. "I think, sir, that it's time for you to leave."

"Sit down, Herr Rothenburg."

Emanuel stared down at Brauner.

"I asked you to sit down," Brauner said. "Please."

Slowly, Emanuel sat. Perhaps, he thought, the man was toying with him—maybe his offer had simply been a bad joke and now they would start again seriously. He could take a joke with the best of them, had always been known around Baden-Baden for his fine sense of humor.

"You still don't understand," Brauner said. "You still don't fully comprehend the gravity of your situation."

"On the contrary," Emanuel said.

"No," Brauner said. "You don't." He paused. "Nor do you understand the extent of my influence, both inside and outside Germany."

Emanuel said nothing, just stared at him. There had been no joke. And there was worse to come, he knew that now, too, as surely as he knew his own name.

"Max Wildenbruch has sworn an affidavit in your favor in New York," Brauner said. "He, above all others, has been a most generous friend, and instrumental in helping you obtain the necessary papers for you and your family. Has he not?"

Emanuel still said nothing, his mind whirling.

"Has he *not*?" For the first time, an ugly tone colored Brauner's voice.

"Yes. He has."

"Wildenbruch asks no payment for himself," Brauner went on. "But the oiling of the system's wheels and the greasing of essential palms has already cost him dearly, has it not? For which you have agreed to pay, have you not?"

For the very first time, Emanuel felt fear, real fear of actual danger, clutch at his heart. This man, this smooth, impeccable stranger, was dangerous to him and to Hedi and the children. He knew that now.

Brauner leaned forward again. "Listen to me now, and listen carefully, because this is your last chance, Emanuel Rothenburg. Are you listening?"

"I'm listening." Emanuel's voice was very soft.

"Those same contacts who would make it possible for me to arrange safe shipment of your works of art to New York could just as easily be persuaded to prevent you, your wife, and your children from ever leaving Germany."

Emanuel's pallor had increased and his heart was pounding.

"Don't you believe me, Rothenburg?" The last pretense at courtesy had vanished. "I think perhaps you do."

"Yes." Emanuel nodded very slowly. "I believe you."

"Good," Brauner said. "Very good." He sat back again. "I think some fresh coffee would be a fine idea now. Perhaps your wife would be kind enough to arrange it."

"Yes." Emanuel got to his feet carefully, feeling ten years older. "I'll ask her."

"Thank you," Brauner said. "And then, if you agree, we can begin our negotiations in earnest. If you do agree."

At the door, still dazed, Emanuel looked back at the younger man.

"I agree," he said. "Of course I agree."

The "negotiations" went on into the evening. Papa escorted Brauner down to the vast converted cellars beneath our house, into the high-ceilinged rooms kept at the perfect temperature and the perfect humidity to safely maintain the valuable canvases and aged papers of the Rothenburg Collection. Papa told Mama later that he had watched Brauner as he had viewed the works, had watched his expression, his dark eyes, his mouth, and he thought he had seen real passion on his face, true lust. Papa saw that the man wanted these works not solely for their value, but for themselves, and whether his yearning was for their beauty or for the prestige with which their ownership might endow him, my father sensed, too, that Brauner's desire was powerful enough to give him almost anything he wanted.

At eight o'clock, we all sat down to the dinner that Brauner had requested. Brauner sat between Mama and Lili, and though at the time, of course, I could not fully understand the situation, I think I can now imagine all too well how my father must have felt during that meal. And how that emotion must have grown later, when Papa himself stood on a ladder in the cellar and took down the Gauguins and the Munch sketches; and when he wrapped them, with love and with real pain; and when he stood at the front door and watched Georg Brauner climb into the back of the black Mercedes that had waited for him for more than seven hours.

Knowing that it would not be long before he came again. Knowing that the blackmail had begun. Not knowing where, if ever, it might end.

FOR ANNIE

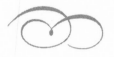

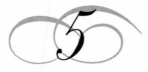

*In the spring of 1987, the three friends were living separate lives in three dif-*ferent countries. Olivia, single, free as a bird, and a skilled linguist—whose preference it had become to travel widely, enjoy life to the hilt, and to interpret, whenever possible, for traveling authors, journalists, and film and television companies—was living in Switzerland, running the Segal Translation Agency out of an office in Geneva. Jamie—free-spirited, gentle, gregarious Jamie—was in Boston, less than sixty miles from the Arias family mansion in Rhode Island, doing what he both loved and excelled at: being an advertising man and running his own agency in partnership with his less than gentle or free-spirited wife, Carrie Beaumont Arias. And Annie, married to Edward Thomas, an English banker fifteen years her senior, with three children, was living an archetypically British, ostensibly joyous life in an Oxfordshire village.

Annie's call for help came at two minutes after ten in the morning, Geneva time, just before Olivia was due to leave her office for a meeting at Gilles-Breque Pharmaceuticals, a corporation for which she had done a number of public relations interpreting jobs. It was only nine o'clock in Britain, and as Olivia picked up the receiver and heard Annie's voice, she registered a brief instant of surprise because Annie was usually much too busy, as a mother of three little ones, to call during the day.

"Livvy?" Annie's tension came over loud and clear.

"Annie, hi. What's up?" Olivia picked up her briefcase, laid it down on the top of her desk, and began stacking papers into it.

"Nothing." Annie paused. "Everything."

"Tell me."

"I can't. Not like this. Not on the phone, I mean."

"The phone's all we have right now, Annie." Olivia stopped filling the case and sat back down behind her desk. "Has something happened? Are you okay? Are the kids okay?"

"Fine. The children are fine." Annie paused again. "So far."

"What do you mean?" Olivia glanced at her watch. "Annie, you've obviously called to tell me something."

"Yes."

Olivia gave it three whole seconds. It was not an aspect of her character that she especially liked, but she had never been overburdened with patience. "Annie, for crying out loud, tell me."

"I need you, Livvy," Annie said, very softly. "I know you're probably much too busy, but I was thinking, remembering the promise we made to each other back in seventy-six."

Olivia felt a sudden chill. If Annie was thinking about their pact after all these years, that had to mean she was in major trouble.

"Do you remember, Livvy?"

"Of course I remember."

As if it were yesterday, the three of them in the room at the hotel near Dukesfield Fell, drinking cognac and trying to decide how they were going to cope with their futures, without each other. *If any of us gets into any kind of a serious jam and needs help, the other two will drop everything and be there to see them through.*

"I didn't know who else to turn to. I'm sorry."

"Don't be a dope. That was the whole point of the pact." Olivia's mind ticked over. She didn't need to check her diary to know how busy she was. If Annie needed her to fly over right now, it would be tough trying to find another interpreter for all her clients, but that, after all, had been part of the deal they'd all agreed to. *Come hell or high water,* she remembered.

"What about Jamie?" she asked. "Have you called him?"

"Not yet. I thought you might."

"Of course I will, if you want me to."

"It's all my own fault." Annie was close to tears. "I'm so weak; I'm such an awful coward—"

"What are you talking about, Annie?" Olivia could hardly believe her ears. "You're amazing—the wonderful life you've made for yourself, the way you are with your children—"

"I'm not amazing at all, Livvy."

Suddenly, Olivia thought, Annie didn't sound like Annie. The woman she knew was a confident, capable person, but right now Annie didn't sound only distraught or depressed. She sounded diminished.

"I'm a mess," Annie went on. "You just wouldn't believe how much of a mess I've made of everything."

Olivia stopped checking the time, stopped even thinking about her meeting. "Is it Edward? Is your marriage in trouble?"

"Not really. Not yet."

She'd said "so far" when Olivia had asked her if the children were okay—Olivia didn't like the way the conversation was going.

"Okay," she said positively. "You want me now, right? I'm not sure if I can actually get over there today. I will, if I can, but—"

"No," Annie said abruptly. "You can't come here."

"So what do you want, Annie? Do you want to meet in London? Or do you want to come here? I'd love it," Olivia added quickly. "You haven't stayed with me in an age." She paused again. "Annie, sweetheart, this is no good—you have to tell me what this is about. If I'm going to be able to help you at all, you're going to have to tell me *something*."

"I'm scared to tell you."

"That's just crazy."

"I'm scared because when I tell you, you'll never feel the same way about me again. Nor will Jamie." Annie sounded close to tears again. "I hate myself so much, Livvy, and I'm afraid you'll hate me, too, when you know."

"Nothing could ever make me hate you, Annie."

"Maybe. Maybe not."

Olivia was growing more alarmed by the second. "Annie, tell me now, right now. Do it real fast, like pulling off a Band-Aid."

Annie was silent.

"Come on, Annie."

"I'm a junkie," Annie said.

Olivia, in shock, said nothing.

"Valium," Annie went on. "Diazepam. They call it being dependent, but that doesn't describe it at all." She paused one more time. "I'm addicted to tranquilizers, Livvy, and if I don't do something soon—if you don't help me do something—I think they're going to destroy me."

Olivia realized awhile later, after she'd called Jamie in Boston and enlisted his help, that until now she had pretty much fallen for the image that Annie Aldrich Thomas had wanted her friends to have of her life in England. Namely that it was just about as perfect as anything could be.

Married to Edward Thomas, a man she loved, with three children—Sophie, aged five, William, aged four, and Liza, aged three—a golden retriever named Bella, two cats named Leo and Boots, and a stable of horses, living in Banbury Farm House (a three-hundred-year-old house in the village of Stone Bridge, Oxfordshire, with a thatched roof, oak beams, and a glorious back garden), Annie had long since been accepted into English village life. She was, of course, an American, but she had received part of her education in England, and she had, from the beginning, made valiant efforts to fit in. She had no apparent arrogance, she was strong, plucky, and patient, yet she also displayed sufficient humility to her neighbors to encourage them to offer first their help and, later, their friendship. Edward thought the world of her, was consummately proud of Annie's ladylike beauty and calm, of the impeccable way she cared for their home and brought up their children, of the manner in which she had fitted, so seamlessly, into his world.

Olivia and Jamie had observed Annie's new life mostly from a distance through the regular correspondence that Annie had scrupulously maintained, but they had both visited the Thomases from time to time, had even stayed in the pretty guest suite at Banbury Farm House, and though Olivia thought of herself as reasonably intuitive, she knew now that she, like Jamie, had utterly failed to notice that Annie was unhappy. Had utterly failed Annie.

★   ★   ★

It was an accident—the third in a trilogy of minor disasters the previous year, in the autumn of 1986—that had first made Annie wonder if she might, perhaps, have a problem. First, in the second week of September, she had forgotten to tell Edward that it was four-year-old Sophie's first parents' day at Stone Bridge Primary School, and so Edward had been unable to attend, and Annie had had to bear the looks of generously reined-in disappointment on both father's and daughter's faces and to explain to Sophie's teachers and the other parents why her husband was not present. Second, just a fortnight later, on the morning when Annie had been supposed to catch the 8:11 train to London to meet Edward for an important solicitor's meeting and luncheon, she had overslept and missed the train and had not arrived until the meeting was over and the luncheon well under way.

And then there was the accident.

To begin with that morning, Annie had woken up with all the symptoms of premenstrual syndrome: tension headache, sore breasts, and a sense of gloom and irritability. She'd taken a two-milligram Valium—as she did on more mornings these days than in the past—showered, applied her makeup, and dressed, feeling a little better. But then at the breakfast table first Sophie, then William, and, finally, inevitably, little Liza had begun acting up—Annie's children's bouts of naughtiness always started with the oldest and then rolled inexorably down toward the baby like a snowball.

"Sophie, go fetch your blazer, please." Annie stood and picked up her coffee cup and cereal bowl to put them in the sink.

Sophie shook her blond curls, cast her blue eyes downward, and played with the remainder of the toast on her plate.

"Sophie, stop that and go on, please." Tension gripped Annie's stomach.

"I don't want to."

"Don't be silly, sweetheart."

"I don't want to go to school today, Mummy."

Annie stopped clearing the big pine kitchen table. "Why?" she asked, instantly anxious, alert as she always was to the slightest hint of illness in any of her family. "Don't you feel good, sweetheart?"

"No," Sophie said.

Annie came right over and laid a hand on her forehead. "You're cool enough. How don't you feel good?"

"I feel sick."

"You do?"

"Sick and tired," Sophie said, and then grinned hugely. She had begun adopting expressions her parents used all too frequently, and thought it was wonderfully amusing.

"Sophie, you're a naughty girl," Annie said good-humoredly. "You know you should never tell fibs about feeling ill."

Sophie threw her bit of toast at William.

"Hey!" William, three years old but big for his age, threw it back and hit Sophie on the cheek.

"William, stop that." Annie retrieved the toast and wiped Sophie's buttery cheek. Sophie wriggled and pushed her away. "You, too, miss."

In her high chair, little Liza began crying and Bella whined. Annie ignored them both and went on removing dishes from the table and placing them in the sink. The tension that had vanished the instant she'd believed her older daughter unwell, returned, and with Edward away in London all this week and Marie-Louise, their Swiss-French nanny, already on her way to Oxford for her day off, Annie knew from past experience that the whole package was a recipe for a really bad day. She'd probably be better off taking a second pill to prevent things getting out of hand, before she let it get to her. Annie believed in preventive medicine; Grace Aldrich, her mother, had taught her that vitamin C kept colds away. Annie had learned for herself that diazepam kept panic attacks away.

Upstairs in her bathroom—with Sophie in her blazer and William ready for nursery school, both minding little Liza, all downstairs waiting to go—Annie took the small plastic bottle from her mirror-fronted cabinet, shook out a little white pill, and swallowed it.

May make you sleepy. If persists next day, do not drive. She wondered sometimes about that caution, yet Peter Cary—Edward's old family doctor—had told her that it was all right to take the odd pill when she needed it, and he knew that wasn't necessarily at night, and the white printed label on the bottle said "To be taken when required" and nothing about taking only at night. And in any case, the pills never seemed to make her sleepy during the day, just soothed her, smoothed away those knots in her stomach and made her better able to cope.

She had delivered both Sophie and William safely and was on her way to collect some groceries from Tryon's, their general store, when it happened. An ancient Morris Minor stopped just ahead of Annie's Range Rover at the crossroads, waiting to turn into Stone Bridge Road. A large gap opened up, but still the Morris Minor waited, its right indicator sticking out like a yellow Popsicle.

"Go on, Mummy," Liza said from her safety seat behind Annie.

"We can't go yet, Liza," Annie said, glad she'd taken the extra Valium, which was so much better than allowing herself to get edgy and impatient behind the wheel.

"Want to go pooh-pooh, Mummy," Liza said—she was always saying she wanted to go pooh-pooh when she wanted things to move faster.

The Morris Minor started to edge out, then stalled.

"Mummy, *go!*" Liza said, the first note of genuine desperation lengthening the second word.

"Take it easy, sweetheart."

Annie took her foot off the brake and pulled smoothly out, preparing to bypass the Morris in order to get to Tryon's before Liza really kept her promise and poohed in her pants. The traffic to the right was way off, held up by a Royal Mail van while the mailbox outside Dolin's Bakery was emptied. She began to turn right, driving smoothly and sweetly, making a perfect, textbook turn—

"Pooh-pooh!" Liza shrieked.

Reflex made Annie look up into the rearview mirror to see if Liza's round cheeks had gone bright red as they always did when she was really about to go—and the Range Rover's left front fender crunched hard into the United Dairies milk float that had come out of nowhere.

"Oh, my God," Annie said.

Liza shrieked again, much more piercingly than before.

"Oh, my *God!*" Annie pulled up the hand brake and turned around. "Liza, are you okay?" Frantically, she unfastened her seat belt and wriggled herself right around. "Sweetheart, *speak* to me!"

Liza's cheeks were scarlet.

"Pooh-pooh, Mummy," she said disgustedly.

Having exchanged details with the milkman and no longer able to contemplate groceries or Tryon's, Annie headed for home. What she
needed most right now was to get Liza bathed and changed and then to
phone Edward straightaway and confess about the car. Not that he'd
mind; he wasn't that kind of a husband, thank God; he'd only care
about her and Liza. But still, if she didn't tell him this morning, Annie
knew she'd get a bad case of the guilts, which would get worse as the
day progressed, and there was always the possibility that if she waited
until evening when Edward phoned from London, she might forget to
tell him, and then he'd get home and see the damage and he might
think she'd deliberately tried to keep it from him.

For heaven's sake, Annie, she told herself as she turned the Range
Rover into their nice, broad, obstacle-free driveway, *Edward isn't like
that—it wouldn't occur to him to think you'd deliberately hide anything from
him.* But he might, she reasoned as she freed her smelly, tear-stained
daughter from her safety harness, if she didn't call him right away, if she
did other things first and maybe forgot. If Edward got home and found
the dents and she'd said nothing, it would be only natural for him to
think just exactly that.

"Are you and Liza all right?" was all Edward wanted to know
when she reached him at his office in the City.

"We're fine, Edward. Not a scratch, not even a bruise."

"And the milkman?"

"He was fine, too—and he was really nice about it."

"So he should have been."

"The car's a bit damaged, though," Annie confessed, "and the milk
float had a real dent in it."

"That's just metal, darling," Edward said. "Nothing to get upset
about." It was such a relief to hear his gentle, wise voice that Annie felt
much better for a while. But then later on the tension came back and
she started seeing pictures in her mind of how much worse the accident
might have been—and before long it would be lunchtime and she'd
have to go and pick up William, and she really wasn't sure she was in a
fit state—she wasn't calm enough, and she'd thought that the second

pill would have soothed her sufficiently, but clearly it hadn't, so she'd better be sure to have another before she got back into the car again.

That night, Liza, who had appeared till then quite unfazed by the whole incident, woke up screaming, and Annie, dragged horribly from her own heavy sleep by the piercing, terrifying sound of her daughter's distress, was able only with difficulty to glean from the two-year-old's garbled account that she had dreamed they were all in the car and Mummy had made a big bang and everyone was dead—Mummy and Daddy and Sophie and William and Liza, too.

At that moment Annie knew that it was time to get a prescription for a higher dosage of tranquilizers from the doctor, because, after all, her children were her responsibility, and she'd only driven into the back of that milk float because her nerves had allowed Liza to distract her, and she needed to be perfectly calm to drive properly, safely.

To function well, sensibly, *normally*, as she'd been brought up. To keep up appearances. To keep Edward's household running properly. To be a good wife to him. And a good, safe mother. The way her own mother had been.

She had swallowed her first tranquilizer the day Franklin and Grace had been buried. Susan Aldrich, a cousin, had handed her a few tiny white pills and had told Annie they would make things a little easier. "Trust me," Susan had said—and Annie had swallowed one down obediently, and her cousin had been right; the pain had still been there, but the pill had dulled the edges a little. She'd taken an occasional one up until the memorial service, but once that, too, had been endured, Annie hadn't even thought about taking another tranquilizer for several months, until a prolonged bout of insomnia had sent her to a doctor in San Francisco who had immediately written her a prescription for a handful of two-milligram Valium.

"Just to relax you," he'd said.

"Tranquilizers?" Annie had been dubious.

"Better than sleeping pills," the doctor had told her. "And certainly better than not sleeping." He'd looked at her anxious expression and smiled. "Now, don't look so worried. This is just to get your sleeping pattern back on track."

The tablets had done their work, and Annie had been careful not to abuse them, had stopped after a few nights' good rest and had stuck the bottle, still two-thirds full, in the back of her night table drawer, not taking it out again for several months, when another period of insomnia had threatened to become debilitating. And that was all. A prescription drug, as safe and respectable and useful as any antibiotic, used for a specific problem and then forgotten.

★   ★   ★

Meeting Edward, generous, successful, attractive, older Edward, whom she accepted was probably as close a figure to Franklin Aldrich as she'd been able to find, had seemed the greatest blessing to Annie. Edward Thomas, with his intelligent gray eyes, fine, strong bone structure, and silver-templed hair, had turned out to be precisely what he had promised to be; apart from a fondness for pheasant and grouse shooting, which Annie loathed, there was no dark side to him, no hidden agenda, no nasty surprises. He was a kind and decent man, a splendid husband and father, and married life for Annie Aldrich Thomas had, in most ways, worked out just as Edward had vowed it would when he had proposed to her.

And yet as lucky as she now accepted she was, some things still seemed to have taken their toll on Annie. The loss of her parents, her roots, and her safety net. The moving from place to place, the jolting back and forth by circumstances and fate. The anchoring in what had been decreed by her marriage as her new, permanent home, the place in which Edward Thomas's wife was expected to thrive, grow old, and, ultimately, be buried. The pressures that her foreignness exerted on Annie, the strain of concealing those pressures from both Edward and their children and their neighbors and friends. Annie coped well enough with the basics, with learning the rules of cricket and rounders and rugby, and she became adept at making jam roly-poly, which William adored, and Yorkshire pudding, which Edward liked on Sundays. But the really tiny, yet crucial things, the subtle differences in British manners and etiquette and basic thought processes, made Annie—strictly in private—desperately afraid of doing the wrong thing.

Edward and their friends all seemed to think that she was a perfect wife and mother—and Olivia told her more than once how super-competent she was—but Annie looked at their neighbors and acquaintances and at the wives of Edward's three brothers, all living in Oxfordshire or Gloucestershire—and found herself wanting. She thought, perhaps, that she felt something like the way an American tree sparrow might feel living in the midst of a flock of indigenous English birds; her feathers looked ordinary enough—to most people, she probably did look like a regular sparrow—but Annie knew that she neither was nor would she ever be, and instead of rejoicing in her originality, she fretted over it.

Yet she would not, could not even contemplate sharing her problems with her husband or with anyone else. Annie came from the kind of stock who got on with life, who put on a brave face, who acted when necessary, and Annie acted with such excellence that she often believed in her own performance. But increasingly the act had come to require a little more help than before, and where some people might have downed a glass of wine or a vodka martini, Annie, who hated the idea of drinking alcohol around her children, reached for her crutch, the Valium bottle, instead.

Little things had started going wrong long before the car accident. In the past, Annie had had such a good, sharp memory, but over a period of time she realized she was forgetting things, so she began making lists and sticking little memory joggers where she knew she'd be sure to see them—on the fridge, on mirrors, on the windshield. But still things went wrong—the odd arrangement here and there. Edward once told Annie that she had become known in the village for being well organized, but first one week she forgot that it was her turn to do the church flowers, and then she got the time of Sophie's dentist appointment wrong—and once, she dragged William and Liza up and down Stone Bridge Road looking for the car, and William kept trying to tell her something, but she'd got too distracted to listen to him, and it turned out she'd parked it in the parking lot instead. No one seemed troubled by the little things—no one else ever really seemed to even notice them—but Annie did, Annie noticed them, and when she did, she took another pill. It was incumbent on her, she told herself, to be happy, calm, and organized for her family's sake. Her wonderful life was far too precious for her to take risks with. And there was certainly nothing risky about taking the odd tablet given to her by Dr. Cary; she had, after all, started out with two-milligram tablets back in 1976, and even if, these days, she sometimes took three tablets in a day, whereas in the beginning she'd only ever taken one, the prescribed dosage on the bottle was up to three daily, so she knew she was perfectly safe.

★   ★   ★

It was the accident with the Range Rover and Liza's nightmare that sent her to Peter Cary, in early October of 1986, for a supply of five-milligram tablets.

"I don't think I'd be happy to do that," he told her.

Annie sat on the bumpy, horsehair-stuffed chair she'd sat on so many times in the past, in the doctor's cozy, overwarm, comfortingly old-fashioned office, and looked at him in surprise.

"Why not?" she asked.

Peter Cary scratched his white head and looked back at her with eyes that seemed more intent and alert than they had ever been before. Annie had often privately thought that while she was perfectly happy to entrust all the normal family influenzas and childhood diseases to this ruddy-faced old man, she would be inclined to take anything more potentially serious to Andrew Miller, her private general physician in London. Yet suddenly here she was, asking for a slightly higher dosage of what Dr. Cary had unquestioningly been giving her for years, and he was looking at her with these new, curious, watchful eyes.

"Why do you think you need five-milligram tablets, Annie?"

Annie felt flustered. "I just thought—" She stopped, feeling as if she were on trial, as if saying the wrong thing, giving the wrong answer to the doctor's trick question, might result in her being sentenced to no pills at all.

"How many pills do you find you take in a day?" Cary asked.

"It varies," Annie said.

"One? Two?"

"Two, sometimes," Annie said.

"Three?"

"Occasionally."

"How occasionally?"

Annie knew she was floundering. If she told Peter Cary the truth, the real truth, if she told him that she felt she had to have stronger tablets because she was afraid she couldn't go on functioning as a good, safe mother without them, he was bound to want to tell Edward, and Edward knowing about her needing tranquilizers was the last thing on earth she wanted.

She decided to back off.

"Just once in a while," she said. "Mostly it's still just one, or two maximum—but now and again I just can't seem to get to sleep properly with the one at night, and then I end up having to get up and take another pill a couple of hours later, and so I just thought if I took one five-milligram it might help me get a really good night's sleep." She paused. "I guess maybe it's not such a great idea after all."

"I think not," the doctor agreed gently.

"So shall we just leave it as the usual?" Annie asked.

Peter Cary leaned forward over his desk. "Any other problems you want to tell me about, Annie?"

"No," she said brightly. "No problems. It's just me—you know—I've always been a little nervy now and again."

"And you're sure there's nothing else?"

"Nothing at all."

Three days later, on her next visit to London, Annie went to see Andrew Miller, and this time she was more prepared than she had been with Dr. Cary.

"I'm nervous about flying," she told him. "I mean, really scared. And the thing is I have a couple of long-distance trips coming up, and this is the only way I can face them."

"You say that diazepam agrees with you?" Dr. Miller asked.

"Pretty well." Annie smiled at him. He was everything Peter Cary was not: good-looking, young—in his early forties, she guessed—and as slick as his state-of-the-art office.

He nodded. "I can prescribe a few two-milligram tablets for you." He reached for his prescription pad.

"I don't think they'd be strong enough," Annie said quickly. "I really get scared, Dr. Miller, and I'm afraid of panicking on board." She paused. "I lost my parents in a helicopter crash, you know."

The doctor took that in. "You want five-milligram tablets," he said.

"I'd feel happier just knowing I had them," Annie said.

"Don't you have a doctor closer to home, Mrs. Thomas?"

Annie fought to stay cool. "I'm not too happy with him," she said. "And I knew I was coming to London, and you looked after me so well when I had the stomach problem—"

Andrew Miller smiled. "I'm glad I could help." He reached for the prescription pad again. "Would you say ten tablets would be enough?"

"I may have a few flights to get through." Annie made a show of working it out. "Maybe fifteen would be better? It would save me bothering you again."

The doctor nodded. "I'll make it twenty." He started to write. "But I'd suggest you break them in half, take one half an hour or so before takeoff, and see how you go. You may not need the second half."

"That sounds sensible," Annie said.

For a while, just knowing she had them, in addition to her regular two-milligram prescription, made her feel strong enough to tuck them away in the back of her dressing table drawer. Until the end of October, when Edward asked her to help him host a house party—and there were so few things he asked of her that she told him it would be fine—but the planning got on top of her and she began to dread getting the details wrong. And by the weekend of the party, she was gulping down pills like M&M's, and on the first day she made a mistake over the seating plan, and then later that same evening, the main course was badly undercooked and she hadn't noticed. And Annie looked at Edward, just after he'd taken his first bite, and she saw the dismay on his face, and then she saw him cover it up, and he was just as much a gentleman as he always had been.

But before the next week was over, Annie was taking ten milligrams at a time.

"I'm flying into London for three days' work with a Swiss feature writer," Olivia told Annie on the phone a few weeks later, "and a meeting at the Arthur Segal Foundation, but I could snatch about three hours or so on Friday afternoon. Can you meet me in Harrods? We could do some shopping and have lunch."

"I'm not sure." Annie floundered.

"Come on, Annie; I'm longing to see you."

Given more warning, in her current jittery state, Annie would have thought up a decent excuse, but as it was, with Olivia's warm, energetic voice practically dragging her out of the house, Annie simply caved in.

"What time?"

"Twelve-thirty okay for you?"

"Fine," Annie said.

She was already terrified by the prospect.

Apart from a short bout of panic in the crush of people on the ground floor, she was doing okay until they sat down at their table in the Georgian Restaurant. It was something about the change in atmosphere, about the old-fashioned serenity of the long, endless dining room. Annie felt a strange sensation almost immediately, an alarming, inexplicable detachment from everyone and everything in the room, as if her mind were made of cotton wool, her body of lead. She looked across the table at Olivia to see if she'd noticed, but Olivia, thank God, was engrossed in the menu. Annie wondered if she could manage to reach for her bag, to get to her pills, take one more—

"I guess I'll go for the buffet," Olivia said. "How about you?"

Annie had the terrifying sensation of sudden paralysis. Maybe her vocal cords were paralyzed, too? Maybe if she tried to open her mouth to answer, no words would emerge. . . .

"Annie?" Olivia put down her menu. "Are you okay?"

Annie felt the panic rising, felt a new urge either to scream or to run or maybe both, but instead, somehow, she dug the nails of her right hand into her own thigh, and, mercifully, she felt the pain, and if she felt that, then maybe she could at least speak, could find a way to escape from this place, from this moment, without Olivia finding out the truth.

"Annie?" Curiosity gave way to concern. "What's wrong?"

"I don't feel too well." There. Words, real words. She dug her nails into her other leg. "I'm really sorry, Livvy, but I think I'm going to have to leave."

"You feel nauseous?" Olivia began immediately to respond. "Hold on while I get these parcels together—"

"Our drinks," Annie said. "We have to pay."

"Yes." Olivia looked around for a waiter. "I'll take care of that. You get to the ladies' room and I'll meet you there."

Annie stood, not knowing if her new, leaden legs would hold her up, but they did. She felt a little relief and wondered, fleetingly, if she might, after all, be able to sit out lunch. *No,* her mind told her. *Get out while you can.*

"Do you know where it is?" she asked.

Olivia smiled up at her, warm and gentle and calming. "I'll find you."

Annie sat, her head in her hands, in the privacy of the lavatory, and gave in, for a moment, to tears. She knew what she wanted, more than anything. She wanted—she *longed*—to tell Olivia everything. Livvy would be shocked, would probably think her utterly weak and foolish, but she would still know what to do, would take over and help her deal with it. Except that the first thing she would insist on was taking her home and making sure she told Edward everything, and Annie could not bear that.

And so instead of telling Olivia the truth, Annie got another pill out of her handbag and swallowed it there, inside the stall, without water, and when she heard Olivia's voice calling her name, she called back that she was all right now, and then she dried her eyes and checked her face in her compact mirror—and even if Livvy did see she'd been crying, it was natural enough to be upset when you were sick.

"I think I must be coming down with something," she said outside by the basins. "Sophie wasn't feeling good earlier in the week."

"Guess we'd better cut things short," Olivia said.

"I'm so sorry, Livvy."

Olivia put a hand on her arm. "Don't be a goose. You can't help being ill, can you?"

"No," Annie said, deeply ashamed. "I suppose not."

Olivia tucked an arm firmly through hers. "Think you can make it out to the street?"

"I hope so."

"I'll get you out. Just hold on to me."

Annie felt better, almost normal, the instant they were outside the store in the fresh air. There were plenty of black taxis, all waiting in line.

"I'll be okay now," she said. "You go back inside, go on shopping."

"I'm taking you to the station," Olivia said.

"No, you're not. There's no need."

"Maybe not, but I still am."

All the way to Paddington, Annie sat quietly, knowing that Olivia would take her silence for queasiness or weakness, but her thoughts were hammering in her head. She ought to tell her now. *But what about Edward?* This was the perfect moment to tell her. *But what about the children?*

She told her nothing.

With Olivia safely back in Switzerland, Annie began to consider the possibility that perhaps she ought, after all, to speak to Edward about the tranquilizers; not making too big a deal, just a mention, perhaps, she thought, of the tensions that had led her to start down that road. The more she thought about it, the more sensible an idea it seemed to her. Edward would not condemn her. She hadn't wanted to tell him before because she'd hated to upset him, but if she went on much longer, she knew she would end up upsetting him far more grievously, because she had a pretty good idea by now that she was addicted to Valium. Or whereas in the past she had believed she could have stopped taking her pills and survived, now the very notion of existing without them was inconceivable.

She decided to broach the subject that coming weekend. They would be at the London flat together, away from the children, and they were going to a birthday dinner at the Savoy, and it ought to be an easygoing affair, and with a bit of luck and the usual help of her yellow pills, she ought to manage the party well enough, and then she would tell Edward on Sunday morning.

If it hadn't been for Ludovic Brandt, the man whose birthday they were helping celebrate, Annie thought she might have gone through with her plan, but as it was, a few chance words by Ludo, thrown into the conversational ring so casually, so innocently, ruined everything.

"I'm bloody tired, as a matter of fact," he replied to Babs Standish's comment that he was looking marvelous. "Haven't had a decent night's sleep in weeks." He swigged down a generous mouthful of Château Croizet-Bages. "Think I'll ask the quack for some sleeping pills."

"Personally, I'd rather stick to claret," Babs said.

"Anything's better than pills," Edward said.

Annie, seated on Ludo's left, tried not to freeze.

"I don't know about that," Charles Standish said. "Those pills the doc gave me for my blood pressure just about saved my life."

"That's different," Edward said. "I'm talking about the dope kind—sleeping pills, tranquilizers, that kind of rubbish."

Annie thought about the contents of her handbag, the pretty little round porcelain box in which her Valium nestled, their very presence a comfort to her. "Surely they can be very useful," she said to her husband, "to those who need them?"

"People who need such things," Edward answered, with a sharpness that startled her, "are either fools or weaklings." He softened a little. "I think—I hope—I'm a reasonably tolerant man on the whole, but I quite frankly despise people who can't cope with life without resorting to drugs."

Later, alone with him at the flat, Annie found him in his study going through papers at his desk.

"Thought you might like a little nightcap." She held out a cognac snifter.

"Thank you, my love." He took it from her. "Nothing for you?"

"No. You know me." She paused. "Mind if I join you for a few minutes?"

"I wish you would." He sipped at his drink. "Good evening, wasn't it?"

"Lovely." Annie sat down on the chesterfield. The question she wanted yet feared to ask was burning a hole in her tongue. "Edward?"

"What, darling?"

She began carefully. "You seemed so upset tonight."

"Did I? When?"

"When Ludo mentioned sleeping pills."

"Yes," he said.

Annie waited a moment, but he said nothing further. "Why?" she asked.

"Why did that upset me?"

"Yes." She looked at his face, saw an unfamiliar dark look in his eyes. "If you'd rather not tell me, I don't mind," she said quickly. "It's just that things don't usually get to you that way."

"And you were concerned."

"Yes. A little." Annie waited again.

Edward drank a larger swallow of cognac, then set the glass down on his leather-topped desk. "I suppose it's never come up before, has it? Not between us, I mean."

"Sleeping pills, you mean," Annie said, still very careful. "No reason why it should have, I guess."

"Not just sleeping pills," Edward said, not quite looking at her. "Other things, too, as I said in the restaurant. Painkillers. Tranquilizers. Pills to dull you, then get you going. Pills to help you survive."

Annie leaned forward, her hands on her knees. Her heart was pounding too fast. "Edward, you sound as if you're talking about yourself."

"No," he said. "Not myself. Not exactly."

Her palms were suddenly damp. He knew, she thought, in terror. Oh, Lord, he *knew*.

Edward's voice was very soft. "My mother," he said.

It had been the one dark secret of his life, he told her, the only thing of significance he had not shared with her. He had not exactly lied to her about his mother. Sophia Thomas had died of bone cancer, but what Edward had not told Annie was that his mother had also been a morphine addict. The drug had not only destroyed her, but it had also ruined his father's life and wrecked his and his brothers' childhoods.

"We saw our mother euphoric when she'd had enough, and we saw her when she tried to stop—and she did try; I'm sure of that," Edward told Annie, and she'd never heard his voice so laden with sorrow. "She'd shake and sweat, and she'd have such awful pains— pains just from the withdrawal, not even related to the cancer. That came later, and by then it was impossible to tell which was which, not that it mattered, not that it helped her or us. Our mother was in agony, more kinds of agony than you can ever begin to imagine."

"Oh, Edward," Annie said, her voice little more than a whisper. "I'm so sorry. So terribly sorry."

"No need," he said. "Not anymore." He smiled at her anxious

face. "I have you now, and the children, and my brothers have good, decent families, too, and I'm a very, very lucky man." He paused. "But you see now why I feel as I do about drugs."

"Yes," Annie said. "Of course."

She saw how he felt—oh, how clearly she saw that. And she knew, just as clearly, that any hope she might have had of telling him about her problem was gone. That she could never, ever confide in him about that, of all things.

And more than that—worse than that—she had a brand-new fear after that night in London. Her husband had told her that his childhood had been destroyed because of drugs, and so Annie was afraid now— she was *terrified*—that if Edward ever learned the truth about her, she might be responsible for ruining the rest of his adulthood as well. Perhaps even the lives of their own children.

So instead of telling Edward, she went on.

And instead of getting help, she took more.

She survived Christmas and New Year's by keeping herself so madly busy that the sheer discipline, mixed with adrenaline and, as always, her pills, dragged her through. But with the festive season over, reality stepped in with renewed vengeance. Edward was back in London for at least five days of most weeks; Marie-Louise was visiting her family in Switzerland; Sophie, William, and Liza were constantly seeking ways to fill their school-free days. And worst of all, however much Valium Annie took during those post-Christmas days and nights, it never seemed to be enough. She trembled too much, she felt her heart racing, sometimes missing beats altogether, she perspired; her mind wandered, she made her lists, scribbled down her memory joggers but forgot to look at them, forgot she'd even made them, let people down, most often the children; her legs and arms felt strange, her words, once in a while, slurred, and she dropped things all the time.

"I'm sorry," Jane Reece-Smith, the mother of one of William's friends, told her one morning outside school on a day when it was Annie's turn to pick up both boys and take them home, "but I've decided I'd rather collect Michael myself today."

"Oh," Annie said vaguely. "I don't mind fetching him at all."

"I'm sure," Mrs. Reece-Smith said. "But still, I'd rather do it myself."

The unmistakably chilly quality in the other woman's tone cut through Annie's morning fog. "Is something wrong?" she asked.

Mrs. Reece-Smith looked her in the eye. "Frankly, Mrs. Thomas, you don't look up to it."

"I'm fine," Annie said defensively.

"No," Mrs. Reece-Smith said firmly. "I don't think you are. If you don't mind my saying so, Mrs. Thomas, you seem a little woolly to me. A little wobbly, perhaps." She paused. "Are you unwell?"

"No." The other woman's steady gaze unnerved Annie. "That is, I think I may be coming down with something."

"A touch of flu, perhaps," Mrs. Reece-Smith suggested.

"Perhaps."

Nothing more was said, but Annie knew now that her deficiencies were being observed. And if Jane Reece-Smith considered her unsafe to drive her son—which was, more or less, what she had said—then perhaps she was right.

Within twelve hours, Annie had called every other mother in the school car pool and withdrawn her services.

"I've been getting bad migraines lately," she told them all. "I never seem to get warnings anymore—and I don't want to take any risks with the children."

None of the mothers argued. No one was anything but polite, even kind, but Annie felt that she'd jumped just before someone else had pushed her. She was running out of time. The drug that she had always believed had been her helper was wrecking her life. The way morphine had wrecked Edward's mother's.

She had to quit. Before someone told Edward, or before Sophie or William heard a rumor at school. Before something awful happened. Before it was too late.

She made up her mind to quit, no matter how hard it was. She worked out a plan. Mrs. Reece-Smith had suggested the flu, so that was what Annie told her friends and neighbors she had—just a mild case, and she needed no help, just a little peace and quiet. She told Olivia and Jamie she was going out of town, so that they wouldn't call, and she got the children away on sleep-overs for a whole week because she thought she might start climbing the walls or getting sick or having the d.t.'s or something, and if the house was empty, there would be no one to see.

For the first few days, apart from the tension of waiting for something to happen and the fear that her will might not be strong enough to stop her reaching for her pills—she had locked them up, but she hadn't thrown them out; she hadn't been able to bring herself to do that—it wasn't too bad. She felt almost smart, almost vindicated. *See,* she told herself, *it's okay, I'm okay, I can give them up, I'm not an addict.*

But then it started.

It was a nightmare. A real, honest-to-God waking nightmare, a thousand times worse than she had anticipated. She felt physically sick, as if she were getting the flu, but worse. She shook and felt so dizzy that it seemed as if the floor was moving. But the worst thing of all was the despair, so awful, so intense that she wanted to die, and the knowledge that there was only one other way of ending it, and that was getting to her pills. Except that she couldn't find the key to the cabinet she'd locked them into, and afterward she didn't remember doing it, but later—hours later, days later, she wasn't sure—when she was starting to come out of it, she found that she'd torn off the door.

Respectable, neat, clean, golden-haired, blue-eyed little Annie Aldrich Thomas had ripped off the hinges with her bare hands, and she had the cut fingers and broken glass everywhere to prove it.

She thought she might go mad. For a long while now, she had been obtaining her tablets simply by telephoning her two doctors—Peter Cary in Stone Bridge and Andrew Miller in London—alternately, and asking for repeat prescriptions. Suddenly, her supply system had begun to fail her. Both physicians were displaying growing reluctance to go on prescribing for her. Both had suggested, independently, that it was time for Annie to seek psychiatric counseling. And then, just a fortnight after her own secret, futile attempt at withdrawal, Peter Cary threatened to stop the Valium completely unless Annie agreed to see a specialist or to let him talk to Edward, and Andrew Miller told her that he wanted to reduce both the strength and quantity of her prescription.

"To see how you manage," Miller said in his calm, gentle manner.

"I won't manage," Annie told him desperately.

"Then diazepam on its own isn't enough for you."

"It has to be," Annie said.

"Why? Why won't you talk to a specialist, Mrs. Thomas?"

"You know why."

Andrew Miller remained very patient. "And you know, because I've told you repeatedly, that there is no more reason for your husband to learn of an appointment with a psychiatrist than for him to find out you've seen me. We're all equally bound, Mrs. Thomas, by patient confidentiality."

"I know that."

"Then why won't you at least give it a try?"

Annie stared at him across his big desk in total frustration. She'd told him and told him. "Because it would mean lying to Edward, and I've never done that, not really."

"You haven't told him you come here, have you?"

"I don't, often," she said. "They're only pills," she added, trying to explain, to make him understand how she felt. "Like aspirin or antibiotics. Going to see someone would be different."

"Diazepam is nothing like aspirin, Mrs. Thomas. And you don't come here often because you telephone my assistant instead, and she sends you an automatic repeat prescription." Dr. Miller shook his fair, handsome head. "And it's been very remiss of me to permit that to go on for so long."

He did let her get away with it that time, gave her, because of her obvious distress, the five-milligram prescription that she had begged for, but he reduced the quantity and made it clear that she would have to return in person when her supply ran out and that he could not guarantee to go on treating her if she continued to ignore his advice.

She went shopping that afternoon. She went to Fortnum & Mason for Edward's favorite mustard, and then she went to Hatchards in Piccadilly to buy the latest Jeffrey Archer novel for Edward and some books for the children, and from there she walked up to Piccadilly

Circus and went into Boots to have her new prescription filled. She had succeeded until then in blocking the new fears that Dr. Miller's warning had aroused in her, but handing over the piece of paper with his familiar, overly large scrawl to the pharmacist, Annie was assailed by a sudden attack of panic. What if this was the last time? What if he did refuse to give her any more? She was even less likely to be able to fool Peter Cary than Andrew Miller, which meant she'd have to find another doctor, and of course London, and even Oxford, were both filled with doctors, but she didn't think you could just walk in out of nowhere and add yourself to a strange doctor's list. And what if she couldn't? What if she ran out of pills?

She was trembling when she left Boots, and a part of her—the old Annie Aldrich Thomas part—hoped it wasn't visible to anyone else, but another part of her didn't care about that anymore, cared only about where she was going to get another slip of white paper with her prescription for comparative calm, for a semblance of normality, of sanity, if it came to it.

The man was right in front of her before she saw him, practically touching her. He was brown-haired and very pale skinned, clean-shaven and wearing sunglasses, even though it was almost dark.

"Need some help?" he asked her.

Annie was startled enough to stop walking.

"No." She shook her head. "No, thank you." She moved away, looking for a taxi.

The man moved with her. "You don't look too good."

Annie tried to ignore him, stepped right to the curb, and looked decisively to her right, searching for an empty taxi.

"I said you don't look very well," the man said.

She turned her head just a little to look at him, then looked quickly away again back into the traffic. She felt ill with shock, knew now for certain that her inner terrors were on show to the whole world. She longed to get the little Boots paper bag out of her handbag and open the new bottle of pills, felt she needed to swallow one down instantly if she was going to be able to make it to the station, let alone home.

"I can help you," the man said, very close to her ear.

Annie turned and started walking away. The trembling became shaking, the feeling of nausea threatened to become actual sickness. It was a cold, damp afternoon, but she felt perspiration on her forehead and upper lip. She abandoned the curb, afraid she might keel over into the path of the buses and cars, got closer to the shops, to the walls, preferring a solid wall beside her just in case, to stop her from falling.

"I know what you need," the man said.

"Go away," Annie said through gritted teeth.

"I can get you anything," he said, right behind her. "No prescription, no quacks, no questions."

"Go *away*," Annie said furiously, and anger and fear pushed some of the sickness temporarily out of her system, pumping sanity-saving adrenaline into her blood. "Get away from me or I'll call a policeman."

The man was beside her, walking at exactly her pace, and smiling. "Now, why would you do that?" he asked confidently. "I'm just offering to help you, that's all. You need help. I can see that."

Annie stopped walking, right outside a pizza parlor. "Please," she said, and tears filled her eyes. "Please, leave me alone."

"Okay," he said easily. "If you're sure."

"Yes," she said. An awful smell of onion, cheese, and cheap beef swam around her head. She thought again that she might faint.

He smiled again. "Last chance," he said. "Sure?"

"I'm *sure*," Annie said, a sob in her voice.

He nodded. "Right, then."

Annie felt the glass wall of the pizza parlor behind her, felt the weight of her two Hatchards bags anchoring her. About fifty yards away, she spotted a free taxi, wondered if she could make it if she ran.

"If you change your mind, I'll be around," he said, and walked away.

For a moment, Annie closed her eyes. Then, opening them again, she saw that the taxi was still there, stuck in traffic. A man was walking toward it from the other direction, a man in a navy blue coat, carrying a briefcase and an umbrella.

A respectable man, Annie thought. *Not a drug addict.*

Home came into her head then, Banbury Farm House, with its thatched roof, so solid and safe. And Edward. And the children.

Annie opened her mouth.

"Taxi!" It was almost a scream. People around her stared as she launched herself, like a demented diver, toward the street. She reached the cab at the same instant as the man with the briefcase. She saw his

hand reaching for the door handle and flung herself in front of him, felt the bag with the Jeffrey Archer book strike him on the shin, saw his startled, pained expression but experienced no guilt, no shame, only desperation.

She got the door open, threw her bags inside, clambered in, and slammed the door shut again.

"Paddington Station," she said, panting, and lay back against the seat.

The shame, she knew, would come later.

The Valium lasted her for one month. She called Dr. Miller's rooms, tried to persuade his assistant to post a repeat prescription to her, but the doctor had either alerted the woman or placed a note on her file, and Annie was given no alternative but to make another appointment. She was in his office two days later, clammy-handed and full of foreboding.

"No more," Andrew Miller told her, as he had said he would. "Not unless you agree to see a psychiatrist."

Annie looked at him, saw that he meant what he said.

"All right," she said. "I will."

"Good." The doctor opened his black leather address book. "I'll call her now, set up an appointment for you."

"Can't I do it myself?" Annie asked.

"No. I have to make the introduction."

"You mean you don't trust me."

Miller looked right at her. "Probably not, in these circumstances."

"Okay," Annie said. "You call."

"When for?"

"I don't have my diary with me."

"That's a pity," Dr. Miller said lightly.

"I don't. I really don't." Annie reached down to the floor for her handbag. "Look for yourself." She opened it and put it on the desk. "Please, look. I didn't bring my diary with me."

Andrew Miller's smile was kind. "I believe you, Mrs. Thomas. But it doesn't alter my decision. No appointment, no prescription."

Annie sagged. "Tomorrow," she said.

"Fine." The doctor nodded and picked up the telephone. "Though

I'd be surprised if she had a free appointment that soon." He looked at Annie's tightly drawn face, into her despairing eyes. "I'll try my best."

His best was not good enough. Annie was not certain, as she left Miller's rooms, stepped out into Wimpole Street, whether she was more or less distraught because the psychiatrist had been unable to find her a space for another three days. She had seventy-two more hours to fret over how she was going to handle the appointment, what lies she would spin to Edward if she had to, how honest she would be with the psychiatrist. Whether or not she would attend the appointment at all, and if she did, what the outcome would be. Would she come away with the only thing she wanted, needed—her precious yellow pills? Or would she be forced to endure a torture that could only be infinitely worse than the few days of attempted withdrawal she had put herself through in January?

She was not certain, later, much later, how she had reached Piccadilly Circus, whether she had taken a taxi or got on a bus or walked all the way. She could not even remember the final thought that had pushed her into that ultimate, irrevocable decision—that one flash of insanity that had risen and flickered above all the other rambling, incoherent craziness.

Once there, in that hubbub of traffic and rushing flow of people, Annie knew why she was there, what she had come for. She was looking for the man. For him or another like him. For a drug dealer.

"If you change your mind," he'd said, "I'll be around."

Annie waited outside Boots for more than an hour. From time to time, self-consciously, she checked her watch, to make it seem to most people as if she were waiting for a friend. Most people. Not the ones who would see through the facade of respectability, past the Aquascutum coat and the carefully applied, not overdone makeup, to the naked desperation beneath.

"Need any help?"

Annie looked at the man. Not the same one. This one was younger, with close-cropped fair hair, a neat beard, and no sunglasses to conceal his green, sharp eyes. A shudder passed through her, making every hair stand on end, giving her goose bumps, making even her nipples rigid beneath her Rigby and Peller handmade bra.

The man's eyes were on her face, focused hard on her.

"I said, need any help?" he asked again.

Annie became very calm. She and Edward had sailed to New York a few years ago on the *QE2*, and they'd passed through a violent storm from which they had emerged, it had seemed to them at the time, from one moment to the next. Out of surging, tumultuous waves into a peaceful, mirrorlike ocean. That was how she felt at that moment.

"Yes," she answered. "Yes, please."

They walked into Leicester Square, turned a corner into an alley, and Annie told him what she wanted, and he told her that would cost her fifty pounds, but she only had forty-seven pounds on her, plus her return ticket to Oxford, and she calculated—still marooned in that sea of temporary calm—that she needed to keep at least twelve pounds in order to get safely to Paddington Station and then from Oxford back to Stone Bridge. For thirty-five pounds she got only half of what he had been going to give her for fifty. That was the name of the game, he told her.

"Seller's market," he said, not unpleasantly.

Annie did not argue.

She vomited twice, once in the lavatory on the train, once back home in her own bathroom, and then she stood under the shower for a long time, the way she understood victims of rape often did. When she swallowed the first of her new yellow pills, she felt suddenly terrified that they might be poisonous, that they might make her ill or even kill her. But the pill just did what it always did, dulled her nerve ends, took the spikes off her feelings, made her tolerably comfortable; and after a while, she became almost happy, because she knew now that she didn't have to go to see the psychiatrist at all, that she could cancel that appointment, and that she could voluntarily cut down on what Peter Cary and Andrew Miller prescribed for her, and they would be pleased with her, and Edward would never have to know.

And in the meantime, she could have as much Valium as she wanted.

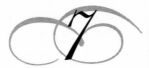

Edward thought she was ill.

"I'm worried about you," he said one rare weekday lunchtime in March—rare in that he was at home—over Marie-Louise's vegetable soup and potato cheese, served at the big pine table in their kitchen. "You look very tired, darling."

"I am a little tired," Annie admitted. It was the first time in a long while that she had been forced to keep up appearances with Edward for so many hours on end, and the strain was proving almost unbearable.

"Could you be coming down with something?"

"No, I don't think so."

"You really don't look well at all." Edward peered at her pale face and shadowed eyes more closely, leaned forward a little across the table, eyeing her over the salad bowl. "In fact you look quite dreadfully tired. Perhaps you should see Peter Cary?"

"I'm not ill, Edward."

"Just for a checkup."

"I don't need a checkup," Annie said sharply. "Please don't stare at me like that."

"All right," Edward said, surprised. "Nothing for you to get het up about." Unpersuaded, he leaned back again. "It isn't like you to get so upset about little things."

"I guess not," Annie said quietly. "I'm sorry."

"No need to apologize, darling."

"Yes," Annie said. "There is." She felt a great urge to cry, to let it all go, to unburden herself. But the memory was still there, like a warning beacon standing in her way, of Edward describing his mother's morphine addiction and the ruination of his boyhood. She could not unburden herself to Edward. Not now. Not ever.

"Annie, love." Edward reached tenderly for her hand. "What is it?"

"It's nothing," she said tightly. "I'm just overtired, as I said."

"Which was why I suggested you see the doctor." Seeing her expression, he held up his left hand. "It's all right; I know you don't want to, though I don't quite understand why. I thought most Americans believed in checkups."

"I haven't been an American for years." Annie forced a smile. "Not a real one anyway. More of a stiff-upper-lip Brit these days."

"What about a holiday?" The suggestion came carefully.

The dropping, at least for the moment, of Edward's threat to speak to Peter Cary about her flooded Annie with relief. "That might be wonderful," she said. The thought of escape flew like a scrap of heaven across her mind's eye. Blue skies, white beaches, no responsibilities, just time alone with Edward might heal her.

"Good," he said, pleased. "Where would you like to go?"

"I don't know." *Anywhere.* "How about you?"

"I couldn't go, my darling," Edward said ruefully. "I wish to God I could, but there's no time, not for a few months at least."

Heaven vanished. "Then I can't go either."

"Of course you can." Edward let go of her hand and helped himself to a second serving of potato cheese. "I expect it would do you the world of good."

Annie put her knife and fork together and stood up. "If we can't go away together, Edward," she said coolly, "then I don't want to go at all."

"Can't you sit with me till I've finished?" he asked mildly.

"No. I have things to do before Marie-Louise gets back with Liza."

"What things?"

Annie felt cornered. "All kinds of things," she said with a touch of aggression. She longed to get upstairs into the privacy of the bathroom and take a pill. She picked up her plate and the fork slithered off onto the tiled floor with a clang. "Damn," she said harshly, and bent to pick it up.

"Take it easy, darling," Edward said, looking surprised.

"I would," Annie responded, "if you'd leave me alone."

"I do," Edward said, stung. "Most of the time."

"Yes." Annie, at the sink, stared down at the globs of half-eaten potato cheese on her plate and felt sick and ashamed and yearning to cry or to go to sleep or to scream. Or to take two pills.

In silence, Edward stood up and brought his own plate over to the draining board and set it down. He looked at her, touched her right arm with one hand, but she wouldn't look back, didn't move a muscle, just went on staring down into the sink.

"I'll leave you, then," he said quietly. "Go upstairs and do some work."

Annie nodded, not trusting herself to speak.

"You're sure you're all right?" he asked one more time.

"Mm," she said, her voice stiff from the effort of holding it all in.

"See you later, then."

"Later."

When Marie-Louise brought Liza home, Annie was deeply asleep on top of their bed, and Edward, who had covered her carefully with an eiderdown, cautioned them not to disturb her. She was quite worn out, he said, and Marie-Louise—who had known for a very long time that Annie took too many tranquilizers, but who had been reminded by her parents in Switzerland at Christmas that so long as the children were being well looked after, it was not her place to interfere—kept silent. Though even Marie-Louise had not the least idea that Annie was heavily asleep because she had taken fifteen milligrams of Valium after lunch, which would in itself have knocked out a normal person for the best part of a day. Except that Annie had already swallowed ten milligrams first thing that morning, not to mention the ten she'd taken before bedtime the previous night.

Early the following Monday morning, Edward drove Annie, who had told him she wanted to go shopping, into London. She had woken up with a head and limbs so heavy that it had taken a long ice-cold shower to allow her to fix herself up sufficiently to pass muster, and what she wanted, more than anything, was to crawl back into bed and sleep forever. But the outing was necessary, even vital, for her pill supply was low, and because Edward had been home for the past week this was the first opportunity she'd had to get to Piccadilly Circus and her lifeline.

"We could have lunch," Edward said as he dropped her off outside Harvey Nichols. "I won't see you till Friday otherwise."

"Oh, Edward, I'd love to," Annie lied. Playing for time, trying to think up an instant excuse, she juggled her handbag and umbrella and the carrier bag that contained a sweater she'd told Edward she needed to exchange. "But there are so many things I have to do." Her mind was too fuzzy to come up with anything better. "Maybe I could call you later?"

"I'll be in meetings all morning." He heard hooting and glanced up into the rearview mirror. "Darling, we're blocking the traffic; I must move." He blew her a kiss as she got out of the car.

"I love you," Annie said.

She wondered, as Edward smiled and drove off into Sloane Street, why she had said that, and thought it was probably guilt. She told the children that she loved them every night at bedtime and often when she was parting from them, even for an hour or two, but it was not a custom of hers or Edward's to exchange loving remarks unless they were making love or engaged in a serious, intimate conversation. *And when did we last do either of those things?* Annie tried to remember as she forced herself into the department store, feeling hemmed in on all sides by tall, slender, daunting, confident young women, knowing that even if she managed no more legitimate shopping that day, she still had to exchange the sweater or risk having to explain to Edward why she had not.

She reached Piccadilly Circus before noon, took up her accustomed position outside Boots, and made all the usual gestures that she felt lent respectability to her pathetic waiting: shifting impatiently from foot to foot, hugging her shoulder bag close in case of snatchers, and checking her wristwatch periodically to indicate that the person she was expecting to meet was late.

When she was approached at last, it was by a young woman she had done business with twice previously. It was hypocritical and quite absurd, Annie realized, yet she remembered feeling a sense of shock and disgust the first time the woman had spoken to her because she had felt so sure that drug peddling had to be a male pursuit. She knew now that was nonsense, and the woman knew precisely what Annie wanted, and Annie knew the price, and all that needed to happen was for the cash and the black market diazepam to change hands.

They were in an alley between Piccadilly Circus and Leicester Square, and Annie was opening her bag, preparing to take out the cash she had brought with her, when the girl glanced up and her expression turned from disinterest to iron.

"Drop me in it, lady," she said softly but violently, "and you're dead."

And then she fled, ran like the wind, pushing past two men standing near the corner, and disappearing into Leicester Square. And Annie, utterly bewildered, just stood there, not knowing what had happened or what to do, and then she saw one of the men turning to follow the fleeing woman. Saw the second man coming toward her.

"Excuse me, madam," he said.

Annie knew, right away, that he was a policeman.

"I'd like a word."

Annie watched him put his hand into a pocket, knew that he was pulling out identification, and there was nothing she could do but watch the hand, watch the wallet thing with the badge and photograph, and she was numb—she was almost always numb these days, but this was different, this was worse. And as the next moments passed and the police officer spoke to her and the other man returned, without the young woman, as they asked her to come with them to the station to answer some questions, even the drug pusher's threat of murder had ceased to reverberate in her mind. One thought and one thought only rolled around and around in Annie's bleak, befuddled brain.

Edward. Edward, who still loved her, would find out the truth about her now. Poor, trusting Edward.

She began to weep soon after they got to the police station, and they were utterly genuine tears, and yet she found herself realizing with sudden and surprising clarity that the crying might just be helping her, for the officer talking to her was gentle and courteous, seemed almost sympathetic. The more incoherent she was, the more incapable of answering the policeman's questions intelligently, the clearer it became to Annie that they weren't really interested in her at all. She was just a pathetic woman with more money than sense, getting what they referred to as her Class C drugs through illegal means; but it wasn't as if she was taking heroin or cocaine or even marijuana, and even through Annie's semipermanent fog of Valium and fear she could see that what they wanted was the woman who had been going to sell it to her. And suddenly Annie Aldrich Thomas, impeccably brought up, educated, honest-as-the-day-was-long Annie, was finding the strength to lie to a British policeman, to tell him that this was a first, that she had never done it before. And she knew even then that he didn't believe her, she thought they might even have watched her before, but she kept to her barely coherent story, kept on sobbing, pleading with the officer not to tell her husband, and she had the sense that she might—just *might*—be going to get away with it.

She ought to have felt relieved. She ought to have felt like the luckiest woman on earth to have escaped with just an unofficial warning. Yet what occupied Annie's mind most as she sat, red-eyed and still shaking, in her first-class seat on the train back to Oxford, was the fact that she was returning to Banbury Farm House without her envelope of pills. All her thoughts of Edward, her fears for Edward and for their marriage, had been pushed right out of her mind now by that one fact, that single, overriding, overwhelming terror. She was going to run out of Valium.

She was going to run out of Valium, and Peter Cary wasn't going to write her a prescription just like that, and she couldn't face having to beg him, to lie to him, and she couldn't get back to London to try to talk Andrew Miller around, or, heaven forbid, to venture back into Piccadilly Circus, where the woman might just be waiting for her with a knife instead of an envelope of black-market drugs. And Annie remembered the agony of withdrawal, and she couldn't face that either, not with Marie-Louise and the children in the house.

She was going to run out of pills.

She thought, perhaps, that she could face anything rather than that.

★ ★ ★

She was standing in little Liza's nursery at four o'clock that morning, gazing almost unseeingly down at her youngest child, when it came to her. She had not yet slept at all, had forced herself to take only half her usual nighttime dose, all too conscious that from now until her next prescription, every precious milligram counted, and so Annie was comparatively calm, not sufficiently doped to be able to rest, but the jagged, fiery edges of the worst of her panic had at least been a little smoothed, damped down.

The words, spoken eleven years before in the hotel room near the hillside where her parents, their parents, had died, came back to her.

"To always being there," Jamie had said, and she had responded: "No matter what." And Olivia, the strongest of them, had drained her cognac in one gulp and added, "Come hell or high water."

They had reminded each other of their pact last summer, at their reunion up on Dukesfield Fell and, later, at Riverdale Hall, but they had spoken mostly of good things, of their achievements, of their separate lives but continuing, constant friendship in spite of their separation. Annie had been taking Valium for years by then, but that reunion had taken place only a matter of weeks before she had driven the Range Rover into the milk truck on Stone Bridge Road, the day before she had made the decision to start increasing the dosage of her tranquilizers.

On the seventeenth night of March in 1987, Annie stared down at her little girl's golden head, at her beautiful dark lashes, at the round, soft cheeks that puffed just a little with her smooth, regular, sleeping breaths, and made another decision.

"There's no place else left for me to go," Annie said very softly, and a single tear, of self-pity and shame and love and regret, ran down her left cheek and fell onto her daughter's soft, pink blanket. "I think— I really think, my beloved—this is my very last chance."

She bent down low and kissed Liza, very gently and carefully, on the top of her head, and then she went just as quietly into Sophie and William's room, and kissed them both, too, and neither of them woke either, for which she was grateful.

And then she went back into her own, Edward-less bedroom, picked up the white telephone, and lay down with it on top of their quilt, on her side, her eyes on the digital alarm clock on her bedside table.

She waited, not sleeping, not moving, even when she heard Marie-Louise getting the children up and ready for breakfast and school, and Edward had asked Marie-Louise not to disturb Annie in the mornings until she was feeling better. Most mornings, Annie liked going into her children's rooms and helping them dress, and then sitting with them at the breakfast table. But this morning, she stayed where she was, still watching the clock.

She waited until one minute past nine.

And then she called Olivia.

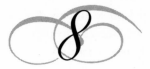

"So," Olivia said, when Annie had, at last, told them everything, "how are we going to tackle this?"

It was a little after ten o'clock at night, and the three friends were sitting in Olivia's living room: Annie, superficially neat as always in a navy cashmere two-piece, but leaning back, exhausted and drained, in an armchair; Jamie on the settee, his body language relaxed enough in jeans, sneakers, and an old Harvard sweatshirt, only the furrow between his dark eyes and the tautness of his mouth betraying his anxiety; Olivia, cross-legged on the carpet in her favorite old Norma Kamali tracksuit, the most focused and determined of them.

Annie had been in Geneva for three days.

"One thing's clear," Jamie said. "It can't be tackled overnight."

"It has to be," Annie said. "Well, not overnight, of course, but in a short time. I don't have any longer." She looked at their perplexed expressions. "I can't stay away too long without Edward finding out."

"Would it really be so terrible if he did?" Olivia asked.

"Yes."

They were in the large, comfortable apartment on the rue du Marché that Olivia had chosen on her move to Geneva as much for its location at the heart of the city as anything. Life in Switzerland was pretty heavenly so far as she was concerned. At home, she had all the comforts and luxuries of a prosperous, cosmopolitan city, yet in no time at all she could be sailing on Lac Léman or skiing at Gstaad or Verbier or crossing the frontiers into France or Italy.

It had taken three days after Annie's cry for help to make their plans and postpone their arrangements. Olivia had found it relatively easy, with the wealth of translation agencies in Geneva, to track down a satisfactory replacement for her clients. Jamie—rather less easily—had talked Carrie, his wife, into taking over two presentations and a host of meetings and lunches at Beaumont-Arias back in Boston. And Annie, racked with guilt, had lied her head off to Edward, telling him the story they'd all agreed on before she'd left home: that Olivia had some major problems of a private nature and needed support—and kind, generous Edward had volunteered to see that everything at home ran smoothly in her absence, making it possible for Annie to gather her Valium and a suitcase of belongings and get herself on a flight to Geneva.

Once Annie had begun to talk that first day, to unburden herself, it had seemed an unstoppable torrent. She'd kept it all inside for so many years, knew now that secretly she had *longed* to talk about it, had some-times even, on those rare occasions when no human being had been in the house, talked to Bella, the dog, and Leo and Boots, the two cats.

"The cats always lost interest pretty quickly," she had told Olivia and Jamie in the soft, pinkish light of Olivia's cozy, comfortingly untidy sitting room, "but Bella used to make me feel better; she used to sit at my feet and listen while I scratched her chest, and if I cried, she put her head on my knee."

"Talking to animals is good," Olivia had said, "but a little limited."

"Better than nothing," Jamie had pointed out. "Or no one."

"Except that Annie did have someone," Olivia said.

They'd all agreed on two rules of play straight off. Here, within these safe walls, while they were all together, there was to be absolute honesty. Annie was going to tell them everything, no matter how long it took and no matter how ugly it was, and Olivia and Jamie were going to talk back whichever way they saw fit. And then somehow, whatever it took, they were going to see to it that Annie's problem was dealt with. Even if the unburdening made her feel better momentarily, there would be no returning to life as it had been. Annie had come this far, and, however painful, neither Olivia nor Jamie intended to allow her to slip back.

★ ★ ★

"Why would it be so terrible if Edward did find out?" Olivia looked up at Annie from the floor, her expressive face even stronger than usual, her green eyes more penetrating. "What do you think might happen?"

Annie flushed. "He couldn't take it."

"Are you sure?" Jamie asked. "Edward's always seemed a particularly strong, stable man to me."

"And me," Olivia added.

"You're both forgetting his mother."

"Not at all," Olivia said. "But you're not his mother, Annie; you're his wife. His partner."

"He couldn't take it," Annie said obstinately. "Trust me."

"He wouldn't like it." Olivia uncrossed her legs, changed to a kneeling position. "He'd hate it—he'd be horribly upset—of course he would be. But mostly, I think, he'd be concerned for you, about you. About getting you right, having you happy and well again."

"Maybe," Annie admitted, "if it were just me and him. But I'm supposed to be the mother of his children."

"You're a wonderful mother," Jamie told her.

"I'm a drug addict. A junkie."

"No, you're not," Jamie argued. "You're dependent on tranquilizers. You've been *made* dependent on drugs by doctors who should know better."

"I'm out of control," Annie said.

"You've never harmed the children," Jamie said.

"I've risked harming them."

"How?" Jamie asked. "From what you've told us, you've taken a thousand precautions—or you did when you realized there might be a risk."

"I've still been taking care of them under the influence of drugs."

"That's true," Olivia said. "But now you want to stop. You do want to stop, don't you, Annie?"

"Yes."

"How much?"

"More than anything."

Olivia wasn't letting her off the hook. "What about withdrawal? You couldn't take it last time. Can you bear it now, do you think?"

"No, probably not," Annie said, softly. "But maybe if I'm not alone, I may stand a better chance."

Jamie stood up and walked over to the window. He pushed back one of the curtains and looked out into the rainy night. It was quiet except for the low sound of car tires swishing over the wet streets.

"We have to get professional help," he said. "We can't handle this alone."

Annie looked frightened. "What kind of help do you mean?"

"What do you think he means?" Olivia said. "We need a doctor."

"A doctor will say I should withdraw slowly," Annie said. "Go home and see a specialist in England. Let my family help me. That's what a doctor's going to say."

"And you don't want that," Olivia said.

"I can't risk it," Annie said. "I won't risk it."

Olivia went next morning, Annie's fourth morning, to visit her own doctor. Dr. Diana Brünli had originally trained in her native England, before marrying a Swiss dermatologist and resettling in Geneva. Olivia had seen the doctor only once as a patient, but they had met again at a seminar that Olivia had attended as Gilles-Breque Pharmaceuticals' interpreter. The two women had sat together at lunch and got on famously, and had since then met at least once each month for pleasure.

"If your friend insists on doing this the hard way," Diana Brünli told Olivia in her spick-and-span blue-and-white office on the rue de Lausanne, "then it really has to happen in a hospital or clinic."

"I don't think Annie wants to go to a clinic," Olivia said. "I know it doesn't make any sense, but she seems to feel that would be a greater betrayal of her husband. She knows she's been lying to Edward for so long, but she feels there are degrees of lies—actually spending time in a hospital without telling him is too much for her."

"And she won't consider telling him?"

"Absolutely not."

"You say the husband is a decent type?" Dr. Brünli asked.

"So far as I know, Edward's a pussycat." Olivia shrugged. "But then, of course, I've believed for years that Annie was perfectly happy, so for all I know, Edward might be a sadist in private."

"But you don't really believe that."

"Not for a minute."

"Which doesn't help us get over the fact," Diana Brünli said, "that your friend seems to be willing to do almost anything to stop him finding out about her dependency problem."

"Or about her withdrawal." Olivia shook her head. "Annie seems to think that with our help, she can go cold turkey and then go straight back home and carry on as if nothing ever happened. I told her—and Jamie told me I was being incredibly tactless, and I guess I wasn't exactly diplomatic—that she was talking about this as if it were a back-street abortion in the bad old days. But this isn't that simple, is it?"

"Not simple at all," the doctor agreed. "Even if Annie can make it successfully through the worst symptoms of rapid withdrawal, that won't be the end of it, not in such a long-term case. Withdrawal could go on for months. She might not feel good for a long, long time. She may never feel as good as she would like to feel. She'll need help."

"So what can you suggest?" Olivia asked. "I don't know who else to go to, Diana."

"To a specialist," Dr. Brünli replied, "who will tell you the same thing as I am—that Annie has two alternatives. Either she goes home to confide in her husband and then begins a carefully monitored long-term withdrawal with his help, or she runs the risk of crashing hard and fast in a clinic." She smiled wryly. "I don't think I have to tell you which alternative I'd recommend."

Olivia was silent for a moment.

"Could it be done at home? In my apartment?"

"The rapid withdrawal?" The doctor shook her head. "Not without risk."

"When you say risk, what do you mean? To Annie's physical health, or her sanity?"

"Both, potentially. Anything could happen; she could suffer a convulsion—it doesn't happen that often, but it does happen, and unsupervised, that can be dangerous. She could try to kill herself—"

"She wouldn't be left alone."

"She could still try, Olivia. You have a kitchen full of sharp objects.

You have windows she could jump out of." Dr. Brünli saw Olivia's shocked expression. "I don't say it's likely, but it isn't out of the question either. She could even attack one of you—aggression can be a symptom of withdrawal."

"I don't think Annie has an aggressive bone in her body," Olivia said.

Diana Brünli's smile was gentle. "But Annie in rapid withdrawal may not be much like the Annie you know."

Olivia went home and told Annie and Jamie what Diana had said.

"I don't want to go to a clinic," Annie said anxiously, as they had known she would.

"It's the only way," Olivia said, "if you want to try and do it the fast way."

"No." Annie was very pale, and her palms were perspiring. "I can't do that. I'd have to give Edward as my next of kin, and they might contact him."

"They wouldn't," Jamie said. "Not if you told them not to."

"You can't be sure of that." Annie shook her head violently. "I want to do it here," she said. "With you two. I know it's an awful lot to ask, but that's why I came to you." Her voice was rising with a touch of hysteria. "If I was going to go into a clinic, I could have done that in England. If Edward finds out that I ran away from him, that I came to Switzerland and lied to him, that'll be the end. I'll lose him and the children. I know it." She paused, and her eyes filled with tears. "I'd rather go home and carry on."

"You'd rather carry on drugging yourself to the eyeballs and lying to him that way," Olivia said bluntly.

"Yes," Annie said.

"I thought you wanted to stop," Jamie said. "More than anything."

"I do."

"Then check into a clinic," Olivia said.

"I can't," Annie said.

She took a pill and rested for a while that afternoon, and Jamie and Olivia sat in the kitchen, where they knew she couldn't hear them talking about her, and racked their brains for the solution.

"There is only one," Olivia said at last.

"Tell me," Jamie said.

"We do it here."

"But your friend said it could be dangerous."

"Not with proper supervision," Olivia said. "If we get the apartment set up carefully enough—if we find a doctor—"

"You don't think Dr. Brünli would go for it?" Jamie asked.

"I don't know. She might, or she might tell us we're nuts, or she might simply have too many commitments. Or she might help to persuade a specialist to help us."

"In other words," Jamie said, "if Annie won't go to the clinic, we bring the clinic here."

"Exactly," Olivia said.

"Oh, yes," Annie said when they told her after she'd woken up. "Oh, yes, please—oh, thank you, Livvy, thank you—"

"It might not work out," Olivia warned her.

"But you're going to try, aren't you?" She sat up on her bed.

"We'll try," Jamie said.

"How long do we have?" Olivia asked Annie. "I mean, how long before Edward starts to get restless?"

Annie swung her feet down onto the floor. "Another week. Maybe longer." She looked at them both, and her eyes were filled with new hope. "Oh, God, do you think we stand a chance?"

"I'm not sure," Olivia said.

"A week's pretty tight," Jamie pointed out. "It might take that long to fix it up. If it can be fixed up."

"It can," Annie said. "Livvy's the greatest organizer in the world. We both know that."

"I'm not so hot," Olivia said. "Just because I manage to get the three of us together every now and then doesn't mean I can set up a makeshift clinic in my home in a day or two."

"The three of us live in different countries," Annie pointed out, still with her newfound optimism. "The people you want to get here are probably all in the same city."

"Well, doesn't that make it nice and easy?" Olivia said ironically.

"You probably can do it," Jamie said. "Annie's right. If anyone can, it's you."

"Me and my big ideas," Olivia said.

It took some doing, but Diana Brünli came through for them, providing them with a doctor and two nurses "on loan" for the duration by the chief professor of a suburban clinic specializing in the rehabilitation of drug-dependent patients. Because the treatment would be carried out on uninsured private property, both Annie, as the patient, and Olivia, as the apartment's lessee, were asked to sign legal documents releasing all concerned from liability.

"It's going to cost a fortune, isn't it?" Annie asked the evening before Dr. Gianni Dressler and his team were due to arrive. Jamie was in the kitchen cooking them dinner. He'd been in there for a couple of hours, ever since he'd had a fight with Carrie, his wife, when she'd telephoned to demand to know what was taking him so long in Geneva. Jamie hated fighting with anyone, Carrie most of all, but he found cooking therapeutic, and the kitchen at home in Boston was where he regularly disappeared to when he and his wife fell out, which they did increasingly often.

"That's all covered," Olivia told her.

"I'm going to pay the bill," Annie said anxiously. "Don't you even think about paying for it, Livvy."

"You can't pay it," Olivia said. "Not unless you've changed your mind about Edward finding out. Consider it a gift from Jamie and me—you know we can afford it."

"That's not the point." Annie was sitting in an armchair in her room, twisting a paper tissue in her hands, shredding it into her lap. She'd destroyed an entire box of Kleenex in a single afternoon.

"Don't worry about the bill, Annie." Olivia, growing edgy, too, was sitting on the side of Annie's bed. "You have more important things to think about."

Annie's small smile was bitter. "You know what I need right now, don't you?"

"If you were me," Olivia smiled back, "it would be a double scotch. As it's you, I guess it's a Valium." She'd got a prescription from

Diana Brünli for some pills to tide Annie over till the controlled with-drawal could begin. "Do you want a glass of water?"

"I shouldn't." Annie's longing was almost palpably obvious.

Olivia shrugged. "If you were giving up cigarettes or alcohol from tomorrow, you'd be entitled to just one more."

"And it would be lovely to think I might sleep at least a little tonight."

Olivia stood up. "When are you calling Edward?"

"Later." Annie flushed darkly. "More lies."

"All in a good cause." Olivia had given up, for the moment, trying to talk Annie into coming clean with Edward. Maybe after the worst was over, she and Jamie had decided, they might be able to talk some sense into her, but right now there seemed little point. At the door, she looked back at Annie. "He still thinks you guys are looking after me, doesn't he?"

"Yes." Annie's voice was very soft. "I'm so sorry."

"I don't mind, Annie." Olivia was gentle. "So long as it helps in the long run. That's all that matters now."

"It has to help," Annie said, shredding the last of the tissues. "It *has* to."

Olivia opened the door. "I guess," she said, "in the last analysis, that's up to you."

Dr. Dressler—young, arrogant, and handsome, with curly black hair and violet eyes—and his nurses took over completely. It was not in Olivia's nature to take so many orders amiably, especially when a strange man was directing her to move furniture in her own apartment, to remove and lock up every pill and potion, every bottle of wine and every remotely or potentially sharp object—even glasses—to go shopping for each and every item he'd written on a list, and to be sure to bring *exactly* what he'd asked for. But Jamie was with her, and Jamie knew Olivia well enough to recognize when she was starting to get mad, and twice that first morning he thought it best to get her out of the way before she erupted, and Olivia was grateful for his help because the last thing she really wanted was to upset Gianni Dressler when it was likely he might be Annie's last chance.

★　★　★

It was a little like getting ready for a small war to break out, Jamie commented apprehensively to Olivia at one point as her windows were closed and locked, but Olivia pointed out wryly that if that were the case, this was one war they'd be sure to lose, since Dressler clearly agreed with what Diana Brünli had said about Annie's unpredictability in the grip of rapid withdrawal and had ordered every knife and fork, every pair of scissors, every hammer and screwdriver—even the needles in Olivia's seldom-used sewing kit—to be locked out of reach.

When all the preparations were complete, Dr. Dressler sat them all down together around the table in Olivia's dining room. In keeping with the precision of his other arrangements, there was nothing casual or relaxed about this piece of planning; it had all the charm and bedside manner, Olivia thought privately, of a corporate strategy meeting.

"All right," he began in the almost unaccented American English he had perfected during his time at Harvard Medical School. "Since we're all going to be in this together, I'm going to run through the kind of thing that may happen to Annie over the next week."

"I think Dr. Brünli already told us most of what to expect," Olivia said.

"Please"—Dressler flashed Olivia a sharp-eyed look of disapproval—"do me the courtesy of allowing me at least to begin before you interrupt."

"I'm sorry," Olivia said, trying to sound as if she meant it. "I was just trying to save time—because we have so little, I mean."

"Preparation," Gianni Dressler told her, still crisply but less harshly, "is all-important in cases like this. The more Annie understands about the symptoms that may affect her, the more easily she may find it to cope with them."

"Forgive me, Dr. Dressler," Jamie ventured, "but isn't there a likelihood of Annie expecting more symptoms just because you've told her to?"

"Perhaps," Dressler replied. "Nonetheless, experience has shown us that ignorance is far from helpful." He turned his face away from Jamie, away from Olivia, and deliberately focused all his attention on Annie. "Forgive us," he said, with sudden and considerable courtesy, "for discussing you as if you were not here."

"I don't mind," Annie said softly. "I really don't mind. It's a relief, in a way, to listen to other people talking about it—about my problems." Her face was pale, but her cheeks were a little flushed. "I've been so secretive about it for so long."

"And how do you feel about my telling you what you may possibly expect?"

"I want to know," Annie said instantly. "Everything. Please." She glanced at Olivia and Jamie, then looked back at the doctor. "Tell me. I need to know everything that's going to help me get through this."

The smile Gianni Dressler bestowed on Annie, Olivia thought, was very gentle and, startlingly, for such an arrogantly efficient man, almost sweet.

"Good," he said. "Now, Annie, you're not—I repeat, not—to be overly alarmed by this list of symptoms. It's extremely unlikely that you will experience all of them. We already know, of course, a little of what to expect from your previous attempt—"

"When I ended up breaking open a locked cabinet with my bare hands"—Annie tried to smile, but her mouth and voice quivered—"just to get at my pills."

"This time," Dr. Dressler said, "there will be no pills to get at." He paused. "Adrenaline can give a person unusual strength," he explained, and leaned forward in his chair. "Think about what your tranquilizers do to your system, Annie. You use them to control your anxiety, to relax yourself, physically and emotionally, to help you sleep, get you through difficult situations. Everything slows down: your heart rate, your thought processes, your movements, your breathing. They dull your senses, they calm you, and your adrenaline levels become low."

"And when you stop taking them—" Olivia, who had started to speak without thought, broke off abruptly. "Sorry," she said. "I'll be quiet."

"It's all right, Olivia," Dressler said, politer now. "I imagine you were going to say that when you stop taking tranquilizers, the opposite happens, and that's exactly right." He returned his attention to Annie. "The big problem we face in your case is that we all know you're going to try to come off your drug much too quickly, which means among other things that your heart and breathing will speed right up, your whole system will start to race, and your senses will no longer be dulled. As a consequence of that, unfortunately, you'll be having to face up to real fear, real emotion, real pain; your adrenaline levels will soar, and you'll probably think you're going out of your mind."

"And will I be?" Annie asked softly.

"No." Dressler shook his head. "Absolutely, categorically, no."

He ran them through the list of potential withdrawal symptoms, studied Annie's changing expressions as he described the more acceptable, more easily tolerable discomforts ranging from nausea and flulike symptoms to palpitations and chest pains, moving downhill to the more horrifying possibilities that might include hallucinations, aggressive outbursts, suicidal feelings, and convulsions.

When he was finished, the room was silent and Annie's face was only minimally paler than Jamie's or Olivia's.

"Any questions?" Dressler asked.

No one spoke.

"Nothing?"

"I have one," Olivia said, and her wide mouth was tightly drawn.

"Go ahead," Dressler said.

"How the hell did a drug that can do this much harm ever get to be prescribed like goddamned aspirin?"

Dressler made a small grimace. "Olivia, I'm afraid we just don't have the time to really get started on that conversation, but if we ever do have a spare few hours, I'll be glad to speak with you at length on the subject. The bottom line is that—used correctly, preferably in the short term—diazepam is a useful, safe drug."

"And if I'd thrown away that very first bottle," Annie said slowly, unhappily, "instead of stashing it in the back of my drawer, I'd be okay."

"Possibly," Dressler said. "Though you might, instead, have turned to an alternative. Drink, perhaps. Which leads me to probably the most important thing I have to tell you." He paused again, his eyes fixed hard on Annie's. "Whatever happens here in the next few days—however successful we are in getting you through the first traumatic stage—withdrawal from a long-term addiction is a long-term, ongoing problem."

"Dr. Brünli told Olivia it might go on for months," Annie said.

"There's no *might* about it," Dressler said grimly. "You know I'm not in favor of this kind of crash program, Annie, but I was persuaded it was, for the time being, the best option available and I'm determined that we will make it work for you. If I didn't believe we could be successful, I wouldn't be here." He stopped again, loading his next words heavily. "But in order for it to keep on working—in order for you to start to put your life back in shape—you're going to have to be very strong for the long haul."

"That's the real problem, then, isn't it?" Annie said, and fear shone out of her blue eyes. "I'm not strong. I never have been. If I had been, I wouldn't have gotten myself into this mess."

"That's not true, Annie," Olivia told her.

"Of course it is."

"No," Olivia insisted, then glanced at Dressler. "May I?"

"Be my guest." He sat back.

"I think," Olivia said carefully, "and Annie, you know it's true because you've told us yourself—that your real problem is not lack of strength, but that you expect too much from yourself. You're just as strong—maybe stronger—than either Jamie or I. The difference is that we both accept that we make mistakes, that we screw up, that there are things we're no good at or things that we hate to do or just *can't* do, period—"

"You can do almost everything, Livvy," Annie said.

"Me?" Olivia smiled wryly. "Don't kid yourself." She paused. "The point is that while I don't enjoy failing—who does?—I can admit to failure, I can even laugh about it, whereas you really beat yourself up about those things, refuse to let yourself off the hook." She shook her head. "For God's sake, Annie, you thought that screwing up a seating plan at one of Edward's dinner parties was a catastrophe, and we all know that Edward probably didn't give a damn and that even if he did, he adores you far too much for it to have mattered for more than a passing minute."

Dressler looked back at Annie. "Does that sound like a fair assessment to you?"

Annie nodded, a small, weak nod of her head. "I guess so."

"Do you believe what Olivia says about you being as strong as she and Jamie are?"

"No. Not really."

"I do," Jamie said quietly.

"And so do I." Gianni Dressler smiled at Annie again, one of his rare, infinitely charming smiles. "I'm not pretending for one instant that your years of deception at home have been either wise or kind. But you have been going through a sickness, Annie, for a very long time, and you have succeeded, for the most part, in continuing about your business in spite of that sickness. You have also succeeded in keeping your secret from your husband. All this you achieved by sheer determination, by a particular kind of strength."

"All you have to do now"—Olivia leaned across the table and reached for Annie's hand—"is channel that strength, that determination, into this fight."

"You can do it," Jamie said. "I know you can, Annie."

Annie was close to tears again. "I hope so."

"Do more than hope," Olivia said, gripping her hand more tightly. "This is your big chance, Annie, and I, for one, am not going to let you blow it."

Gianni Dressler rose from his chair.

"Your friends have said it for me. So, shall we begin?"

Jamie looked up at the doctor. "How do we begin?"

"By waiting," Dressler answered.

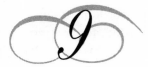

As it had been for Annie the first time she had tried to stop, for the first forty-eight hours, apart from the apprehension she felt and they all shared, nothing much of consequence happened to her.

"The diazepam is still in your body tissue," Dressler explained to Annie. "You've been taking such large doses for so long, and it's still working in your system. We have to wait for it to be gone, for the reaction to start."

"Maybe it won't," Jamie said.

"It will," Dressler said.

"Ever the optimist," Olivia commented.

"You're the linguist," Dressler said, unruffled. "I'm the doctor."

Until that day, Annie had called Edward each evening to let him know that she was well and to find out about him and the children. Tactfully, always diplomatic, Edward had asked after Olivia's invented problems, and Annie had kept her answers noncommittal, as if Olivia were in the room and might hear her. Each time he asked her those gentle, concerned questions, Annie's face grew hot with shame and guilt, and when she put down the receiver her hands were trembling and her palms sticky with perspiration.

"I'm such a liar," she had said to Jamie after one of the calls. "I'm such a terrible *liar*."

"Only because you don't want to hurt him." Jamie had tried to reassure her. "That doesn't count—it's more of a white lie."

"You don't believe that any more than I do," Annie had said.

"Sure I do," Jamie had said, but they had both known he was lying, too.

"I think it's time we switched on the answering machine," Dressler said to Olivia on the third morning. "Once Annie's symptoms start in earnest, she won't be able to handle a normal conversation with her husband."

"All right," Olivia said, her stomach sinking, and went to turn it on. They had all agreed in advance that when the time came, Jamie would field all telephone calls, would cover for Annie, explain to Edward that his wife was off somewhere outside the apartment, taking care of Olivia.

Annie became restless before lunch that day, complained of a headache, paced a good deal, asked for windows to be opened more than once so that she could breathe properly, went to the bathroom over and over again, fretful and acutely embarrassed that the key to the door had been removed, wanting privacy and solitude one moment, needing company and reassurance the next.

Edward telephoned at nine o'clock that evening, Annie not having rung him. They all heard his voice taping, calm, deep, and English, and right after the click that signaled his replacing the receiver at his end, Annie had her first full-blown anxiety attack during which she shook so hard and for so long, her teeth chattering violently all the while, that Olivia and Jamie both silently feared that she might never stop.

"Can't you do something for her?" Jamie asked Dressler.

"It will pass," the doctor answered.

"But she's so distressed," he whispered.

"There's nothing he can do," Olivia said softly, taking Jamie's arm and leading him out of the room, leaving Annie with Dressler and one of the two nurses he had now called in to assist.

For the next twenty-four hours they had their work cut out for them. The symptoms hit Annie one after the other, sometimes more than one at a time, buffeting her physically and emotionally like a kind of internal tornado. It was the way Olivia imagined it might be watching a loved one taking a beating from a gang of thugs with one's own arms tied behind one's back. Annie gasped for breath. Her speech became garbled. She ran back and forth to the bathroom, needing to pee again almost as soon as she'd gone, then suffering bout after bout of diarrhea. She paced faster and faster, grew frustrated and angry, struck at walls with her fists, kicked at a wardrobe door, splintering the corner and badly bruising her toes, yet unable to sit still long enough to allow Dressler or the nurses to look at her foot. Assailed by despair, she went into the bedroom and flung herself down on the bed, facedown, sobbing quietly for a while, and neither of the nurses seemed able to console her, so Olivia and Jamie went in, ignoring Dressler's words of caution, and sat down on either side of her. Olivia held her hands, Jamie put his arms around her, and they saw that they weren't quite reaching Annie, could still do nothing to help her, yet they thought, they hoped, in spite of her desperation, that she felt their love.

"Which might make us feel a little better," Olivia said afterward, outside the bedroom, "but does her damn-all good."

"It may be what makes all the difference in the long run," Jamie said quietly. "It's love she's going to need more than anything."

"Annie's never been short of love," Olivia said, "but it didn't stop her getting into the state she's in now."

"I know." Jamie shared her wretchedness. "God, don't I know."

The telephone rang again, and this time it was Carrie, her voice extra cool and clipped because Jamie hadn't called her all day and she still didn't know when the hell he was coming back to Boston, and perhaps if his *friends*—she underlined the word with sarcasm—could spare him five minutes, he might find time to call her at the office?

"Maybe you should call her right back," Olivia suggested, seeing Jamie's anxious face.

Jamie shook his head. "She's in the mood to fight," he said. "I'm not."

"Things not so great with you two." It was not a question.

"Things aren't easy," he admitted.

"Have they ever been?"

"No." Jamie mustered a smile. "But I still love her."

"Then she's a lucky woman," Olivia said.

"I'm not sure she'd agree with you."

"Then she's also a fool."

★   ★   ★

Annie slept for a while that night, fitfully, waking up each time escaping from the clutches of some black, not quite identifiable nightmare. Alternately she shivered and begged for blankets, then sweated, drenching her nightdress and pleading for the windows to be opened. Olivia and Jamie took turns sitting with one of the nurses, while Dressler slept on the couch in the living room.

A little after five in the morning, she got out of bed, heading for the bathroom, but the walls seemed to close in on her and the floor was tilting, and she cried out and stumbled to the floor, and Olivia and the nurse helped her back to the bed, and Annie started to weep, and Olivia realized, with the most intense pity, that she had wet herself, and she was thankful beyond words for the nurse's calm presence, because though she would not have minded one scrap changing Annie's nightdress and bed linen, she knew that Annie could not have borne it.

"She seems more comfortable this morning," Jamie said to one of the nurses, a young Swiss woman named Ruth with blond hair and blue eyes who reminded him a little of how Annie had looked in her late teens. "Or is that just wishful thinking?"

"I know you wish it," Ruth said gently. "And it's true, at least for now."

"But that doesn't mean it's over."

"No," she answered. "I'm sorry." She paused. "Martina, my colleague, told me it was not a good night for Annie."

"No," Jamie said. "It wasn't too good."

"Annie has very fine friends," Ruth said, and smiled at him.

"Thank you," Jamie said.

Twenty minutes later, Annie walked into the kitchen, where Olivia was drinking a cup of coffee.

"Hi," Olivia said, looking up at her.

Annie didn't answer. If she had been pale before, now she was almost as white as chalk. Even her lips seemed bleached to cream. Her eyes stared at Olivia, but Olivia felt she was not seeing her.

"Annie, what's wrong?" She put her cup down on the table and stood up, moving slowly, sensing she needed to be very careful. "Annie, what is it?"

Annie went over to the sink, put out her right hand, and touched the stainless steel with her index finger. Then she took away the hand and gazed at the finger.

"Annie?" Olivia felt uncertain what to do. Gianni Dressler was on the telephone in her bedroom and she hadn't seen either Ruth or Martina for a while. She had believed one of them had been with Annie.

"It doesn't feel like me." Annie spoke at last in a hushed, scared voice.

"What doesn't?"

"This." Annie held out her hand. "Or this." She reached up and touched her own cheek. "Nothing feels like me."

"You mean you're numb?" Olivia asked gently, trying not to let her own fear show. "What do you mean, Annie?"

"I don't know." Annie was still staring the same vacant stare. "I don't *know*." Her eyes wandered around the kitchen, then seemed to fix on the wall facing her. "I was sitting down, and I think I was asleep for a while. And then I woke up and I wasn't me. I wasn't inside myself anymore."

"Okay," Olivia said. "It's okay, Annie." Still moving slowly, she went over to her friend and took her arm. There was no response. "I know what this is, and so do you." Gently, she pushed Annie over to the table and down onto one of the chairs, meeting no resistance. "You remember when Dressler told us the things that might happen—you remember, Annie?"

Annie shook her head.

"There was something called depersonalization—I think that's what it was called." Relief flooded Olivia as she remembered what the doctor had said. "It's very common when your anxiety level goes too high. It'll stop, it'll go away when you calm down again."

"I'll go away," Annie said softly, but the fear was still there. "That's how it feels, like I've gone away."

"No, Annie," Olivia said more firmly. "That's not what I mean." She looked over at the door, wondered if she should call for help, decided that would only panic Annie more. An idea struck her. "Give me your hand." Annie did not budge, so Olivia took the hand herself. "You feel me touching you?"

Annie gave a tiny shrug.

Olivia pinched the skin on the back of the hand. "You feel that?"
Annie blinked. "I think so."

Olivia put down the hand again, then reached up and suddenly, quite hard, pinched Annie's cheek instead.

"Ouch," Annie said.

Olivia smiled.

"See?" she said. "You're still here."

"I thought I was going crazy," Annie said to Dressler a little later. "I've had similar things happen to me before, but never nearly as frightening." She looked weakly at Olivia. "A long time ago, when you and I were having lunch in Harrods, I had a panic attack that was a little like that—remember, I told you I was ill?"

"Sure, I remember," Olivia said. "I only wish I'd known what you were really going through."

"It's a normal effect of withdrawal," Dressler told Annie. "It's unpleasant, as I warned you it might be, but you have to try to remind yourself that it is perfectly normal under the circumstances, and you are not going crazy."

"Maybe I shouldn't have pinched her," Olivia said.

"Why not?" Dressler asked easily. "It didn't really hurt her, and it worked, didn't it?" He gave a small smile. "I shouldn't make a habit of it, though."

The telephone rang, but Olivia, having grown accustomed to not answering it, stayed where she was.

"It's Edward," Annie said, even though they couldn't hear the machine from the kitchen, where they still were.

"Could be anyone," Olivia said. "Could even be for me."

"It's Edward," Annie said positively.

"He won't call again till this evening, will he?" Olivia asked.

Annie stood up. "I want to talk to him."

"If it was him," Dressler said, "it'll be too late."

"I want to talk to Edward." The despair was back in her tone. "I want to see Edward."

"Are you certain about that?" the doctor asked her quietly. "If you are, I'm all for it."

Annie sat down again. "I miss him," she said. "I miss my children."

"I know," Olivia said.

Annie stood up again. "I'm going to call him."

Olivia was startled. "You're going to tell him?"

Annie stared down at her, and her eyes were suddenly cold. "I want to talk to my husband. Why don't you want me to do that?"

"I do." Olivia glanced uncertainly at Dressler, who gave her the smallest, hardly perceptible, shake of his head. She thought he was reassuring her, but she wasn't sure. "Of course I want you to talk to Edward, Annie. It was you who wanted him kept in the dark."

"I don't know what you're talking about, Olivia." Still, the same coldness. "I only know I want to speak to him." She began to walk out of the room.

"Annie?" Olivia stood up, looked down at Dressler for help.

"Let her go," he said.

"But what if she calls him? This isn't really Annie, is it? It's part of the withdrawal, isn't it? If she calls him, it'll all be for nothing."

"It's certainly another part of withdrawal," Dressler agreed. "But if she calls him, I'd say it was the best thing in the world, for her and for him. For the whole family."

Olivia sat down again. "You're right, of course."

Annie did not call Edward. Halfway to the telephone, she experienced another attack of dizziness, felt as if she were choking, felt violently nauseous, and had to be helped to the bathroom by Ruth and Jamie. By the time she had recovered again, not only had the desire to speak to her husband left her, but she was utterly appalled that she could even have thought about calling him.

"Please," she begged Olivia, clutching at her arm, "please don't let me call him. You mustn't let me talk to him—I don't care if you have to lock me up."

"Okay," Olivia soothed her. "We won't let you call, not if you don't want to. You don't have to worry about Edward—he's fine, and the children are all fine, too. Jamie spoke to him last night, remember?"

"He didn't tell him anything, did he?" The naked fear was still in Annie's eyes. "Oh, God, he mustn't tell him."

"Jamie knows that. He hasn't told him anything except what we arranged. Stop worrying about Edward, Annie. There's nothing to worry about."

"I just love him so much," Annie said.

"I know you do," Olivia said.

Just before three o'clock that morning, Annie woke up out of a shallow, restless sleep and saw a large coiled snake, dark brown and gleaming, lying on the big square pillow beside her face. She screamed so loudly that not only Martina and Jamie, who were with her in the bedroom, but also Olivia and Dressler, both camped out in the living room, came running.

"Take it away!" she pleaded piteously, on her knees over by the window, cowering, covering her eyes. "Oh, God, please take it *away!*"

Jamie, beside her on the rug, tried to put an arm around her shoulders, but she shrieked again and flung his arm away as if it had burned her. "Annie, sweetheart, what is it? What did you see?"

"The *snake!*" Her hands still covered her face. "On the pillow—get it away from me, please!"

"It's gone, Annie." Dressler, grim-faced but calm, spoke loudly and firmly. "Annie, uncover your eyes and look." He waited. "Annie, uncover your eyes right *now.*"

It was the first time any of them had heard him raise his voice, but it worked. Annie took her hands away from her face, and her eyes were as huge and saucerlike as a small, terrified child's as she stared disbelievingly at the bed and saw that there was, indeed, nothing there.

"Where is it?" she whispered.

"There was no snake," Dressler told her.

"There was." Annie's breathing was rapid, painful sounding. "It was right beside me, there on the pillow."

Dressler went over to her, indicating with a small nod to Jamie that he should leave her side. "There was no snake, Annie," he said again. "It wasn't real. It was just a hallucination." He sat down on the floor beside her, cross-legged and easy, like an old companion. "Remember I told you you might get hallucinations."

Annie looked at him. "But it was so real."

"I'm sure it was." The doctor smiled at her. "With some people, it's spiders, with some it's monsters. Many people just see weird faces hovering over them while they're lying in bed." He paused. "Want to talk about it?"

She shook her head and shuddered.

"How about some warm milk, then?"

Annie looked back toward the bed, became more conscious of the others in the room, saw Olivia's pale, concerned face. "Has it really gone, Livvy?" she asked, still childlike, needing more reassurance from someone she knew better than the doctor.

Olivia went to the bed, picked up the two white pillows, held them up for Annie to see, turned them over, then drew the quilt back so that she could see the clean white sheets beneath.

"Okay?" she asked. "Nothing there."

Annie nodded slowly. "Okay."

Dressler got up, helped her to her feet, and she stumbled and almost fell down again because her legs were so weak, so like jelly, and her stomach was churning and the relief at knowing there was no snake was already gone, and in its place was the most intense shame.

"Don't do that," Dressler told her quietly.

"Do what?" Annie asked.

"Feel embarrassed or ashamed," he said.

She looked at him. "How can I not?"

"Feel proud instead," he said simply.

"Proud?" She was incredulous.

"That snake was a symptom of withdrawal. You're in withdrawal because you've quit, because you've stopped taking the drug. That's good reason for pride."

Annie considered being proud of herself for about ten seconds. And then she made a dash for the bathroom and threw up instead.

"What next?" Olivia asked Dressler later, after Annie had been persuaded back to bed and had, at last, fallen asleep.

"Couldn't say."

"More snakes?" She ran a hand abstractedly through her thick dark hair.

"Maybe. Or not."

"Might the worst be over?"

"I doubt that very much."

Olivia found herself mentally rerunning the symptom list Dressler had gone through six, or was it seven, days ago? It seemed to her that Annie had already endured far more than her fair share of what had been on that list, yet suddenly she realized there might, after all, be a lot more to come.

"Tell me again, Doctor," she said. "Annie doesn't have to go through everything you described, does she?"

"Of course not." Dressler looked tired. "And I think, if you don't mind, that you could call me Gianni."

"Okay," she said. "You look tired, Gianni."

"So do you."

"Do you think it would be okay if we slept for a while now?"

Dressler glanced at his wristwatch. "I'd say that was a good idea. Jamie and Martina are still in there with Annie, so she's perfectly safe." He paused. "He should get some rest, too."

"The snake thing really freaked Jamie," Olivia said, and gave a small smile. "He hates them, you know. I think it made him even more protective of Annie, which was why he refused to give up his shift."

"He's a very good friend," Dressler remarked. "He's obviously intelligent and articulate, yet he knows when to be silent and lend support." He glanced at her. "Is there something going on between you two?"

"Between Jamie and me?" Olivia was startled. "Of course not."

Dressler shrugged. "Why not? You're both very attractive people, and you seem unusually close."

"He's married, for one thing."

"Not especially happily, though," Dressler said.

"Not all the time, maybe," Olivia said, "but he still loves Carrie."

Dressler was right, of course, in a way. She had always, all the way back to their school days, found Jamie attractive, but she hadn't thought about him in that sense for years. Jamie had fallen hard for Carrie, and Olivia had never suffered from a shortage of available or eager male companionship, but even if Jamie had remained single and free, she had long since resolved that the closeness of their particular friendship was too precious to take risks with.

"Do you think we are doing the right thing for Annie?" Olivia asked Dressler, her thoughts returning to the grim situation they were all enduring, fresh doubts and weariness suddenly threatening to over-whelm her. "I mean I know you and Diana both said this isn't the ideal way."

"It's a lousy way," Dressler said bluntly. "But the only one there was."

"What really scares me—" Olivia stopped.

"Yes?"

Olivia looked at him. "What's going to happen when Edward finds out? I mean, he will find out somehow, sometime. They do have a close bond. At least I always thought they did—Annie says they still do."

"You're afraid he might not forgive her?" Dressler asked.

"Of course." Olivia shook her head. "If it were me—if it were my marriage, and if I found out that my partner hadn't had enough faith in me, hadn't trusted me enough to share something so—so *crucial*—I don't think I could forgive. Or maybe I could forgive, but I'd certainly never forget."

"You're not Annie's husband," Dressler said.

Olivia looked at him curiously. "What about you? If it were your wife."

"I'm not married," he said.

"But if you were."

"I'm not sure." Dressler took a moment. "I know more about this kind of problem than most men, so I should have greater under-standing. Yet if I'm candid with you, Olivia, if I were in a relationship I believed entirely honest and open, I think I would find it hard to get over."

"And you're a doctor." Olivia's heart sank. "Edward's just a man."

"And an Englishman at that," Dressler said.

Through the daylight and twilight hours of the seventh day, Annie saw no more snakes, faced no specially traumatic assaults on her sanity. She had a bad pain in her jaw, which Gianni Dressler explained was a com-monly experienced kind of neuralgia severe enough sometimes to have patients begging dentists to extract all their teeth; if it became unbear-able, he told Annie, he could give her something to relieve it, but Annie told him no, partly because having got this far she wanted no more drugs, and partly because the pain, at least, was real, not imag-ined—was something tangibly bad for her to focus on, for her to fight.

"It's the first symptom I've had that hasn't made me feel as if swal-lowing a Valium might take it away," she explained, holding the left side of her face with the lightest possible touch, since anything firmer made it worse. "I know it's happening because of the withdrawal, because you tell me it is, but it doesn't feel that way. Does that make sense?"

"Perfect sense," Dressler said. "And it's a good, healthy response, Annie. More reason to be proud of yourself."

Annie managed a tiny smile, then winced as the pain bored through her jaw again. "How long does it usually last?" she asked. "I wouldn't want you to think I'm that brave, or some kind of masochist."

"It shouldn't last too long, hopefully."

"This isn't the most exact of sciences, is it?" Annie said ruefully.

They might all have preferred it if the pain had gone on. But instead, just after nine-thirty that evening, Annie had a convulsion. They were all in the sitting room—Annie with her feet up on the bigger of the two sofas, Jamie and Ruth on the other, Dressler in the armchair closest to Annie, Olivia on the rug—watching CNN Headline News. Annie had found some relief for a while from the neuralgia by applying an ice pack to her jaw, but then she'd become shivery and complained of the cold, so Ruth had covered her with a blanket. There was a sense of comparative peace in the room for the first time. They all felt it, were all tentatively optimistic, even Dressler.

"I'm so hot," Annie said suddenly, and kicked the blanket away.

Ruth started to stand up, but Dressler stopped her with a gesture.

"You okay, Annie?" he asked her from where he sat, his tone easy, calm.

"No." Her voice was fretful, like a sick child's.

"What's up?" Olivia asked her gently, taking her cue from the doc-tor, trying not to overreact despite the warning prickle on her spine.

"How about some water?" Jamie asked.

It happened so swiftly. Annie gave a single sharp cry, then tumbled from the sofa onto the floor, twitching and jerking. Jamie and Olivia both leaped to their feet in alarm, but Dressler and Ruth were already at her side.

"It's all right," Dressler told them. "Nobody panic."

"She isn't breathing." Jamie stared down at Annie's chest, saw that it wasn't moving. "Doc, she isn't *breathing.*"

Olivia got down on her knees, trying to reach Annie, but Dressler pushed her away.

"Keep clear." It was an order. "She'll be fine."

"Do something!" Olivia felt her own heart pounding. "Her mouth—shouldn't you stop her biting her tongue?" Dressler ignored her. "For God's sake, Gianni, why don't you *do* something?"

The jerking stopped. Annie's whole body seemed to slump into relaxation, and Olivia and Jamie watched a stain forming on the back of her dressing gown as she urinated involuntarily.

"Oh, God," Olivia said softly, and Jamie turned away.

Dressler pronounced Annie safe and well, and aside from a feeling of confusion and disorientation and a slight headache, she did seem to have suffered no serious ill effects. But less than three hours later, she had a second convulsion in the bedroom, no longer, no more superficially harmful, but this time, when Dressler emerged from the room to speak to Jamie and Olivia, they could see that his expression had altered.

"I'm concerned about her."

"Why? What's wrong?" Olivia asked.

"Two seizures in such a short space of time. I don't like it."

"But you told us she might have convulsions," Jamie said anxiously. "What's worrying you?"

"I told you that convulsions can happen in rapid withdrawal," Dressler agreed, "and neither of these were prolonged—" He paused. "I've decided to admit Annie to my clinic."

"You can't," Olivia said. "She doesn't want that."

Dressler's violet eyes were keen and clear and decisive. "If Annie were to have a more prolonged seizure," he said, "without prompt emergency treatment, it could be fatal."

"Shit," Jamie said, and looked at Olivia.

Olivia thought about Annie and her greatest fears of all, of Edward finding out, of losing his confidence, his trust, his love. Of losing him and even her children. And then she looked at Gianni Dressler and his last four words jangled in her head. *It could be fatal.*

No contest, she thought.

"What are we waiting for?" she said.

10

*E*dward *arrived the following evening.*

No one had told him. The admission to Dressler's clinic had gone smoothly; Annie's insistence that her husband not be informed had been respected. But in all the panic, Jamie, whose role it had been to see that all Edward's calls were returned and the sham continued, had forgotten to phone England, and shortly before ten that morning Edward had rung again. The trouble was that Olivia—fresh from the relief of knowing that Annie was safely tucked up in a hospital bed and of having her apartment to herself again—had picked up the telephone without waiting for the machine to take over.

"Olivia?" The man's voice had sounded surprised.

"Yes." It had taken her a full two seconds to realize who it was. Her right hand flew to her mouth and she screwed her eyes shut in anguish at her stupidity and carelessness.

"Olivia, it's Edward Thomas speaking."

Olivia took her hand away from her mouth. "Hello, Edward." She knew her voice sounded strained. "How are you?"

"I'm very well, thank you. How are *you*, more to the point?"

"I'm fine." *Oh, Lord,* she thought. She was supposed to be the one with problems, the reason Annie was in Geneva. Her mind raced. "Actually, I'm not that great, really."

"So I gathered from Annie."

Olivia waited for the next, the obvious question.

"Is Annie there, please, Olivia?" Edward asked.

"No, Edward." *Shit,* she thought. "Not at the moment."

"Only I haven't spoken to her in days, as you know."

"Yes." Her brain, usually reasonably agile, seemed to have turned to mush. Guilt, she decided. She had never been much good at telling lies.

"In fact, the only person I've spoken to has been James Arias."

Olivia knew he was onto them, onto something, anyway. "Jamie's been the only one here, Edward." She paused. "You know, because of the problems I've been having."

"So Annie has been with you, has she?"

"Yes. Of course. She's been great."

"Annie's very fond of you, Olivia," Edward said. "I hope she's been having a bit of a break, too. She was exceptionally tired before she left, you know."

"I know." At last, here was something to latch on to. "That's why she's not here this morning," she said quickly. "She's having some time to herself."

"Good. Shopping, I imagine."

"I expect so. Probably buying presents for you and the children. How are they?"

"They're wonderful," Edward replied, then paused. "I'm glad to hear you sounding so well, Olivia. I rather had the impression from Annie that you were quite under par."

"I was." Olivia thought about Annie in the clinic. She had not the slightest idea yet how long she might be there, whether she would be coming back to the apartment with Dressler and his nurses, or whether that was all over now for keeps. "I still am, a little," she added for good measure.

"Anyway," Edward said, wrapping the call up, "will you ask Annie to call me as soon as she gets back? I'm in London."

"I will," Olivia said.

"Tell her I miss her," Edward said. "I mean, I want her to take the time she needs, but I do miss her very much. So do the children, especially Liza—well, all of them, really."

"I'll tell her," Olivia said, guilt making her feel slightly sick.

"Thank you, Olivia." He paused again. "You'll make sure she calls me, won't you, please?"

"Of course. When I see her."

"Good talking to you again. I wish you well."

"Thank you, Edward."

Olivia hung up. *Hell,* she thought. *Bloody, bloody hell.* He was already suspicious. If he didn't hear from Annie by lunchtime, he'd know that something was up. Christ, she felt so *ashamed*—of lying to Edward, of not lying well enough. Most of all she felt ashamed of letting Annie down so badly.

She looked down at the telephone, thought about the nice, caring, sensible, clever man at the other end. *If it were me,* she thought, *I know what I would do.*

He came after leaving two more messages on the machine and receiving no response, from his wife or from Jamie or Olivia. Instinct drove him to organize his plane reservation, to leave one final message in a strong, clear voice, telling whoever might be listening that he would be flying to Geneva that evening—instinct and sudden fear, though he was uncertain exactly what he was frightened of. Something was wrong with Annie, he knew that much, though what he did not know. She might be ill. She might be having an affair. She might be wanting to leave him and be working out—with her two old friends and, perhaps, some Swiss lawyer—the best way of going about it. She might simply be sick of living with him. Edward didn't really believe that was it—for all the strain he had noticed in her face recently, for all the weariness one of his sisters-in-law and some of their neighbors and friends had remarked on, he had continued always to observe the love in Annie's eyes. Not just for Sophie and William and little Liza. It was still there for him, too, he was certain. Almost certain. He suspected, somehow, that his first fear was the right one. And the worst.

Annie, his beloved Annie, was ill.

"How could you?" he asked Olivia at the airport, when she had told him, as gently and carefully as possible, that Annie was in a clinic but that she was in no danger. "How could you even *dream* of not telling me my own wife was ill?"

He was walking fast, sweeping toward the exit, desperately upset but crisp and determined that nothing and nobody was going to keep him from Annie for a single moment more than was absolutely necessary.

"Edward, please listen." Olivia strode beside him and tried to take his arm to slow him down, but he shook her off. "Edward, there's more you don't know—things you have to know before you see her."

"More?" He ground to a halt, his eyes filled with new fear. "What more?"

"Can we sit down somewhere? Have a cup of coffee?"

"Coffee?" Edward laughed harshly. "If you think I'm going to waste time drinking coffee while my wife's lying in some hospital bed, you must be mad." He started walking again, then stopped abruptly and took hold, quite roughly, of Olivia's left arm. "How ill is she?" His gray eyes bored into hers. "Tell me the truth, Olivia. I need to know the absolute truth."

"I agree," Olivia said softly. "But we have to go somewhere and sit down quietly so that I can tell you everything. It can't be done in the back of a taxi on the way to the clinic." She paused. "And I swear to you, Edward, on everything that's ever been important to me, Annie is not in danger—not in the way that you think, anyhow." She saw the confusion, the fresh alarm in his face. "Come on," she said very gently, "and I'll tell you."

"Oh, God," he said when she'd finished. "Oh, my God."

Olivia said nothing, just sat back against the vinyl seat and watched his devastated expression in the dim light of the bar. Edward had downed a malt whisky while she had been speaking, and she was pretty sure he needed another, but she thought she should keep silent now, knew that she had said enough. More than enough.

"I don't know what to say," he said very softly. He looked at Olivia directly for an instant, and she saw that there were tears in his eyes, and then he looked away again. "If it's any help to you—" He stopped and cleared his throat, blinked hard and began again. "If it's any help to you, I don't blame you or Jamie—I accept—I think I can accept—that you thought you were doing the right thing by Annie."

"No," Olivia said. "We didn't think we were doing the right thing at all. We just came to see that it was the only possibility she would consider. All the others were even worse, even more dangerous."

"Like telling me, you mean." Bitterness arrived in Edward's tone.

"No, Edward. That was never a possibility. Not in Annie's eyes."

"Because she thought she might lose me."

"Yes."

"How could she think that?" He shook his head, still dazed. "How could she think such a thing about me?"

"I don't know," Olivia said. "But I'm afraid she did." She hesitated. "I think—"

Edward looked piercingly at her. "Yes?"

"Nothing."

"Olivia, what do you think? Tell me. Please."

She took a breath. "I think it might have had something to do with your mother."

They went together to the clinic. Edward saw Gianni Dressler first, spent ten minutes with him, then went to Annie's room. Jamie was sitting in a chair between the bed and the window. He rose as Edward walked in, put out his right hand with automatic courtesy, then dropped it back to his side as the other man gave him the briefest of nods and passed him.

Olivia, at the open door, caught Jamie's eye, gestured to him to come out into the corridor. And then she saw Annie's face. It was almost ghostly white with shock, and her blue eyes, catching Olivia's for a second, were loaded with condemnation.

Jamie came out, and they closed the door. Dressler was a few feet away, watching them.

"It's the best thing," he said to them both. "You know that, don't you?"

"You didn't see her face just now," Olivia told him.

"It's still the best thing," Dressler insisted. "Believe me."

"I thought she knew," Jamie said. "I've been sitting with her for more than two hours, and she never asked where Olivia was, never asked after Edward, and she never really slept, hardly even dozed. I was convinced she realized he was on his way. But then, when he walked in—"

"Annie's been keeping this secret from him for virtually their entire marriage," Dressler said, "and now she's been found out. This has been

her greatest nightmare, along with what may or may not happen next."
He paused and gave them a smile of great warmth. "Whichever way it
goes, you two good friends, you two very nice people, it's still Annie's
only realistic way forward."

"I guess we knew that anyway," Olivia said.

"That doesn't make it any easier for Annie, though, does it?"
Jamie said.

"How are you feeling?" Edward asked Annie, sitting on the side of the
high hospital bed, holding her icy right hand in both his.

"Not too bad." Annie's voice was so quiet it was almost inaudible.

"Dr. Dressler tells me you're doing very well."

"He tells me the same thing."

"He seems a good man."

"He is." Annie swallowed hard. "You mustn't blame him. He
wanted you to know. I wouldn't let him tell you. I wouldn't let Olivia
or Jamie tell you either."

"No. I know." Edward paused. "I don't blame any of them."

"Just me," Annie said.

"Just myself," Edward said.

She was appalled. A tinge of color crept back into her cheeks.
"You can't, Edward. You can't possibly think that you have anything
to blame yourself for."

"I'm your husband," he said simply. "We've been married for six
years. We have three children. Yet you've felt unable to share your
pain with me. I'd say that means I have rather a lot to blame myself
for."

"No." Annie took her cold hand from his, saw its tremor, tucked
it, ashamed, beneath the covers. "Please, Edward, don't do this to me.
Not on top of everything else."

"Do what?" He was newly confused. "What do you mean?"

"Don't try taking my guilt away from me."

"But you have no reason to feel guilty."

"Edward, please." Her eyes filled with tears. "Please let me."

"Let you what, darling?" he asked. "I don't understand what you
want."

"I want—" She broke off, her mouth trembling, swallowed down the sob building in her throat, tried again. "I've waited too long for this moment. I need it."

"What do you need, Annie?"

"I need you to blame me, Edward. I need you to blame *me*. Not yourself. I'm the guilty party here—*me*. This is all my fault. All my doing. My weakness brought me here, my pathetic weakness and my deceit." She gathered a little strength. "Suppose I'd been hiding a lover all these years instead of bottles of pills. Imagine I'd finally plucked up the courage to try to dump him for the sake of our marriage—"

"There's no comparison—"

"Edward, please, let me," she pleaded. "It isn't so very different— well, of course it is, because there's never been anyone else. I've never *wanted* anyone else and I never will—but still, try and listen to what I'm saying."

"I'll try."

She gritted her teeth despite the nausea that was threatening to overwhelm her again. "Imagine that I'd come here to ask Livvy and Jamie to help me get over my lover, and let's take it a step further— imagine I'd found it too hard, too unbearable and maybe I'd done something really stupid—taken an overdose or something—and you'd come and found me here in this clinic now." She paused. "Would you still feel you were to blame?"

"No, of course not." Edward shook his head. "But Annie, darling, you can't—you really, honestly can't compare taking too many tran- quilizers with taking a lover."

"I don't just take too many tranquilizers, Edward," Annie said, quite brutally. "I'm an addict."

"Valium's not exactly heroin, Annie."

"I've bought it from pushers on the street," she said. "I've even been arrested for it." She saw the horror on his face. "I was never charged—they weren't all that interested in me really. But still."

They were both silent for a few minutes. Annie stared down at the white hospital quilt covering most of her body. Edward looked at the wall, seeing nothing, isolated with his thoughts.

"Can I ask you something?" he said at last.

"I wish you would. Ask me anything you want."

"Did my telling you about my mother make a difference?" He

paused. "You were going to tell me about the pills, weren't you? Before I told you about her morphine addiction."

Annie could not look at him. "I might have. I was planning to."

"And I made you afraid to," Edward said quietly. "Oh, dear God."

He stood up and walked over to the window. The curtains were drawn, and he lifted one back a little way and stared out into the night. His thoughts, Annie's words, seemed to be roaring in his mind, filling his brain, overloading it. He was, had always been a controlled man, but suddenly he felt as if he wanted to weep, even to scream.

"Edward?"

He heard her voice, weaker suddenly, desperately afraid, but he did not, could not seem to, turn around.

"Edward, what is it?" She was newly frightened. "What have I said?"

"Nothing," he said, with an effort, then turned back to face her. "Nothing at all, Annie."

"Yes, I have." She was staring up at him, curiously, fearfully. "I've upset you somehow. Talking about your mother. You don't want to talk about her, obviously, otherwise you would have done so years ago. I'm sorry, Edward, I just wanted to try to explain. I need to at least *try*—"

"I know." He came and sat down on the bed again. "But you're very tired now, darling. I can see it, hear it. You have to rest—you have to sleep. The doctor told me not to exhaust you and I'm afraid I have."

"No," Annie said. "I mean, yes, I am tired, but I don't care about that." Her eyes sparkled with tears. "I've missed you so much. I thought I had to do this without you—you have to believe I thought I had no choice."

"I do believe that." He stood up again. "You have to sleep now, Annie."

"I will." The fear was still there. "Where will you be?"

"At the Des Bergues."

"And you'll come tomorrow?"

"Of course I'll come." His face was full of reassurance as he bent to kiss her, first on her forehead, then on her mouth. "Try not to fret too much, my darling. Tomorrow we'll speak to Dr. Dressler together, and he'll tell us exactly what we have to do to get through this, how to get you completely well again."

"It might take some time," Annie said.

"I imagine it might," Edward said. "But we have the time."

She lay back against the pillows, tried desperately to muster a smile for him, but failed. "I'm sorry, Edward," she said, very quiet again. "I'm so very sorry for everything."

"Me, too," he said.

Olivia slipped back in to see Annie after Edward had left. Jamie had offered to go with him to the hotel, and Edward had thanked him but told him a little stiffly that he could manage very well on his own, so Olivia had asked Jamie to go back to her apartment and rustle up something simple to eat because she didn't think she could face a restaurant that night.

Annie was still awake, and though she told Olivia that Edward had been wonderful, Olivia could see that she was still fretting about something.

"I'm not leaving until you tell me."

"Oh, Livvy, there's nothing to tell. Nothing real, at least. Just more of my imaginings."

"Share them with me anyway," Olivia encouraged gently.

Annie sighed. "We were talking about it, or trying to, and then—"

"Then?"

"We talked about his mother."

"And?"

"And it was all right, for a moment or two anyway. And then suddenly he got up and walked away, over to the window, and he seemed to shut down. It was as if he couldn't bear to talk anymore, not just about her or his childhood, but about anything."

"He was probably exhausted," Olivia said.

Annie smiled wryly. "That's why he said we should stop, because I was too tired to go on."

"He had a point. You look wrecked."

"I guess I am."

"And Edward's had a tough day." Olivia looked at Annie's frightened eyes. "Oh, Annie, sweetheart, don't give yourself such a hard time." Olivia felt a stab of the greatest pity for her friend. "Edward's right about you being exhausted. You're still in the midst of early withdrawal and you've had to confront what you were most frightened of. What you need right now is to go to sleep, and I mean real sleep, not just lying there with your eyes closed."

"Olivia's absolutely right," Gianni Dressler said from the doorway.

"I don't think I can sleep," Annie said.

"Then we'll do something to help you," Dressler told her.

"I thought you said no drugs," Olivia said.

"I don't want to go backward," Annie said anxiously.

"And I don't intend to let you," the doctor reassured her.

"You really do need some proper rest," Olivia said to Annie, standing up.

"Leave that to me," Dressler told her, then turned to Annie. "And you can trust me not to set you back. All right?"

"Yes," Annie said softly. "Thank you."

"Olivia?" Dressler looked back at her. "With the greatest respect"— he smiled at her—"please get out of here."

Olivia smiled back at him. "I'm leaving."

"Now."

Olivia blew Annie a kiss and opened the door. "Call us in the morning when you're awake."

"Go," Dressler said.

"I've gone."

Olivia set her alarm clock for seven-thirty and called Edward at the Des Bergues, asking if she might meet him for breakfast before he went back to the clinic. They met in the Pavillon restaurant and ordered coffee and croissants.

"What can I do for you, Olivia?" Edward asked her.

"I wondered if there was anything more I could tell you, that might help you take care of Annie." Olivia paused, trying harder than usual to be tactful, still well aware that she and Jamie had overstepped the bounds of friendship, had usurped Edward's own role. "Anything, I mean, that might have gone on in the last week that perhaps you ought to know about."

"Other than the fact that my wife has been trying to withdraw from a serious drug addiction, you mean?" Edward's words were cutting, despite the lightness of his tone.

Olivia put down her coffee cup and looked at him candidly. "Edward, we've been through the apologies, and I honestly don't think it's going to help Annie or you or your family for us to start all over again. You know why we did it, right or wrong."

"Yes." Edward was softer. "I'm sorry."

"No need." Olivia hesitated only briefly, then plunged back in. "I went in to say good night to Annie last night after you'd gone. She seemed upset about the way your conversation had ended."

"Olivia—" Edward leaned in toward the table. "I know you mean well—believe me, I really do know that—but there are certain things—"

"I know"—Olivia interrupted—"I know. They're none of my business, and Annie didn't say much—believe me, Edward, she's much too discreet to say too much. But she used the words 'shut down' when she mentioned the way your talk last night had ended, and that worried me."

"I'm sorry you've been worried—"

"Oh, Edward, don't be so stuffy." Olivia jumped back in. "It doesn't matter a bit whether I'm worried or not. I just thought you might want to know that it had worried Annie. Upset her. Because anything right this minute that upsets Annie is important. And that doesn't mean," she added quickly, "that she isn't to be upset, because that's not real life."

"I know what you mean," Edward said, relenting. "You mean that things that upset her need to be dealt with, not pushed under the carpet."

"Yes," Olivia said. "That is what I mean."

"And what you're skirting around"—he managed a smile at her—"which is rather unlike you, if I may say so—"

"I know it is." Olivia smiled back at him.

"What you're skirting around is the subject of my mother."

Olivia said nothing.

Edward's eyes were darkening again, but he kept going. "Olivia," he said quietly, "I've coped with that particular subject all my adult life by doing what I did last night with my wife. By shutting it off." He paused. "I'd had a bit of a shock yesterday, one way and another, and I suppose there came a point when I couldn't take any more." He paused again. "I told myself that nothing was going to make me dredge it all up again. There was nothing to be gained by it. I'd proved that, after all, hadn't I? I'd bottled it up the way they claim these days is so bad for you. I walled up all those awful memories, entombed them, if you like, and I went on with my life and did pretty well in spite of them."

"Yes, you did," Olivia said. "Clearly, you have dealt beautifully with your life. You're a very successful man with a lovely family."

"And a deeply unhappy, drug-addicted wife."

"Yes," Olivia said softly.

"In other words, what was good for me may not have been so good for Annie." Edward picked up the coffeepot, poured some more into both their cups. "And my sealing off the darker side of my own life made it harder for Annie to approach me about her own troubles."

"It certainly contributed," Olivia agreed. "I sincerely doubt that it's been all that's kept Annie silent."

"No," Edward said. "I expect that's true." He took a breath. "I have a question. Though it's one I don't think you'll be able to answer."

"Shoot," Olivia said.

"How could I not have known what was wrong with Annie? How in God's name could I not have seen how much my wife was suffering?"

Olivia looked at him, saw how tortured he was, how genuinely wretched, and her heart went out to him. Yet in order to most effectively answer his question, to give Edward and Annie their best chance of repairing the damage, she knew that she had to be honest, to tell it how she saw it.

"No one's blaming you, Edward," she said. "Least of all, Annie."

"But?" Edward's mouth quirked again. "Surely, there's a but."

Olivia nodded. "But there is something you have to realize. You've always believed that Annie was doing fine. You saw what she wanted you to see, but I also think you might have seen what *you* wanted to see—and by the way, so did I, so did Jamie."

"You weren't living with her," Edward said somberly.

"That's true, but Annie's a good actress—I never realized that before, but I do now. And she's also very brave, even if she sees herself as a coward and a liar."

"So what do I do now, to help put things right?"

"You're going to have to stop accepting Annie at face value," Olivia answered. "You're going to have to take a sledgehammer to that outer shell of hers—you're going to have to break through and keep on breaking through to the *real* Annie."

"I'm not sure," Edward said, "that I'm much of a sledgehammer type."

"No," Olivia agreed, "I'm sure you're not. But I expect you'll find a more tender, gentle way of cracking Annie's shell, if you really try. And let's face it, Edward, the only chance you have of helping her—of helping you all—get through this mess, is by facing it together. Dealing with it together."

Annie stayed at the clinic for another week, with Edward coming in every day to see her and to participate in some of the counseling sessions that Gianni Dressler recommended they take together.

She was already looking better. She accepted that she had a long way to go, that it might be several months before she was entirely over withdrawal, that perhaps she might never feel as good, as invincible, as she might choose to feel. But she would, ultimately, be taking control of herself and of her body and mind. She would need help, had to learn, now that she had begun, to keep on asking for that help. She would need to keep busy, to feel useful and productive and to be patient with herself. Exercise was highly recommended, together with work, general activity, and love.

"What can we do now? Jamie and I?" Olivia asked Dressler at Au Fin Bec, a popular and friendly restaurant on the right bank.

They'd planned dinner for three on Jamie's penultimate evening in Switzerland, but Jamie had backed out at the last minute, with urgent business to take care of.

"About Annie, you mean?" Dressler asked.

"Of course."

"Nothing," Dressler said. "You do nothing."

"But they're going home the day after tomorrow."

"Don't you think they should?"

"Of course I think they should," Olivia said impatiently. "But Jamie and I are both anxious about abandoning Annie back in England where all her troubles started."

"You're not abandoning her. She'll be with Edward and their children."

"You know what I mean, Gianni."

"Of course I do." His eyes were warm. "You have to leave them to it, Olivia. You'll stay in touch, naturally, let Annie know you're there for her, just as you've always been."

"But she waited six years before she told us anything was wrong."

"That was before. This is now." Gianni paused. "I know it's a hard thing for you to walk away from Annie while she's still so vulnerable."

"You admit she is still vulnerable."

"And will be for a long time. Perhaps always. But Annie's no fool, Olivia. The toughest thing for her was her dark secret, the hole she'd dug herself into. Now that she's on her way up out of that particular hole, I'll be surprised if she lets herself fall back in without giving a good, loud yell first." He smiled. "Annie knows you and Jamie are a telephone call away. But you have to let her tackle this next stage by herself."

"So?" Annie was the first to ask the following evening at Olivia's apartment. They were dining alone, Edward having understood that he was simply not invited, that this was a special occasion for the three friends. "How was last night with Gianni?"

"Good," Olivia answered.

"What do you mean, good?"

"Not bad."

"You're aggravating Annie," Jamie chided her. "She's not supposed to get aggravated, remember?"

"Gianni never said that," Olivia said. "He prescribed 'real life.' Being aggravated by me has always been part of real life for Annie and you."

"Don't we know it," Jamie remarked.

"I want to know about last night," Annie insisted.

"Pleasant," Olivia said. "Enjoyable, in fact."

"Livvy, that won't do," Annie said. "I need details. Romance is good for my soul—my drop-dead-gorgeous doctor says so."

She knew she was babbling a little, that the euphoria of being released from the clinic and of feeling almost well would not, could not, last; but tonight, at that very moment at least, she did not care.

"So go get some romance," Olivia told her.

"I'm an old married lady," Annie said.

"So get some with your husband."

Annie looked at Jamie. "She's not going to give anything away, is she?"

"Doesn't look like it."

"You know they're going to have an affair, don't you?"

Jamie made no comment.

"Enough." Olivia poured wine into Jamie's glass and refilled her own.

"Olivia Segal"—Annie wasn't ready to give up—"this man is every red-blooded woman's fantasy."

"He's arrogant," Olivia said. "A successful, handsome doctor, and Swiss-Italian—I'm surprised his ego made it through my front door."

"Olivia has a point." Jamie grinned. "Two egos that size might be a tight squeeze, especially in this little apartment."

"So you do think he's handsome," Annie said.

"I'm not blind," Olivia said dryly, ignoring Jamie's crack.

"So you are going to have an affair with him?"

"Nothing's impossible."

The pause that followed was long and awkward.

"I'm scared," Annie said abruptly.

"Of going home?" Olivia asked, gently.

"Yes." Annie shook her head, angry with herself. "I want to go back more than anything—I feel I'll go crazy if I don't see Sophie and William and Liza for one more *day*." She paused again. "But it's where it all began, isn't it?"

"That's not really true," Jamie said. "I'd say it began eleven years ago when that helicopter crashed."

"Jamie's right, Annie," Olivia agreed.

"But it all came to a head in Stone Bridge," Annie maintained.

"And it's all still there, waiting for me. The house to run, the children to look after, the community to fit into."

"But one important thing has changed, Annie," Olivia said. "The two most important things of all, I should say."

"Edward knowing, you mean," Annie said.

"Yes," Olivia said. "You have Edward to share your problems with now. And you don't have to fight them all by yourself anymore."

Annie was smiling. "I'm going to miss you both so much," she said softly, and felt tears beginning to threaten.

"We're going to miss you, too," Jamie told her, and reached for her hand.

"We'll be calling you a lot," Olivia said. "We're probably going to drive you crazy, checking up on you."

"Feel free," Annie said. "And come whenever you can."

"I'd come now," Jamie said, "if I thought it would help."

"We both would," Olivia agreed. "But Gianni says you have to deal with the next bit yourselves—you and Edward, not you alone."

"I know," Annie said. "And you've done more than enough for me, both of you."

"We failed you, Annie," Jamie said.

"You've never failed me." Annie was vehement.

"We ought to have known," Jamie insisted.

"That's how Edward feels," Annie said. "But I know he's wrong, that you're all wrong about that. I know what a great liar I've been—" She held up one hand, fending off protests. "You can call it acting, putting up a facade, whatever you like. But if part of getting myself straight again is acknowledging the truth about myself, then let me at least be honest about what I know." She paused. "I lied. To myself, and to everyone who loved me. And I almost let it go too far."

"Thank God you didn't," Olivia said.

"Thank God I had you two," Annie said.

Olivia spent a long time at the airport next day, first with Jamie, seeing off Annie and Edward on their British Airways flight to London, and then, a little later, seeing Jamie off back to Boston.

"Give my love to Carrie," Olivia said, then grinned. "If she can stand it."

"Carrie doesn't hate you, Olivia," Jamie said earnestly.

"I'm not exactly her Woman of the Decade."

"She's jealous of you."

"I know she is," Olivia agreed. "What I've never understood is why."

"She must have her reasons."

"She does know we've never been anything more than friends, doesn't she?" Olivia looked at Jamie, at his beautiful soft dark eyes and sleek hair. "Though maybe, if I were Carrie I might feel that way too about an unattached female who got too close to you."

"I doubt that," Jamie said.

They strolled slowly toward passport control, taking their time, making the most of every remaining minute they could share.

"Be safe," Olivia said when they got there.

"You, too."

"And be happy. Don't let Carrie get you down."

"She doesn't, Olivia." Jamie paused. "I wish you two got along better."

"It's not just me though, is it? She doesn't like Annie much more."

"You're not being quite fair, are you?" Jamie wasn't being critical, just frank. This was old territory; they'd trodden it before and would do so again. "Carrie's always known neither of you liked her, right from the start."

"I guess that's true," Olivia admitted. "And I am sorry for that, Jamie. I do wish I could have loved your wife. I meant to."

"I know you did." He picked up his travel bag, then hesitated and put it down again. "If you do get involved with Dressler," he said, "watch yourself, won't you?"

"Sure I will," she said lightly. "You know me. Easy come, easy go."

"Like hell." Jamie took her hand. "That's just your front, Olivia—we all have facades, not just Annie."

"Don't worry about me," Olivia told him.

"I can't help worrying about you. I always have."

"I know. Me, too."

They embraced. Olivia felt his slender strength, smelled his old familiar fragrance, and thought how important he was to her, how fundamental his and Annie's friendship had become to her whole life.

"Love you," Jamie said softly, against her ear.

"Love you back," Olivia said.

And then he was on his way, stopping for just one more instant to look back and wave at her and blow her a kiss, and then he was gone, out of sight. And Olivia turned, when she was sure he wasn't coming back, and began to walk toward the exit, heading for the garage where she'd left her car. And she had the strangest feeling, reflecting bemusedly on those parting words of love, words they'd spoken to each other almost every time they'd said their farewells over the years, that this time, for her—she knew and accepted that it had only been for her, not for Jamie—there had been a curious difference.

She thought—she was not certain, she didn't think she *wanted* to be certain, because not only was it wrong, it was also out of the question, utterly and entirely impossible—but she thought perhaps that she had meant it.

And not just as a friend.

OLIVIA'S BOX

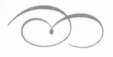

By the summer of 1938, fifty-five thousand Jews from Germany and Austria had escaped to the United States of America, but not a single member of our family was amongst that number. My father, who had once been so confident that his high standing, wealth, and contacts would mean that he could, if sorely pressed, arrange safe passage for us all at comparatively short notice, now knew better. The emigration paperwork that his old friend Max Wildenbruch's affidavit ought to have ensured had mysteriously failed to materialize; the essential arrangements taken care of by Max's lawyers that ought to have enabled us to travel to America had repeatedly and inexplicably fallen apart. Papa, after one call to New York, said that Max had sounded perplexed and upset; he had done the same for Ferdy Steiner from Nuremberg, and the Steiner family were now safely ensconced in an apartment on Seventy-third Street in Manhattan. It made no sense, Max Wildenbruch said, when all they heard was that the Nazis were encouraging Jews to get the hell out of Germany.

It made perfect sense to Papa, Mama, and to me, though we all kept our fears from Lili and Trude. As time passed and the Nazi terror had gathered strength and savagery, Brauner's blackmail had grown ever more systematic and brutal. Mama and Papa had seen him at the outset as nothing worse than an opportunistic collector; now we knew he was an unscrupulous thief. With deadly efficiency, Brauner had ransacked our cellars and by now the bones of Papa's cherished Symbolist Collection had been picked almost clean. What had begun, seemingly, as a rather one-sided business deal to make it possible for us to leave Germany with at least a small percentage of our pride and possessions intact, had become a bargain for far higher stakes. If Papa continued to cooperate, Brauner had told him in the early months, he would use his influence to allow us to remain, unmolested, in our home. If Papa went on quietly handing over his treasures, Brauner had said a few months later, he would see to it that we were allowed, eventually, to leave Germany for America. But all that had long since changed. Brauner no longer bothered dangling carrots of help; now he simply used his personal power to threaten us all. Brauner had friends in high places, he reminded my father repeatedly; all he had to do was to inform on Papa, implicating him in anything from race defilement to some fictitious anti-Nazi plot, and then Papa would at the very least be sent to the concentration camp at Dachau, near Munich, or, more probably, be executed.

It had taken three years. Since the autumn of 1935, Brauner had come and gone eleven times, his visits irregular and unpredictable, and we all suspected that Baden-Baden might be only one of his ports of call, that he might be trawling around Germany, cold-bloodedly reaping his once-in-a-lifetime artistic harvest.

All that remained in our cellars by September 1938 were a small group of works by Hodler, Redon, and Ibels. My father had learned from Max Wildenbruch that out of the one hundred and thirteen paintings that had left the house, only nine had reached him: six during the first year of their arrangement, just three in the second, when Papa had still clung to the vain belief that Brauner was, to some paltry degree—because it suited him—keeping his word.

"What happens when the cellar is empty?" Anton asked Emanuel late one September evening as they walked together in the garden.

"Who knows?" Emanuel said softly.

Emanuel knew better by now than to actively lie to his son. Anton was seventeen now, and infinitely more mature than a young man his age ought to be. There was little purpose in lying, for the boy knew as much as his parents did about the ever growing dangers facing the Jews of Germany and—since March that year—of Austria.

"I suppose Brauner will skulk back to wherever he came from and never come back again," Anton said quietly as they walked in the dark.

"I suppose so," Emanuel said.

"What will happen when they've taken the house and find the whole collection gone?"

"They may not take the house," Emanuel said.

"They will, Papa. You know they will. The laws have all been passed. Everyone knows it's only a matter of time before they throw us out."

"Perhaps."

They walked on in silence for a while, thinking. About what had befallen the Viennese Jews almost overnight after the *Anschluss*: all rights immediately taken away, physical assaults and humiliation. About the burning down of the main synagogue in Munich in June, and in Nuremberg in August. About the arrests that had begun in the summer all over Germany and were still going on. About the rumors that kept filtering through, slowly and terrifyingly, of the fate that had befallen those arrested.

"And after they've thrown us out"—Anton was unable to leave it—"what will they do to us then, Papa? When they open up the cellars. Everyone knows about the collection—they won't be able to pretend it never existed." He paused. "What if they say we plotted with Brauner to rob them?"

Emanuel patted his son's shoulder. "You mustn't worry so much about things that may never happen," he said gently. "Things we can do nothing about."

"But he's made so many threats, Papa."

"Only to keep us doing his bidding," Emanuel said with an ease he did not feel. "Once he has all the paintings, he won't need us anymore. He'll simply be finished with us."

They walked a little farther. The gardener had mown the back lawn that afternoon, and the scent was sweet.

"Surely," Anton said after a while, "he might see us as witnesses."

"Witnesses?"

"He's a criminal, isn't he?" Anton paused. "A foreigner, smuggling art treasures out of the country. And we know what he's done."

"I don't think we need worry about that," Emanuel said tightly. "Brauner has friends in high places. He's told us that often enough."

"Mama says that just means he's bribed a few Nazi officials here in Baden-Baden."

"And I say we don't have to worry about his crimes," Emanuel insisted. "When he's finished with us, our papers will come."

Anton stopped and stood very still.

"Do you really believe that, Papa?"

Emanuel went on walking.

"I have to believe it," he said.

Papa did not, of course, believe it. He knew as well as Mama and I did that his small, blissful empire of beauty and peace was gone forever. He would go on scrabbling around his swiftly dwindling network of contacts day after day, trying desperately to find a means—*any* means—of safe exit, at least for Mama, Lili, and Trude and myself, if not for himself. But I don't think he any longer had any real faith that he would succeed.

Our family had been taken in, taken over, and then betrayed by the man who called himself Georg Brauner. We had been at his mercy for three years, and before much longer, our usefulness to him ended, he would, we realized—looking at it in the best of lights—abandon us completely. Though if my fear was right, and if Brauner did see us as witnesses—if he did regard our presence as some kind of personal threat—there was, of course, no telling what he might do.

We heard that Dachau and the newer concentration camps were filling up with every passing week. We and countless other families much like us who had waited too long to leave our homeland were now waiting, like helpless chickens in a broken coop, to be devoured by the Nazi fox. And with all possible exits continuing to be blocked to us, Mama, Papa, and I knew that we and the girls were, to all intents and purposes, trapped. We did our best to wear our bravest faces for Lili's and Trude's sakes, and even at night, after they had gone to sleep, we seldom voiced our true feelings. Mama and Papa were doubtless keen to spare me what little they could.

But I think—I know—they were as terrified as I was.

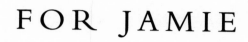

FOR JAMIE

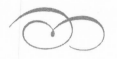

12

"*It's crazy,*" *Annie said, after Olivia outlined her plan for getting back at* Carrie Beaumont Arias. "I mean I love it, in a way, but it's completely, absolutely crazy, and it scares me."

"Why?"

"Because it's so off-the-wall."

"It's perfect," Olivia said.

"But it seems so—immoral."

"We're dealing with an amoral person, Annie. It's the only way to really get to her. To hit her where it hurts."

"You really hate Carrie, don't you, Livvy?"

Olivia thought about that for a moment. "I wouldn't say I hate her. I don't think I've ever hated anyone—actually *hated* anyone—in my life. But I do most certainly despise her."

"We could never pull it off," Annie said.

"If I didn't think we could," Olivia answered, "I wouldn't be suggesting you get involved."

It was January 1990. They were sitting at Annie's kitchen table at Banbury Farm House. Almost three years had passed since Annie had swallowed her last Valium, and she often felt like a completely different woman, as if that whole nightmare had happened to someone else. That was one of the aspects, if she was totally honest, that she appreciated most about the plan Olivia had just shared with her. As recently as a year ago, Annie doubted if Livvy would have considered her strong enough or tough enough to participate in anything like this. It was, she realized, a tribute to her recovery that they were sitting there today, working out ways to help Jamie.

"But are you sure it isn't wrong not to tell Jamie?" Annie asked Olivia. "After all, we'd be doing it for him. Doesn't he have a right to know?"

"No." Olivia shook her head definitely. "For one thing, knowing Jamie, he'd never agree to go along with it." She looked down at the notes she'd made, and her green eyes glittered at the thought of what was to come. "And for another, this whole thing is only going to work—really work—if Jamie doesn't know a damned thing about it."

If Olivia's parents, she sometimes thought, had lived to see their daughter become an adult, they might, she hoped, have been proud of her, but they were also bound, she was certain, to have been perplexed because she was so unlike either of them. Arthur Segal, her father, had been born in Berlin in 1933 to Jewish parents who had made it to the United States one year after his birth, aided in their quest for a peaceful, safe existence by Arthur's mother's affluent brother, already living in Manhattan. Arthur had become a well-respected art dealer and philanthropist, his own collection of paintings—much of it directed to him by old Max Wildenbruch in New York and including some of the great French Impressionists at the top end and a large number of works by young, up-and-coming artists at the other—both admired and envied. His collection had, in his lifetime, spent more time out on loan to public galleries than hanging on its owner's own walls; Arthur firmly believed that art was created to be seen and enjoyed, to be shared, not hidden away. That had also been his general philosophy on life, which was why he had become something of a slave to his fund-raising activities, and why he had regularly given substantial sums of money to so many charities.

Arthur had often claimed to have been shamed into doing his good works because of Emily, his wife and the driving force in his life. Emily Segal was a pediatric heart surgeon, and no man could have been prouder of his wife than her husband. Emily, a truly selfless person, loved her family and respected her Jewish heritage, but it had always been understood that her work often had to come first—before birthdays, before regular Friday night dinners, before even the high holy days if a child was sick and needed her help. She was fortunate in that she was naturally pretty and slender, but unlike most of the other wives in the Segals' social circle, Emily had no time or patience for shopping or beauty parlors. Where was the sense, after all, Emily asked, in buying great clothes or hairstyles when she spent most of her life in white coats or sterile overalls with her hair scraped off her face and covered?

Unlike Olivia—who skied regularly to downhill racing standards and who had, over the past decade, also gone scuba diving, backpacking, hang gliding, and horse riding in the Grand Canyon—neither Arthur nor Emily had been especially physical folk. Their vacations—at the rare times when Emily could get away—had been restful affairs, usually in France or Israel or occasionally in Italy, with unadventurous swimming and gentle strolls their only exercise. They had shared an abiding passion for each other's bodies, but neither would have claimed to have unusually powerful sexual appetites. They were two immensely successful, worthy people, yet they were also highly conventional. Emily, the child of two doctors, had grown up believing fervently in the liberation of women, yet she had wanted marriage and children as much as Arthur, though a ruptured uterus had forced them to stop at one daughter.

Olivia sometimes thought she might be a throwback to some forgotten relative, some irrepressible, unbridled Jewess—probably on Arthur's side, she mused, some Russian girl who had not toed the conventional line, a fellow spirit. Not that Olivia was particularly bold compared to some young women she had encountered on her travels; she only seemed adventurous when she compared herself to her mother or father. Perhaps, she reflected in the odd, rare, guilty moment, she was trying to compensate for being such an unworthy successor to the Segals, was trying to make up for her undoubted inadequacies by making her life as action-packed as possible. She worked hard and played hard, she tried to be decent, was not an unhelpful or particularly unkind person, was certainly not a bad all-round human being, but compared to her parents, Olivia did sometimes feel useless. She wondered if she might have taken a completely different road if Arthur and Emily had lived, thought she probably would have. They had known

about her plans to go to the Sorbonne in the fall of 1976 and they had
not expressed disapproval, yet Olivia suspected they might have urged
her on to higher things if time had allowed. As it was, she had her
qualifications—was, she supposed, a comparatively distinguished linguist—and her business, and she also knew how to have fun better than
most people she met.

Olivia's affair with Gianni Dressler, which had begun in earnest within
a week of Jamie's and Annie's departure from Geneva in the spring
of 1987 and had continued with considerable passion into the summer, had run its course by autumn of the same year. There had been,
since then, a number of other men. It was not in Olivia's nature to be
alone for long. Not that she minded being alone; in fact, she cherished
her independence, enjoyed her own company, and greatly valued
her women friends. But Annie had once told Olivia that there was a
spark in her green eyes that ignited in the presence of attractive or interesting men.

"It isn't deliberate; I know that," Annie had said. "But I've watched
it drawing them to you, and then they seem to find it impossible to pull
away again."

"God, Annie," Olivia had said, "you make me sound like a vamp."

"Not at all," Annie had said. "But you do have that spark."

"And how on earth"—Olivia had laughed at the notion—"would
you describe this so-called spark?"

Annie had thought for a few moments.

"It's a promise," she said, "of fun, adventure, and warmth."

Later, on reflection, Olivia had thought it was not a description she
found either unflattering or displeasing.

The men drawn in and out of her life since the violet-eyed, dynamic
Dressler had all been interesting, intelligent, and attractive in one way
or another, but only Gianni had pointed out to Olivia, more than
once, one of the very few things she had ever, if she was honest with
herself, tried to bury in her mind.

"You realize, of course," he had said on the evening they had
agreed, mutually, though not without a degree of regret, to end their

relationship, "that whatever you say and however much you deny it, you're in love with Arias."

"Don't be absurd," Olivia had said. "Jamie's one of my best friends, I've told you."

"Friendship doesn't rule out love," Gianni said.

"It does in this case." She was adamant. "As does marriage."

"To a woman you dislike."

"What does my dislike have to do with it?"

Gianni smiled. "That depends on why you dislike her."

"I dislike Carrie for reasons that are none of your damned business," Olivia said irritably. "And just because I never fell in love with you, Gianni Dressler—"

"Nor I with you," he countered charmingly.

"—does not mean I must be in love with anyone else." She shook her head impatiently. "Honestly, Gianni, I thought you were above this kind of chauvinistic crap."

"Surely not." He grinned again. "How could a Swiss-Italian male surgeon possibly not be a chauvinist?"

"That's true." Olivia softened slightly. "I guess you can't help it."

"Just as you can't help being in love with your Jamie," Gianni said. "You're forgetting I've seen you together many times."

"You've seen two old friends. Dear friends."

"And I repeat, since when does friendship preclude love?"

Olivia sighed. "You really are full of shit, aren't you?" she said, more good-naturedly now, aware that he was deliberately goading her to get a reaction.

"If you say so." Gianni paused. "So why do you dislike Jamie's wife?"

"And I repeat," Olivia said, "none of your business."

For all that it was true that Olivia had instinctively disliked Caroline Beaumont from the first time they had been introduced—and if she and Annie were perfectly honest, they had certainly been guilty of mistrusting her even before they had met her—she had quickly enough grown to see that Jamie's happiness with Carrie in the early days of their marriage was genuine.

Whatever life had thrown at Jamie Arias, he had remained the same charming, gentle man, in private and in public; and even in his working world of advertising, an industry populated by any number of cutthroat types, Jamie had become known as much for his old-fashioned courtesy and innate empathy as for his considerable talent for copywriting.

Jamie was permanently, guiltily aware that his late father, Carlos Arias, had anticipated that he, like his older brother Peter and their cousin Michael, would automatically enter the family's shipping business. Had Carlos lived, Jamie, who had adored his father, suspected that he might have felt compelled to do just that. As things were, he had prepared himself, when the moment of truth came, for a battle royal with Michael, the head of Arias Shipping, but to his great relief his cousin—who had elected to rule from their New York offices, an easy flight in a private jet from the Arias family compound at Newport— had given way gracefully, had said that he thought that what Carlos would have wanted, more than anything, was for his sons to be contented men.

"If you prefer the plebeian buzz of advertising," Michael said, grinning at his young cousin, "to the splendor and power of your own shipping company—and I have to tell you that neither Peter nor I even begin to understand why—it's your decision to make."

After all, Michael pointed out, Jamie's personal share of the family fortune was his, safe and sound, with no strings or conditions attached. Jamie, however he might choose to spend his time, was an immensely wealthy young man. He might just as well be a happy one too, Michael Arias reasoned.

Jamie chose advertising. His swift, creative, agile brain, his hunger to learn at least *something* about almost everything he happened upon in his daily life, his eager, still boyish fascination with other people's lives and businesses—what they did, what they liked, what made them tick—made him an ideal candidate for the industry. He had told Olivia once that though his education had been a fine one, he believed his real schooling had come via television; he claimed he had been far more stimulated over the years by what he had watched on that small, much-maligned box of tricks—from news and documentaries through feature films right down to cartoons and even children's programming—than by most of his teachers or tutors.

"I can watch *Dallas*," he told Olivia, "and I know I'm watching grade-A junk, but I'll catch a snippet of conversation between J.R. and another oil baron, and in a second I'll be reaching for a reference book or searching for a database on my computer—you can really get quite an education watching soaps."

Jamie Arias could be told one afternoon about a new merchandising campaign up for grabs, and by next morning he was likely to know more than anyone in any other agency about the new product, how it had been created and why and for whom, and then his real talent, his natural gift for writing hard, sharp, incisive, witty, and, above all, unforgettable copy, would come to the fore. Since leaving Harvard in 1980, he had worked for eighteen months at Ogilvy & Mather as a copywriter—a period he had loved with a passion; for Leo Burnett first as an account supervisor, then as an account executive—two of the most frustrating years of his life; and then, given an opportunity by a man named Norman J. Kane for which he would be forever grateful, as a creative director for the small, high-flying Kane Agency. Kane, a middle-aged, rough, gruff, Brooklyn-born New Yorker, had started calling Jamie his pet whiz even before he'd won the agency its first Clio, and when Jamie showed no signs of offense at being referred to that way, Kane told people gleefully that was because Arias was a true gentleman. And though he'd been born and raised an American and denied being descended from the Spanish aristocracy, Kane knew that class was what gave him his edge.

"I'm forever telling him it isn't true," Jamie told Annie one day on the phone, "but he doesn't want to know, so I've stopped arguing."

"Maybe you are an aristocrat compared with him," Annie suggested.

"As far as I'm concerned," Jamie said, "they don't come any more aristocratic than Kane."

One of the things that Norman J. Kane loved so much about Jamie Arias was his seemingly limitless capacity and desire for learning. Kane was tickled to death when his beloved agency won its Clio for Jamie's innovative dog food campaign, but what pleased him infinitely more was the fact that the pet food manufacturers reported that their sales curve was moving steadily upward. Jamie understood that Clios and Andy Awards were great ego trips but did not necessarily equate with long-term success for the client, the creative team involved in the campaign, or the agency. Jamie accepted that sheer hard work on the basics, getting the bedrock of a proposed campaign as solid and immaculately researched as humanly possible, looking way beyond the high of a big award—flattering as it certainly was—was just as fundamental to success as the near orgasmic joy of hitting the occasional, inspirational big idea.

It was while he was working for Kane at the end of 1984 that Jamie first met Caroline Beaumont at a party thrown by his boss, who wanted to get a closer look at Beaumont with a view to asking her to join the agency. It was, on Jamie's part, adoration at first sight. Carrie Beaumont was everything he was not: she was tough, intensely ambitious, and too fiercely focused to even know what being free-spirited was. But she was also the loveliest woman Jamie had ever met, and from the first moment on he pretty much threw himself at her feet, blown away by the sparkle of brilliance in her cool blue eyes, by her smooth, pale skin and natural spun-gold hair and by the low, crisp snap of her Bostonian voice.

The luck of it [Jamie wrote to Olivia] *is that Carrie seems to have fallen in love with me, too.*

I don't see anything lucky about it [Olivia wrote back to Jamie] *since falling in love with you can't be exactly hard to do, given that you're probably one of the most eligible bachelors living in Manhattan.*

Not relevant [Jamie wrote back joyfully] *since if anyone's the catch in this relationship, it's Carrie. The Beaumonts have just as much money as the Ariases, and Carrie's a lot shrewder than I am, more sophisticated and practical than I am—definitely a lot more desirable than I am—and a real whiz at advertising.*

Carrie, who was also five years older than Jamie, turned down Norman Kane's offer flat and, instead, snatched her brand-new fiancé straight out of Kane's arms. She had plans, and she'd been coasting along in New York for a while now, gathering experience and contacts and biding her time until she could have exactly what she wanted. What she wanted was her own small but perfectly formed agency, based in her hometown, Boston.

"I know you'd probably rather stay in New York, darling James," she told him, preempting any arguments, "but your family does live in New England, after all, so you must understand why Boston really is the only city I feel truly, entirely comfortable living in." She took a short, efficient, aerobics-trained breath and swept on. "And I know I'm a bit of a spoiled bitch in that I do tend to go after what I want, and I apologize for that, James, I honestly do, but I know what I want now, *really* want, for the first time in my life." The wide blue eyes passed lovingly, lingeringly over his still shell-shocked but delighted face. "I want you for my partner. In business, in marriage, in life."

She got no arguments from Jamie.

"I think she really does love him," Annie told Olivia during a telephone call in the early spring of 1985.

"Well, why wouldn't she?" Olivia said acidly. "As I told Jamie, he's handsome, he's clever—he is richer than she is, whatever he might prefer to believe—and I'm beginning to think he's hers to command."

"Why don't you like her?" Annie asked her, then instantly corrected herself. "Why do we both dislike her when we haven't even met her?"

"I talked to her once," Olivia said. "When they were both at Jamie's place and I asked him to put her on so I could say hi."

"And?"

"And she was cool. She was polite enough, and she said the right kind of things about looking forward to meeting me, and how much James—you know she calls him James, for Christ's sake—"

"That's not so bad, surely?" Annie said mildly.

"No, it's not *so* bad, but it isn't Jamie, is it? Anyway, she said all the usual stuff about how much James had told her about us, and what wonderful friends we sounded."

"But you didn't think she meant it?"

"I *knew* she didn't mean a word of it."

"Still," Annie said carefully, "maybe we ought to suspend final judgment until after we've actually met Carrie—it might be fairer."

"I dare say it would be," Olivia said.

Annie smiled into the telephone receiver. "But you just don't like her."

"She was cool, Annie. Too cool. Jamie Arias is not a cool person."

"No," Annie agreed. "He isn't."

Olivia and Annie flew together from London to Boston in the first week of June, five days before the wedding. Jamie came to Logan Airport to meet them. He looked fit, relaxed, and undeniably happy.

"I have to admit," Olivia said without delay, "I don't think I've ever seen you looking better."

"You, too," he said, hugging her, then embracing Annie on his other side. "And you look just wonderful. Motherhood certainly agrees with you."

"Think so?" Annie grimaced. "I think it makes me fat and tired."

"Well, if it does, it doesn't show." He picked up both their travel bags and began walking them toward the exit.

Olivia looked around. "So where is she?"

"Carrie couldn't make it," Jamie said. "She sends her apologies, but with less than a week to go she just has so much to do."

"Of course she has," Annie agreed. "I didn't really expect her to come."

"When are we meeting her?" Olivia wanted to know.

"This evening," Jamie said. "If you're up to it, not too jet-lagged."

"We'll be up to it," Olivia said definitely. "Or I will, anyway."

"I wouldn't miss it," Annie said.

"Where are we eating?" Olivia asked.

"It'll just be drinks, I'm afraid, at the Ritz-Carlton." Jamie looked apologetic. "Carrie and I have to go to a dinner with a potential client tonight."

"Sure you can manage drinks?" Olivia didn't bother concealing her irony.

"Come on, Livvy," Annie said. "I remember how impossible it was managing my time when it got close to our wedding."

"I'm really sorry," Jamie told them both. "And so's Carrie."

"I'm sure she is," Olivia said.

"She can't wait to meet you."

★   ★   ★

If they'd disliked her unfairly before they'd met Carrie, they positively loathed her when they did come face-to-face. She was beautiful, she was charming, she was welcoming, and, as she had on the telephone, she said all the right things, but Olivia felt Carrie's own distaste for her and for Annie lapping over her like sour waves.

"She's jealous of us," Olivia said to Annie later at Durgin-Park as they waited hungrily for their broiled lobsters.

"Don't be silly."

"It may be silly but I'll bet the rent I'm right."

"You don't mean jealous because we're women." Annie grinned. "She certainly couldn't be jealous of me."

"Why not?" Olivia said. "You look fantastic."

"But I'm married with three children."

"And still beautiful, and Jamie loves you." Olivia paused. "Seriously, Annie, Carrie's definitely pissed that we're here. She's certainly jealous of our closeness to Jamie."

Annie drank some Perrier. "Maybe," she said thoughtfully, "I would be, too, if I were her."

"I doubt it."

"No, honestly," Annie insisted. "I do remember that before Edward and I got married, he had a couple of good women friends. They used to lunch together, had the odd dinner, but that began to peter out when we got engaged, and after the wedding it stopped completely."

"Because you wanted it to stop?"

Annie shook her head. "No, I never said a word. But I do think I'd have minded if it had gone on."

"Even if they were just friends?" Olivia looked surprised.

"I'm afraid so, yes." Annie grinned ruefully. "I guess it's not the way we're meant to be these days—I guess I should know better—but that is how I felt." She paused. "So if Carrie is jealous, I think I can understand her a little, especially in your case."

"Because I'm single."

"Single and beautiful and smart, and yet the absolute antithesis of her. And sharing more past history with Jamie than she ever will."

"I guess," Olivia said.

"So maybe we should go easy on her."

"Play things her way, you mean?"

"Maybe."

"Playing things Carrie's way," Olivia said, "would probably mean us going home. You want to go home, Annie?"

"No."

"Nor do I." Olivia spied their lobsters heading their way, and raised her glass of chardonnay. "Here's to our darling Jamie," she said warmly. "May Carrie make him as happy as he deserves to be."

The marriage had been okay to begin with—better than okay, because they were in love and sex was good—sensational, sometimes, if Carrie was in the mood to let herself go. And they were both thriving on building a new home—the charming town house in Beacon Hill that Carrie had found while Jamie was still in New York—and a new business—Beaumont-Arias Advertising on Newbury Street—together. And they still, most important of all, respected each other. But that was the element that went first, and after that it was the start of a long downhill slide to hell on wheels.

The trouble was, whereas Jamie had recognized Carrie's greatest character flaw long before they had married (he knew that she was a little compulsive about being in control: of herself, of business, of the people she surrounded herself with, and especially of a prospective husband) and had realized that he loved her enough to put up with it, Carrie, who had zeroed in on Jamie's faults just as swiftly, had decided, instead, to eradicate them. Jamie's faults, as Carrie saw them, began as dear little blemishes that she, with her accustomed efficiency, would soon wipe away. But the gentleness that she had assumed would make him a most biddable husband was of a genuinely moral kind more deeply rooted than she had at first suspected. Jamie was a truly tender-hearted man, yet he was not a docile one. Though modest, he was neither self-effacing nor unaware of his assets or his talents. He was far from egocentric, but he did like himself, was happy in himself, and so once he recognized Carrie's intention of changing him, the same strength of will that had allowed Jamie to draw away from the Arias family's might began to manifest itself in this new situation as a mild-mannered, light-hearted obstinacy.

Carrie liked her way in most things.

"James, darling, you can't wear that tie tonight," she said when they were getting ready for dinner with her family at the beginning of the second year of their marriage.

"What's wrong with it?" He glanced at the mirror over the fireplace in their bedroom. It was a perfectly nice tie, pure Italian navy silk with neatly designed flecks of vivid pink enlivening it. "I bought it this afternoon."

"Did you?" Carrie peered carefully at her face and gave it a final fine-touched brushing of translucent powder. She was, she realized, a borderline obsessive about her own physical perfection. There was no question that natural-born beauty was a trial, almost as much of a curse as it was a blessing. After all, she reasoned, a plain woman had lower expectations of herself and aroused far fewer in others; a beautiful woman had to be constantly on the alert for imperfections. Which was why Carrie, however busy her schedule—and she was a workaholic—always made time, and bullied others into making time for her, for her facials and workouts and massages and other treatments. She still remembered the instant when Jamie had first seen and fallen in love with her, and she was under no illusions that he, or any of the other men who'd ever been in love with her—and there'd been a few—would have felt even remotely the same way had she been homely. Jamie was, of course, hers now, and she knew that he really didn't mind, scarcely even noticed, if her hair was less gleaming than usual or if she had even the slightest *trace*—heaven forbid—of a zit, but Carrie's standards regarding her appearance were as rigorous as they were about most things in her private or professional life.

"Where did you get it?" She returned to the subject of Jamie's tie, touching Chanel No. 5 to her wrists and behind her ears. Carrie had strict rules about perfume. She had no objection to wearing more recent creations like Chanel No. 19 or perhaps the new Givenchy perfume, or even, at a pinch and at the *right* kind of gathering, Giorgio, but when they were seeing her parents or other bona fide Bostonians, only the true classics like No. 5 or Houbigant would do.

"A little place down the street." He was deliberately obtuse.

"Which place?" Carrie stood up. "If you tell me, I can change it for you."

"Why would you want to do that?"

"Because it's awful." She smiled at him fondly. "You know your taste isn't always quite what it might be."

Jamie looked back in the mirror again. "I like it."

Carrie sighed. "Oh, well, if you like it that much—"

He knew she'd left the last sentence up in the air in the hope that he would cave in and tell her that she was probably right, and that anyway, if she didn't like it there wasn't much point in his wearing it. He knew that six months ago he most likely would have said exactly that, and if it came to it now, he didn't actually give a damn about the tie itself—he liked it well enough, but it was just a tie, after all—but there were principles at stake here, so he said nothing more and kept the tie on.

Carrie liked having things her own way at Beaumont-Arias as well as at home or when they were traveling together. Usually light-heartedly, Jamie tried to point out to her that he had never regarded marriage as an end, for either of them, to personal choice; to make her see that the differences in their tastes and in their characters were a bonus, that different attitudes were positive and healthy, would keep them both on their toes and stop their relationship from becoming dull. But as time went on, Carrie's desire to control all the decision making in their partnership grew more intense; she wanted to approve everything Jamie wore, drove, and did, inside and outside the house, and when Jamie was less than pliable, she stamped her beautifully shod feet and created hell.

Not in public, of course. Carrie Beaumont Arias's public face was of the contented, serene woman who had been fortunate enough to find a way to keep her brilliant career and discover the most wonderful husband and partner in the universe. To friends and acquaintances and colleagues, she and Jamie were an idyllic blend, a marriage created in heaven and staying there. But when they were alone, the face became increasingly ugly, for Carrie was more than spoiled, more than obsessive about perfection, more even than simply manipulative; Carrie was a full-blown control freak. And once she began to see clearly, after about a year of marriage, that Jamie was still not hers to control, Carrie began to do what she had always done with people who crossed her and with whom she could not immediately or easily dispense. She put him down.

"You know you made yourself look absurd this afternoon, don't you?" she told him in the spring of 1986.

They had just sat down in their cream and chintz, soothingly decorated and furnished drawing room with a couple of dry martinis. Jamie had removed his jacket, loosened his tie, and unfastened the top button of his shirt, and was just contemplating kicking off his shoes.

"Which particular part of this afternoon?" he asked, staying amiable.

"At the presentation, obviously."

"Which particular part of the presentation?"

"Every part that followed the opening niceties," Carrie said.

"Ah." Jamie sipped his martini. "So that bit went okay."

Carrie set her own glass on the side table next to her armchair. "You just refuse to learn, don't you, James? You really don't want to know."

"Know what, Carrie?"

Jamie was tired, he knew that much. He'd slept fitfully the previous night, and then the pitch to Ralston for their new light beer account had begun badly because big Fred Ralston had started the proceedings by declaring that he'd never really liked their mainstream Ralston Beer campaign in any of its subtly evolving forms, and if their sales curves were still healthy it had everything to do with their beer and fuck-all to do with Beaumont-Arias's work. Jamie and Carrie had taken what Ralston had thrown at them in their stride, had done what Jamie had regarded as a fine job of smoothing big Fred's ruffled feathers so that Maggie Carmichael and David Baum, their top creative team, had been able to begin their new pitch from a position of reasonable strength. The Ralston jury was out, but Jamie was cautiously optimistic. He was also in no mood for one of Carrie's viper sessions.

"I'm very tired," he said.

"And you think I'm not?"

"No, I'm sure you are."

Carrie returned to the subject of the Ralston presentation.

"I said that you made yourself look absurd this afternoon because of the idiotic way you built up Baum and Carmichael to Fred Ralston."

"What would you have had me do?" Jamie took a bigger swallow of his drink.

"Obviously," Carrie said, "you should have sacrificed them on the spot." She looked at his startled expression. "For goodness' sake, James, Ralston as good as demanded their heads—he said he had no confidence in them—"

"In our campaigns," Jamie corrected her. "Not in Maggie and David. In any case, you knew he was only bitching because he likes throwing people off balance."

"What Ralston wanted," Carrie went on crisply, ignoring him, "was for the two of us to take over and give his ego a good stroking. He knows perfectly well that we're still the real number one creative team at Beaumont-Arias."

"I didn't think that was what he wanted at all," Jamie argued, going on drinking. "And given the terrific job Maggie and David did today—"

"Baum and Carmichael did an okay job today," Carrie insisted, "and nothing more. I'm not too sure about you right now—not with your attitude—but I know that I could have taken those same ideas and left Fred Ralston thinking he'd been dealing with geniuses instead of mere adequates."

"You know I won't play that kind of game, Carrie," Jamie said. "It's immoral and ruthless and rather short-sighted."

"Are you accusing me of immorality, James?" Carrie's eyes flashed a sudden cold lightning blue. "Because I'm more capable than you of recognizing what a client needs, or of admitting when a team is on the wane?"

"Carmichael and Baum aren't on the wane, Carrie. You've just decided you don't like Maggie anymore, though I'm not quite sure why."

"You're the last person to cast that particular stone, since you know very well that you insist on running your whole life—our business included—by surrounding yourself with only the people *you* like."

"Trust," Jamie said calmly. "Not necessarily like." He met her eyes.

"Meaning what precisely? That you don't like me?"

"Not very much. Not at times like this."

"I'm not sure if I care whether you like me or not," Carrie said softly. "What I find much more disappointing is the fact that I find myself not respecting you anymore." She paused. "And what, frankly, worries me even more than that is that I've noticed I'm not alone in that."

"Ah, Carrie," Jamie said.

"What does that mean?"

"It means, what are you trying to do? Pick another fight?"

"I can't see the point in fighting, unless it's for the pleasure of making up, and I have no desire for that tonight."

"So it's just malice," he said, hating the thought.

"If you say so. I'd prefer to call it honesty. A few home truths." Carrie paused. "I'm sorry if they hurt you."

"They don't, on the whole," Jamie said quietly. "I don't, on the whole, believe they have much to do with truth."

"That's a pity," Carrie said. "But then again, not accepting what others think of you is part of what's wrong with you."

He tried, for a long time, to laugh it off. He was a modest man but he still knew his own worth, and so he tried to make Carrie see that he thought her accusations ridiculous, and then, as she became more aggressive, to let her know that it did both upset and anger him. But Carrie was becoming masterly at the arts of spite, mockery, insinuation, and sneering. She could be subtle when she wished, tiny pinpricks or hurtful banter, or she could be barbaric, locating a nerve and drilling it over and over again till her victim—whether a new secretary or a salaries clerk or a copywriter like Maggie Carmichael—was about ready to scream. But with Jamie, her greatest challenge was in finding a suitable nerve. When Carrie wanted to get at her husband, she criticized everything about him: his lovemaking, his decisions, the way he looked, his softness, his creativity. But nothing rang true, because Jamie just went on being Jamie, working successfully, being popular, being so goddamned fine at whatever he liked doing—and that was the worst of it from Carrie's point of view: her husband *did* like what he did, and he liked himself, had no deep-seated dark shames or angsts. The only two abiding guilts he'd ever suffered from were the sense that he'd let down his late father first by choosing advertising over shipping and then, even though Jamie had long since lapsed, by marrying a non-Catholic.

It was love that provided Carrie with her greatest weapon. Jamie did still love her. In spite of her. He had thought, when her attempts to denigrate him had first begun, that he could see through her hardness to a softer interior, had fancied that if he could only find a way to penetrate the steel, he might uncover a nicer, gentler person. But then he had realized that he was playing Carrie's own game—wanting to change her—and so he had forced himself to stop thinking that way. If he loved her, Jamie rationalized, he had to love her as she was, even if it was tough to do.

It became tougher. In the late spring of 1987—shortly after Jamie had answered Olivia's call and flown to Geneva to help Annie with her addiction nightmare—Carrie fell pregnant and insisted on a termination. Displaying real vulnerability for the first time in a long while, she begged Jamie to understand, told him it was simply too soon for her to think of having a baby, that continuing to build up their business was just too important to her. And in spite of a startling deep stab of Catholic guilt, Jamie did almost understand that, though he also suspected that her decision had been made because pregnancy would make her fat and imperfect and out of control; but he thought he could understand that too, and it was, after all, her body, and mostly therefore her decision to make, and they were both still young and there was plenty of time. Six months later the same thing happened, with the same result, but this time Carrie laid all the blame for the unwanted pregnancy on Jamie.

"You're a careless, callous, selfish fool," she ranted at him in the clinic, and then she lay back in the high white hospital bed and began to weep bitterly, and Jamie's heart went out to her because whatever she said, he thought that in spite of her reasons for aborting the pregnancy she was still mourning the loss of her child.

But then, less than two months later, Carrie went, without consulting him, without ever raising the subject, to be sterilized. The first Jamie knew about it was when she called him from the clinic after waking up from the anaesthetic.

He waited for two hours, trying to clear his head, to calm himself, before he went to see her.

"How could you do this?" He asked the question quietly, almost gently, though he knew as he spoke that finally, at that moment at least, he hated her. "Tell me, please, if you can."

Carrie was pale but composed. "Oh, I can," she said.

He waited. "Go on."

"Are you sure you can take the truth?"

"Yes," Jamie said. "I can take it."

"All right." Her eyes were on his face. "The truth is that I found I couldn't contemplate having your child, James." She paused. "That if you had been less of a disappointment to me—as my husband and as my partner—I might have gotten over my own fears and gone through with it."

He got up from his chair and walked out of the room and went down in the elevator and out into the street, and he took a cab and went home to Beacon Hill and packed a suitcase and went to the Meridien Hotel on Franklin Street, the site of the old Federal Reserve Building.

He stayed for two nights, going into the office as usual, knowing that even Carrie was likely to be out of action for at least a day or two. He was, for the very first time in his life, desperately lonely. He wanted, very badly, to talk to Olivia, but each time he reached for the telephone something—pride, he thought, with a kick of shame—stayed his hand.

Carrie called him early on the second morning and asked him to come home.

"I don't think so," Jamie said.

"Please," she said, her voice soft and unfamiliar, "come back."

"I can't."

"I need you to."

"Why?"

"I need my husband," she said simply.

Jamie looked around the empty, lonely hotel room. "I wanted babies," he told her. "I wanted children."

"I know," she said, and there was real sorrow in her voice. "Me, too."

"Then why?" Jamie shook his head. "For God's sake, Carrie, why did you do this? Just to spite me? To punish me? *Why?* I need to understand this."

"No, you don't," Carrie said.

"Yes, I do." He paused. "If there's ever to be anything between us again, I do need to understand why you did this thing."

Carrie sighed. "Of course," she said. "You're always the same. The ever understanding, long-suffering Jamie."

He frowned. "You never call me that."

"No."

"So why now? And why make it sound like a term of abuse?"

"Because I married a man named James Arias, not a boy called Jamie," Carrie replied. "Olivia and Annie's friend."

She came to the Meridien that night and asked if he would have dinner with her. They stayed inside the hotel, went to Julien—a grand vaulted affair of a French restaurant that had, in the days of the Federal Reserve Building, been the boardroom—and sat in wing-back chairs, both pecking disinterestedly at their food to the chagrin of the maître d'hôtel and waiters.

Jamie asked Carrie how she felt, and she said she felt fine, and he had to admit that she had seldom looked more beautiful, or softer, or more vulnerable. All through the meal she was quiet and distant, yet it was not, he felt, a deliberate, calculated remoteness, but a distance created by depression and, he thought, fear. Jamie could not remember ever having seen Carrie really afraid before.

She asked, near the end, for a very fine Armagnac.

"I'm going to do something now," she said when the waiter had brought it to her, "that I've never done before in my whole life." She paused. "I'm going to beg."

"Don't," Jamie said, appalled.

"I have no choice," Carrie said. "So I'm begging you, James, to come back to me."

"Why? What for?"

"Because I need you. I'm alone, and I feel as if I've lost you, and I suppose I deserve to lose you. And I know what an eighteen-carat bitch I've been—will probably go on being—"

Jamie almost smiled then, admiring her, in spite of everything, for her honesty.

"—but I do need you, James. I find—and it does surprise me a little, I have to say it does—but I find that I really do need you."

Jamie thought about his father again then. Carlos had never questioned the faith handed down to him by his own father; he would have found the terminations hard enough to accept, and the sterilization almost impossible. And yet, at the end of it all, Jamie knew that Carlos would still have held to his marriage vows, would never have contemplated divorce.

Jamie was not like his father, nor was Peter. Cousin Michael, who strongly resembled his own late father, Juan Luis Arias, was the one who had taken on the mantle as head of the family and Arias Shipping, and who, though sadly childless, had remained a good, staunch, unquestioning Catholic. If Jamie did stay with Carrie, he would not lie to himself and pretend it was because of his faith, but it might perhaps, in part, be because of the guilt he had always felt about having failed Carlos in the past. He did not want to fail him in this, too.

He looked into the eyes that had so often lately looked at him with such disdain, such diamond-coldness, but that seemed suddenly to reflect a naked, raw insecurity torn from its hiding place deep inside her. And he sighed, and he knew that he would go back to her because, Carlos aside and despite all she had done to hurt him, he still saw in her now what he had once loved.

And because he thought that, despite her hardness and callousness and the bravado that would, almost certainly, return within days, perhaps even hours, Carrie was probably, deep down, like most people, genuinely afraid of some things: of being left alone against her will, of losing her perfect beauty, of growing old—or maybe even, though Jamie doubted that, of losing him.

And he felt pity for her.

13

In March of 1988, Olivia, on a visit to Boston before relocating from Geneva to Strasbourg (her restless, nomadic nature had drawn her to Alsace and the attractive old city, which buzzed these days with international activity, making it a perfect base, at least for a while, for the Segal Translation Agency) was disturbed by the changes in Jamie. He seemed tired and, she thought, not exactly depressed, but his joie de vivre had vanished along with the natural, easygoing contentment that had always been such an essential part of him.

It was not difficult to see the cause of the changes. A few of Carrie's digs at Jamie were public these days, though with other people around, her fault-finding took on a more indulgent, patronizing face. But in Olivia's company—a woman Carrie had never liked, who she knew had never liked her, and for whom, in a crisis, Jamie was maddeningly likely to drop anything at a moment's notice—Carrie hardly bothered to put on an act at all. After all, she reasoned, the more unpleasantly she behaved toward Jamie in his old pal's company, the more uncomfortable she was likely to feel. And so far as Carrie was concerned, the sooner Olivia Segal left Boston, the better.

"Why are you putting up with this?" Olivia demanded one day over lunch in the sushi bar at Agatha on Berkeley Street. "It's not as if you're blind to it—you've told me you hate the way she behaves. Why don't you leave her, for Christ's sake?"

Jamie drank some sake and smiled wryly. "You make it sound so simple, but then I guess you always do."

"It seems pretty simple to me." She paused. "It's not some deep-seated Catholic guilt, is it?"

"No," he said, and smiled again. "Not entirely, at least."

"Carrie doesn't love you, Jamie," Olivia said bluntly. "If she did, she couldn't treat you the way she does. She's using you—your talent, your good nature, your wealth. Let's face it, you're still a beautifully presentable and useful husband."

"Carrie's just as talented as I am—perhaps more," Jamie answered quietly, "and she doesn't need my money."

"Because she has enough of her own?" Olivia was scathing. "Everyone knows that two fortunes are better than one." She had listened to Carrie's sniping and observed her attempts to undermine Jamie for six days now, and she'd started out with a degree of diplomacy, just a smidgen of delicacy, but now she was growing desperate to get through to him. "She's hurting you, Jamie. She's *damaging* you—can't you see that? Of course you can, you're not a fool, or you never used to be."

"I'm not a fool," Jamie said.

"So why not leave her?" Olivia looked into his eyes, saw how wounded he was, and wanted to weep for him, wanted to wring Carrie's slender neck. "Don't you know how much better you are than her?" she asked more gently. "How much better you deserve than this?"

"Maybe," Jamie said.

Their sushi was laid out before them, and more hot sake. It all looked wonderful but neither of them moved to touch it.

"I'm not ready to leave Carrie," Jamie said a moment or two later. "I know it seems strange to you, I know that if you were in my place you might walk out—"

"If I were in a marriage where my partner put me down every time he opened his mouth, you bet I'd walk out."

"It isn't always like that."

"You mean she behaves like a halfway decent human being occasionally?" Olivia couldn't keep her sarcasm down. "I'm impressed. Let's give her the Humanitarian of the Year award."

"Shut up, Olivia."

Olivia blinked at the harshness of his tone.

"If I tell you that Carrie doesn't always act the way she has this past week, then it's up to you whether or not you believe me."

"Of course I believe you."

"Then please"—Jamie smiled at her—"try and stop interrupting me every time I try to tell you how it is for me." He paused. "For me, not you, okay?"

Olivia nodded. "Okay. Of course."

"As I said, it may seem strange to you, but I have this thing about marriage vows—not just because I was born a Catholic. But my parents did feel the same way."

"Your parents *were* good Catholics, and they had a good marriage."

"Olivia, shut up," Jamie said pleasantly.

"I'm sorry."

"You're right, of course, up to a point. My parents were both religious, and they did have a good marriage in the long run, but my father once told me that it was pretty rocky for a while. They could have separated without divorcing, but my father said it never occurred to either of them to do that."

Olivia waited a second. "I expect they still loved each other."

"And maybe Carrie and I don't anymore," Jamie said softly. "I don't deny that. As you said, I'm not a fool. But I do still care for her, about her, and I do happen to think, hard as it may be for you to believe it, that she still needs me."

Olivia looked at him for a long moment.

"As a matter of fact," she said very gently, "it isn't so hard for me to believe that Carrie needs you." She waited another instant. "But I do find myself hoping—and I'm sorry if this hurts you—you know the last thing in the world I want to do is hurt you, Jamie—"

"I know."

"But I do find myself hoping that the time will come when you realize—without too much pain, and without any guilt—that you don't need her."

Everything changed the following autumn. Until now, despite their differences, both husband and wife had remained faithful: Jamie

because he had no wish to stray; Carrie partly because infidelity, if discovered, would have tarnished her image, and partly because Jamie,
whatever his failings, had seemed a safe haven of sorts in this new era of
AIDS and herpes and God knew what other inhibiting horrors.

Suddenly, though, Carrie had found someone else. Someone even
more suitable than James Arias. Wealthier, older, worldlier, tougher—
arguably even more attractive. Certainly more ruthless, more like herself. And the supreme irony was that Jamie had brought them together,
had invited the other man into their home, had believed that, of all
men in the world, this had been one of the two he could trust with his
life, certainly with his wife. Except that Jamie had forgotten Carrie's
powers of seduction and persuasion, those same powers she had used to
ensnare him just a few years before. And now Peter Arias—Jamie's
own older brother, recently separated from Daisy, his wife, somewhat
ashamed of himself but just as crazily in love with Carrie as Jamie had
been in those early, heady days of 1984—was set to replace him.

Michael Arias, as head of the family, came to Boston to see Jamie. He
was forty-five years old and an impressive man to be around, distinguished and handsome, less gentle perhaps than his uncle had been, but
proving himself a clever, measured, and effective leader.

"Is she here?" Michael asked when he arrived at the house one
Sunday morning in late October.

"No."

Jamie walked ahead of his cousin into the library. It had always
been one of his preferred rooms, but now he favored it especially
because Carrie had spent less time in there than any other part of the
house and so now it reminded him of her less, did not have the faint
whiff of her scent that much of their home seemed to be pervaded by.

"Where is she?" Michael asked, sitting in one of the leather
armchairs.

Jamie shrugged. "You tell me." With Peter based with Michael at
Arias Shipping's head office in New York and Carrie's dedication to
Beaumont-Arias undiluted despite the breakup of her marriage to
Jamie, the lovers were tending to spend their weeks apart, sharing alter-
nate weekends in Boston or Manhattan. "I only know that she's not
here. I imagine she's with my brother."

Jamie did altogether more imagining than was good for him. Images kept flashing through his mind, of his wife and his brother, naked between silk sheets—the kind Carrie liked, the only kind she would have in their house. Peter had sworn to Jamie that they had never made love in the Beacon Hill house—"What do you take me for, for Christ's sake?" he had asked indignantly, and Jamie had not cared to answer the question truthfully. He took Peter for exactly what he was. A traitor. A stranger whom Jamie would have liked to beat to a pulp. He had always been a gentle man. He did not feel gentle anymore.

"I've spoken to Peter, of course," Michael said.

"Of course."

"I found it hard," Michael went on, "to express my feelings."

Jamie looked into his cousin's face, searching, he realized, for a point of contact, of familiarity, of sure, solid ground. "How do you feel?"

Michael's dark eyes, a rich velvety color like Jamie's own, seemed almost black. "Deeply angry," he answered quietly. "Shocked." He paused. "More disappointed, I think, than I can ever remember feeling."

Jamie experienced a semblance of comfort, of reassurance. "Thank you," he said.

"What for?" Michael asked, wryly. "I didn't stop it from happening."

"Did you know about it?"

"No, of course not. But perhaps I should have."

Jamie thought back, suddenly, to his childhood, simpler times spent in the magnificent Arias home on the cliffs at Newport. He remembered a time when he was still just a little boy of around four, a day in summer, not long after Juan Luis Arias, Michael's father, had died, when the whole family had been there in the gardens. Carlos sitting in a white cane chair beside Barbara Arias, Jamie and Peter's American mother. Jamie recalled her beautiful, pale face and her dark hair, still lustrous then, before the cancer had turned it dull and stolen her away just a few years later, from her sons, from her husband. Jamie remembered Peter, at about ten, teaching him how to kick a ball around, and he remembered being hit by the big ball, full in the stomach, and going down and crying with the shock of it. And he remembered Michael, his big, grown-up cousin—eighteen or nineteen back then, Jamie guessed—picking him up and checking him over and soothing him until the tears had gone.

"Pedro, for God's sake," he remembered Michael scolding Peter, "you must be more careful." At home in those days, Carlos had called them all by their Spanish names—Miguel, Pedro, and Jaime—and his sons and nephew, who, like most young people, preferred conformity outside in the real world, were happy enough at home with the sense of individuality—even, the two older boys felt, of exclusiveness—that those private identities seemed to give them.

"Jamie"—Michael's voice broke into his thoughts—"are you all right?"

Jamie smiled. "I'm fine. I was just remembering."

"Carrie?"

"No." Jamie shook his head. "Us. As a family." He looked at his cousin. "You were always protective of me."

"You were very young," Michael said, shrugging it off.

"You were always like a brother to me," Jamie told him, and smiled again at another memory. "You know, Olivia once said that when the three of us were all together, we reminded her of the Mafia."

Michael raised an eyebrow. "Did she?"

"Olivia's always had a vivid imagination."

"Has she? I don't really know her all that well."

"I guess not," Jamie said. "Not well enough." He paused. "She's my closest friend."

"Closer than Annie?"

"Sometimes, maybe." Jamie thought about them. "Annie's more like my little sister."

"And Olivia?" Michael asked.

Again Jamie smiled. "Olivia's different."

Michael stayed for lunch, cooked by Jamie himself since their house-keeper had the weekend off. It was not the most relaxed of meals. So long as they were talking old memories, reliving the distant past, the conversation went easily and the atmosphere between the two cousins was warm, but whenever the present intruded, the contrasts between them became emphasized. Aside from blood and memories, they had little in common to discuss, especially now that any mention of Peter was a grinding of fresh salt into Jamie's wounds. Michael asked, over coffee, if Jamie wanted to fly back to Newport with him where he and Louise, his wife, had been staying the weekend, but Jamie declined, claiming that he had too much paperwork to get through before Beaumont-Arias reopened in the morning. It was only half true, and he felt that Michael probably knew that, but if he did, he showed no sign of being offended.

"I'll try tackling Peter again this week," Michael promised before he left. "Though I get the impression there won't be much I can do to cool things down." He paused at the door. "Would you take Carrie back, if she and Peter ended the affair?"

"No," Jamie said, and found that he meant it. "Never."

"Good." Michael reached out his right hand and laid it on Jamie's shoulder. "You know I'm with you a hundred percent on this, don't you, little cousin?"

Jamie nodded. "I know. And I appreciate it. It does help."

"You know, too," Michael went on, a little uncomfortably, "that that doesn't mean I can turn my back on Peter. Maybe I should be able to do that, to take the ultimate religious or moral high ground, but I find that I can't." He scanned Jamie's face anxiously. "I hope you understand."

"I do."

"It isn't easy for me," Michael said. "Seeing Peter every day at the office, knowing what he's done to you—what he's doing." His eyes were very dark. "I'm very angry with him. I try to imagine what your father would have said to him—or my own father, come to that."

"I'm glad they don't have to know about it," Jamie said.

"That's something, I guess," Michael said. "Not too much, though, from where you're standing."

"No," Jamie agreed. "Not too much at all."

Once Carrie saw that Jamie was not going to ask her and Peter to end their affair, nor, under any circumstances, to beseech her to come back to him, she began, with considerable relish, to rub his nose in her dirt. His brother was the better man, she told Jamie, exhilarated by her newly heightened capacity to wound—Carrie the picador, piercing her husband with the lance of her magnificently ill-chosen infidelity, paving the way for the kill.

"I want a divorce," she said right after the second Monday morning campaign meeting that November, just after the last account executive had left the boardroom. "And I intend to have it on my terms."

"I hardly think you're in a position to lay down conditions," Jamie said.

"Oh, I disagree."

"How can you possibly disagree?" Tiredly, Jamie began to stack his folders, getting ready to leave.

Carrie got up from her chair at the opposite end of the oval table and came to Jamie's end, pulling out the chair to his left and sitting down.

"Because morally," she answered, slowly and carefully, smoothing down the skirt of her new pink Versace suit, confident for the moment in her appearance thanks to forty-eight hours of alternate sweat and pampering at her favorite spa, or "fat farm," as Peter had teasingly referred to it (which had led to their first really big fight), "at the end of the day, I doubt if anyone would blame me for going to another man."

Jamie looked up. "And how do you figure that?"

"Easily." She paused. "Once people knew what had driven me away from my husband, out of our marriage bed."

"And what exactly did drive you, Carrie?" Jamie found that he felt as calm as he sounded, like a weary nurse calming a delusional patient. Any moment now, Carrie would presumably tell him how patronizing he sounded. He supposed, maybe, that he felt patronizing, among other things.

"Your own sick little affair drove me," Carrie said.

"My affair?" Startled, he stopped sorting his papers.

She smiled at him. "Not so little, perhaps, on reflection."

"Just who am I supposed to have had an affair with?"

"With your two friends, of course."

Jamie grew very still.

"Did you imagine I didn't know?" Carrie asked, looking directly at him, her blue eyes very large and clear.

For a long moment Jamie stared back at her. And then he laughed.

He leaned back in his chair and threw back his head and laughed, deep and long. And then, when all the laughter had gone, he sat forward again and his eyes, fixed on her face, were almost black.

"You must be mad," he said quietly.

"Must I?" Carrie stood up, returned to her original seat at the far end of the table, and picked up her own files. "I think not, James," she said. "I think you would do well to understand that I'm not in the least bit mad. And that if you make any fuss about my divorce terms—if you offer even the slightest resistance to my demands—I will not only smear you with every last glob of mud I can find, but I will also drag both your beloved friends through the dirt with you."

Jamie watched her turn her back, go to the door, open it, and walk through it without glancing back at him, watched the door close behind her. Her words were repeating themselves inside his head, over and over again. In all his thirty years, he was not aware of having ever heard anything more patently absurd, more open to ridicule. More outrageous. Especially when it came to Annie. He could maybe *just* have comprehended a hint of jealousy of a gorgeous single woman like Olivia, though Christ knew there'd never been anything of that nature between them, not even back in their school days when he'd thought Olivia the most attractive girl he'd ever known. But Annie—of all people, *Annie*. And Jamie knew that Carrie's accusation had nothing whatsoever to do with jealousy; it was entirely down to poison, nothing else. And he felt a rage growing within him, greater, more powerful even than the fury he had felt when he had learned about her infidelity with Peter.

"How dare she?" he muttered, unaware that he was speaking aloud. "How *dare* she?" His fists were so tightly clenched on the armrests of his chair that even his short, neatly clipped-back fingernails cut into his palms. He stayed in the chair, allowed the rage to rise and rise, filling him, consuming him, conscious even in the midst of its heat that it was safest to do that, to let it take him over here, in this room, where there was no one to see him. No temptation to allow it to fire fully, to be directed at the man and woman whom he knew now that he hated, honestly, truly *hated*, with all his soul.

It passed. He had no awareness of how long he sat there, his Jamie

Arias, Gieves & Hawke–suited outer shell containing and controlling that inner explosion of loathing.

"Okay," he said quietly to himself. "Get a grip."

He closed his eyes, took a deep, composing breath, then opened them again. The white-hot fury had gone and only a dark, bottomless contempt remained. And a great sadness. Carrie had taken the best, perhaps the purest, thing in his life, his friendship with Olivia and Annie, and had tried to soil it, to pollute it with her own special brand of filth.

He would not let her. He could not let her. Even there, in the aftershock of his rage, still seated at his end of the boardroom table, Jamie was clearheaded about that one thing. No matter how he felt, no matter how close to murderous he might feel, no matter how intense his desire for revenge, Jamie knew that it was more important to protect Olivia and Annie. He doubted, when all was said and done, if Carrie would go through with her threats, because that kind of exposure might end up backfiring on her own image, and maybe—just maybe—Peter might have retained enough shreds of decency to make her draw the line somewhere. But Jamie could not be sure of either of those things, could not be certain that Carrie might not be so obsessed with malice that she would willfully kill Annie's marriage and destroy Olivia's professional life.

He could not risk that. Olivia was probably tough enough to withstand anything that Carrie could throw at her, but Annie was still fragile, still needed to be protected, and Edward had already put up with so much and Jamie was not going to endanger that family's hard-earned happiness.

At least, he reflected wryly as he rose at last, calm enough to put together his folders and leave the boardroom, there were no children for Carrie to use as bargaining chips in their divorce. He sighed. Even if he did ultimately have to give in to most of her financial demands, at the end of the day it was really only money, and Jamie had the rare, privileged consolation of knowing that he would still have more than enough.

He saw Peter just once during the next three months, while their respective lawyers were battling it out. It was an accidental meeting in

January of 1989, capricious fate leading them both, at the same hour of the same day, into the electric train department of F A O Schwarz in New York.

Jamie was buying some rolling stock to add to the collection he had begun last year for William Thomas, Annie's six-year-old son. He didn't notice Peter until he'd handed over his American Express card and was waiting for his parcels to be wrapped. His brother was standing near one of the big fully operational German electric sets, but he wasn't looking at the distinctive green train just gliding past him; he was looking across at Jamie and it was clear from his expression that he had been debating whether or not he might make his escape before being spotted.

Jamie nodded at him curtly, and Peter began to walk toward him. His face was taut, his handsome mouth a straight, compressed line.

"Hello, Jamie."

"Peter."

They had not seen each other since the last of several heated encounters in the period immediately after Carrie had first told Jamie about their affair. The passion and the rage had gone out of Jamie now, squeezed out by the relentless litigious process and the increasing tedium of seeing his adulterous wife every day at the office. Jamie would never have thought it possible to regard Carrie and her savage tongue as tedious, but he found that she had now ceased almost entirely to wound him. He fancied that he had grown a new, protective outer layer, an uncharacteristically thicker skin that carried him through research meetings, campaign strategy meetings, luncheons with clients, presentations and corporate dinners—all those occasions when Jamie accepted that for the sake of Beaumont-Arias and its employees, he and Carrie had to perform together as smoothly and effectively as possible.

"Unlikely place to meet," Peter said.

"Indeed," Jamie said.

"I was looking for a birthday gift for Andy."

Peter and his ex-wife, Daisy, had two young sons, Andrew and Paul, and Daisy Arias, Jamie had heard on the ever fruitful grapevine, was so disgusted with Peter's behavior that she was talking about trying to cut back on his visitation rights to the boys.

"I've already organized his gift," Jamie said quietly.

"So the trains aren't for Andy?"

"No."

"I only ask because that's what I was thinking of for him."

"No," Jamie said again. "They're not for Andy."

The sales assistant returned at that moment and handed back Jamie's American Express card. "Is this zip code correct, sir?"

"It's a British post code," Jamie said, glancing at the delivery address on the invoice. "That's fine."

"And can I just check the name again, sir?" The woman gave Jamie an apologetic smile. "My pen was fresh out of ink when I wrote it down." She bent over the counter. "It looks like William—?"

"It's William Thomas," Jamie told her.

"Thomas, that's it." She smiled again. "Thank you, sir."

"You're welcome," Jamie said.

"That must be your friend Annie's boy," Peter said behind him.

Jamie looked at him. "It is."

"Nice for him," Peter said, "having such a fond—" He gave a small, amused-looking grin. "—uncle? Does he call you Uncle Jamie?"

"He does not," Jamie said, and a little of the rage that he had thought all squeezed out or simply under control came back, tightening his throat. He looked at his brother with distaste. "Good-bye, Peter," he said.

Peter smiled again, a knowing, ugly smile. "Be seeing you."

"As seldom as possible," Jamie said.

14

What irked Jamie far more than the financial settlement was the fact that Carrie was insisting not only that he remain her business partner—thus ensuring that Beaumont-Arias held on to the clients won through Jamie's personal talents—but also that he become, in terms of major decisions, a silent and, thereby, impotent partner. It was not that Carrie was trying to ignore the scandal that her brother-swapping exercise might create. On the contrary, she was contriving, with considerable panache, to turn it into an enthralling bonus.

"Peter and I have suppressed our feelings for years, you know," Carrie was telling people, oh so confidentially, oh so discreetly. "It was simply a case of James and I having married too quickly—we found that out pretty early, I'm afraid to say—and we've all tried so very hard, but finally I guess we had to give in. And we're all on such good terms, it's all so civilized, and that must be obvious to everyone because otherwise how could we even *think* of staying in business together?"

Jamie moved out of the Beacon Hill house that March into a duplex condominium on Rowes Wharf overlooking the harbor, bought a trim white sailboat called the *Joie de Vivre*—Carrie hated boats—and tried to enjoy his regained bachelor status. It was good to be an individual again, wonderful to be free—at least at the start and end of each working day—of his wife's savage tongue, yet he was a million miles from being even close to happy. He felt that he had failed in every way that counted. Before Carrie, he'd been so confident, his only sense of failure that to his late father, but here he was, not yet thirty-one, and he'd screwed up his marriage, as good as lost his brother, all but abandoned control of his business, and put his two dearest friends in jeopardy. Oh, sure, Olivia and Annie would both say that it was all down to Carrie, none of it his fault, but Jamie knew it all came down to two basic flaws of his own. He was weak, and he was a damned fool. He had provoked Carrie during the years of their marriage by seeming to be strong enough to withstand her, strong enough to keep loving her. Yet at the end of the day he had capitulated, and now he was left with nothing that he really valued—except for Olivia and Annie, and Lord knew Carrie had done her best to taint even that.

Olivia and Annie came to visit him in May, Annie for just a few days. She was in great shape, hair newly bobbed and full of pride and enthusiasm for a new project recently embarked upon.

"I'm studying reflexology," she told Jamie and Olivia. "I know some people turn up their noses and think it's all trendy nonsense, but it was one of the alternative therapies that really helped me with my stress levels after I first kicked the tranquilizers—and they're doing so much serious research into using it as a pain management technique."

"I've done some reading about it," Jamie said. "It all seemed to make pretty good sense."

"Anyway," Annie went on, "I'm doing a lot of the written work by correspondence, and I go to evening classes during the week when Edward's in London and Marie-Louise is home with the children." She was flushed with excitement. "I've been told that I have quite an aptitude for it, and a couple of our neighbors have said that they'll let me treat them when I qualify, and it would be so great to feel useful outside the house."

"Did you get that?" Olivia asked Jamie. "She said *when* she qualifies, not if, or maybe, or she probably won't be good enough and even if she is, the neighbors will back out at the last minute."

"It's okay to mock." Annie was laughing.

"Not mocking," Olivia said, "just teasing."

"I think it's fantastic." Jamie squeezed Annie's hand. "Edward must be very proud of you."

"I'm proud of me," Annie said softly.

"So you should be," Olivia told her.

Annie went home after four days, but Olivia said she could stay on in Boston for another ten, and Jamie was grateful for that, for already he felt a little more like his old self, felt some of his confusions coming into clearer focus.

"I have some things to say," Olivia said to him just after breakfast the morning after Annie had flown back to London. "Things that Annie wasn't sure I ought to say to you just yet, but which I'm going to anyway. Okay?"

"Sounds ominous."

The remains of their juice, croissants, and fresh-brewed coffee were on a low table between them, and they were sitting facing each other on the two soft leather settees that Jamie had installed into the glass-surrounded alcove off his sitting room. The alcove jutted out over the wharf below, giving the sensation of hanging directly above the harbor, blue and sparkling this morning and already alive with gulls and sailing boats and commuter and tourist ferries.

"Right." Olivia drained her coffee cup and set it down. "First, I'd like to get one thing straight in your head. You are *not* a failure, and if I ever hear you saying or even feel you starting to *think* that way again, I will fly straight back here from wherever I am and beat the crap out of you. Clear?"

"Clear enough." He smiled, deciding that her own chic new shorter hair emphasized her marvelously mobile face, made her, startlingly, even more feminine than before.

"I think, maybe," Olivia went on, more slowly, more thoughtfully, "that Carrie's got you confusing basic decency with weakness." She looked into his face, saw his vulnerability. "Don't you realize that your decency and your gentleness and your kindness are your special strengths, Jamie? They're the reason Annie and I both love you so much—part of the reason, at least—and I'm pretty certain they're part of the reason for your success with your colleagues and your clients."

"For what that's worth," he said wryly.

"Oh, come *on*," Olivia said, exasperated. "You're thinking failure again. Falling in love with a superclass bitch like Carrie wasn't a failure—just the aberration of all time. And getting the hell *out* of your marriage has got to be the best thing you've ever done, whatever it's costing you."

"If all it was costing me was money—" Jamie stopped.

"You mean the business," Olivia said.

She and Annie had both asked him about his clearly unsatisfactory arrangements with Carrie at Beaumont-Arias, but Jamie had been reluctant to talk about that and so they had both withdrawn from the subject.

"I still don't understand," she went on now, "what's going on there. It's the only part of your divorce proceedings that I think you're crazy to be going along with. I mean, surely it's insane for you to go on pouring even one ounce of your talent or effort into Carrie's and Peter's coffers."

"Peter doesn't figure in this," Jamie said.

"The hell he doesn't," Olivia retorted. "He's still sleeping with your wife, isn't he? They're still talking about getting married, aren't they?"

"They are."

"So how long do you plan to go on helping Carrie pay her bills?" Olivia threw up her hands. "And don't start telling me again that she doesn't need your money. We all know she's never really needed it, and you've always said that she didn't need your talent either, but it hasn't stopped her using both, has it?"

"Have you finished?" Jamie asked quietly.

"For the moment."

"Good." He paused. "Do you really think I'm unaware of what you're telling me?"

"No. Of course not."

"And do you think I'm enjoying the way things are at Beaumont-Arias?"

"No, I don't," Olivia said. "But that doesn't explain why you're putting up with it."

"I have my reasons," Jamie said.

"Which you won't tell me."

"That's right." There was no way on earth that Jamie was going to tell Olivia about Carrie's threats. He hated the thought of Olivia feeling pushed away or excluded, but he knew he had no choice, because if she found out the truth, she would very likely blow sky-high, and then Lord knew what shit would hit the fan and it was probably Annie who would end up suffering, and Jamie was still not prepared to risk that.

"May I ask another question?" Olivia asked.

"Could I stop you?"

"Are you planning to find a way out?"

"Ultimately, of course," Jamie replied. "But there's a lot to consider."

"Losing some of your clients," Olivia surmised.

"Losing them wouldn't be the biggest issue," Jamie said. "But if I left Beaumont-Arias, I might be forced to walk out on them, to abandon them to Carrie. I see that as morally indefensible."

"If that's true," Olivia said slowly, considering, "then surely what you have to do is find a way to get the best for them and for yourself."

"Easier said," Jamie told her.

"Easily done," Olivia argued. "If you want it enough." She paused. "You're a brilliant man, Jamie. A creative man. Isn't it time you started using those gifts to your own ends? And if that does mean learning how to be a little more devious and a little more selfish, surely it's worthwhile if it's the only way you can really cut loose?"

"And regain my own self-respect, you mean?" Jamie asked softly.

"There's not a single reason on earth for you to have lost that," Olivia said. "Believe that, Jamie, even if you believe nothing else."

It was so good for him, having her there with him, having her strength and audacity and capacity for both luxurious and simple pleasures. Olivia was keen to share some of the energy and satisfaction she was finding in her own life in Strasbourg. Yes, she confessed in a quiet moment, living alone was sometimes lonely, but most of the time she enjoyed her own company, and there were, of course, a couple of new men—one a young Canadian lawyer, the other a French music teacher—neither of them serious relationships, both of them just good, light-hearted company, people with whom to lark about generally and to share all that rich Alsatian food.

"It's what you need," she told Jamie on her seventh evening in Boston.

"I'm okay as I am," he said.

"No, you're not. Which is my main reason for being here. To remind you—before it's too late and you fossilize—what it's like to have fun, *real* fun."

Jamie was wary. "Am I up to this, I wonder?"

"Take a few days off and find out," Olivia said. "I have almost a week left. We could make some real plans."

"I can't," he said. "I'd love to, but it's impossible." He looked at her face, and saw her disapproval. "Not because of Carrie—or not in the way you're thinking—not because she mightn't like it but because she probably would, and I won't leave town right now because I don't trust her."

"Okay," Olivia said. "That makes sense." She smiled at him. "Guess we'll just have to find ways of squeezing some fun into your schedule."

"Guess we will."

She made it a week to remember. Tossing aside her guidebooks and seizing instead upon two or three groups of students and a couple of tutors around Harvard Square, grilling them for Boston know-how, Olivia the organizer set about cramming their days and nights with activities ruthlessly designed to get Jamie back on the road. His heavy commitments at Beaumont-Arias might have dampened a less determined spirit, but having extracted from his secretary a schedule of Jamie's appointments and meetings for the next seven days, Olivia mapped out her own agenda, which entailed whipping Jamie in and out of the Newbury Street office several times each day.

She turned him into a tourist, led him by the hand from tavern to tavern, to The Bell in Hand, the oldest in the country, to Clarke's, one of the sportiest in the city, to The Black Rose, the most fervently Irish. She took him to lunches and dinners at The Salty Dog, the Union Oyster House, Locke-Ober's and the Ritz-Carlton dining room. She took him to listen to jazz at Saffi's and the Regatta Bar and Ryles, and she took him dancing at Spit and the vast, noisy, neon Metro. During the day, working around meetings, business lunches, and cocktails (that week, at least, Jamie had no official dinners to attend), she took him on a swan boat ride on the Public Gardens lagoon and for a picnic on the Common: Carrie's face when she saw Olivia carrying in the wicker hamper she'd filled with everything from cold lobster to chocolate-dipped stem cherries from Bailey's, was a picture both Olivia and Jamie would cherish for years to come.

"You realize you're killing me," Jamie told Olivia on the day of the picnic, after he'd had to run back to Newbury Street for a presentation rehearsal between courses. "By the time you go back to Strasbourg, I'll either be on my knees or flat on my back."

"No, you won't." Olivia fed him a cherry. "I've figured out that this is like dragging someone into aerobics classes every day until the endorphin high gets to them and then they just go on and on."

"Until they drop dead."

"Until they realize that life is richer and more alive and just plain *better* when it's being lived to the fullest."

She took him to the children's petting zoo at Franklin Park, prodded him up the spiral pathway through the huge New England Aquarium. She paid through the nose for tickets for a Celtics game at Boston Garden, bribed someone to let them and a stash of hot dogs into Fenway Park, even though neither the Red Sox nor any other team was playing. She got him to jog with her along the Esplanade beside the Charles River. And, no less than three times, she got him out onto the water in his beloved, barely baptized, pure white *Joie de Vivre*.

She was due to return to Strasbourg the following Monday.

"Michael called," Jamie said to her on Friday evening, on their way to dinner. "Louise suggested we might like to come out to the Newport house for Sunday lunch. Daisy's going to be there with the boys—Michael said that if the weather holds they'll probably be barbecuing."

"No Peter, I take it," Olivia said.

"Definitely not."

"Sounds like fun."

"Are you sure? I mean, it's going to take over an hour getting out to the cottage, and lunch is bound to take at least the same amount of time—and then there'll be the trip back." Jamie's eyes were teasing. "All that for just one ordinary family lunch."

"I daresay I'll find us something more to do while we're there," Olivia said, playing it straight.

"As long as it's not jogging," Jamie said.

Olivia had only been inside the Ocean Drive mansion once before, and had found it attractive from the outside, raised it as it was on a small hill, overlooking the ocean: a white, handsome house with a Spanish tile roof and delicate verandas. But once inside, she found it too large and, perhaps, a little too overbearing for her personal taste. Her own early childhood homes, first on Riverside Drive and then on Park Avenue, had been pretty splendid by Manhattan standards, and the Aldriches' family house in San Francisco had been nothing short of exquisite both in style and dimensions; but the Arias mansion had been more than grand enough even before Michael and Louise had added a new wing, and she knew that Jamie had never liked the changes, would have preferred his father's and uncle's fine home to have remained unadulterated.

Still, Olivia had to admit, if the proportions of the house were too grandiose for her liking, the collection of art that hung on the majestic walls was eclectic, impressive, and fascinating. On the way to Jamie's suite of rooms alone, she saw a Bonnard, two Picassos, a portrait by Delgado, and a large, melancholy painting by Puvis de Chavannes on the staircase, and a Dalí in the small dressing room attached to the marble bathroom. She thought about her father then, and how he would have admired and enjoyed many of the works here, remembered what Arthur had once told her about the way great paintings, whether famous or not, could transcend their settings, carry with them other lives, other atmospheres, sometimes even other worlds. Olivia felt that way now, here, inside this mansion that was a part of Jamie's heritage but in which he seemed, to her at least, so out of place, yet she could look at the Picassos and the beautiful little Bonnard and the bizarre Dalí and think about Jamie's father and uncle assembling them over the years, and the house itself just melted away, and there was the connection, and any lack of harmony had ceased to matter.

★   ★   ★

"Anyone want to join us for a bike ride?" Olivia asked later when they'd finished eating. The gardens in which they sat fell away in glorious abundance from the house, shaded by oaks and elms, willows, chestnuts and firs, and, on this warm and sunny late spring afternoon, vivid with all the colors of the rhododendrons.

Jamie groaned. "I knew it was too good to last."

"Sounds too energetic for me," Louise Arias said, "after all that food."

"I'm too tired from cooking," Michael said.

"First time he's done more than switch on the espresso machine since last summer." Louise looked benevolently at her husband.

"How about you, Daisy?" Olivia asked.

"I haven't cycled since I was fourteen," Daisy Arias said, "and found the exercise was overdeveloping my calves."

"I've always been proud of my muscles." Olivia smiled sweetly at Daisy. "Especially my thighs."

They were sitting in an imperfect semicircle of white cane chairs on the lawn of what Jamie called their second layer of garden. It was very warm for May, but with a pleasant breeze. Michael wore a British panama hat and, with his eyes shielded by dark glasses, Olivia thought he looked like some impenetrable, old-fashioned spy, though earlier on, at work on the big stone barbecue, he'd been every inch the classic American family man, and she had to admit he'd served up some of the best steaks, ribs, and hamburgers she'd ever tasted. Louise, his wife, auburn-haired, hazel-eyed, svelte in slender cream wool pants and perfectly toned sweater, had started out, Olivia thought, a little uptight—which, given the awkward mix of company, was very understandable—but several glasses of Chablis on, she had relaxed into a genuine Sunday afternoon peaceableness. And then there was Daisy, Peter's ex-wife, pretty, blond, and soft featured, long since over the infidelity that had first split them up and glad to let her boys maintain contact with their uncle and cousins, yet always still just a little uncomfortable in the presence of the Arias family, more so now than ever before in the face of Peter's awful betrayal of Jamie.

"I shouldn't have come," Jamie said in a lull before lunch, when he and Olivia had been fleetingly alone. "I think poor Daisy's embarrassed."

"I don't see why she should be," Olivia said. "She's hardly responsible for what her ex-husband gets up to." She gave a sudden grin. "Unless, of course, she's hoping that you two might get together."

"For God's sake, Olivia—" Jamie looked around, appalled.

"It's not so unusual," Olivia said. "The two aggrieved parties—that kind of thing—all that lusty mutual outrage—"

"Olivia, shut up."

"You're much better looking than Peter, and younger, of course." She checked him over appraisingly. He was wearing blue jeans, sneakers, and a cricket sweater; he looked, she thought, stirred, like a dark-haired Gatsby.

"I hardly think she'd want to go from one brother to the other."

"It didn't stop Carrie," Olivia said, and walked away.

"I guess the boys are too young to come biking," she said now, lunch over and the coals on the barbecue dampened down. She glanced over to where Daisy and Peter's sons were kicking around a pair of footballs at the foot of a copper beech tree.

"Paul can ride a bicycle," Daisy said.

"Where were you thinking of riding?" Michael asked Olivia.

"Cliff Walk, I thought," Olivia said.

"Paul can't ride there," Daisy said quickly. "It isn't really meant for cycling, Olivia, just for walking."

"It is pretty rough in parts," Louise said. "And steep."

"We'll be careful," Olivia reassured her.

Jamie sighed. "You really want to go, don't you?"

"I'd love it," she said. "I've been starved of the ocean for so long."

"We've been out on the boat three times in a week," Jamie said.

"Not enough. I need more."

He stretched his long legs out lazily in front of him. "You realize this is the first peaceful hour I've had all week."

"You realize it's my last day with you," she countered. "This way I can have you and my last fix of ocean."

"See what I'm up against?" he said to his cousin.

Olivia looked at Michael. "Has Jamie never told you what a pushy broad I am?"

"Not exactly." Michael smiled at her. "But we're learning."

"Would you like to join us?" she asked him.

"I think I'll pass," Michael said. "But thank you for the offer."

It was a gorgeous afternoon. The bicycles that Jamie had unearthed for them in one of the garden sheds were old and rusty and harder to ride than the modern, lightweight bikes that Olivia had ridden for the past several years, and Jamie grouched for the first fifteen minutes about aching legs and no respite and how he was beginning to think he might be glad to see the back of her. But then the rugged splendor of their surroundings and the invigorating quality of the air began to work their magic, and Olivia's intermittent gales of laughter as she veered to avoid bumps and narrowly missed coming off altogether were too infectious for him to continue bellyaching; and in any case Olivia had taken no notice, so there seemed little point, after all, in complaining about a few aches and pains, and they paused every now and then to look away from the ocean back to the famous Vanderbilt and Astor mansions and, especially, at Rosecliff, Jamie's old favorite, regarded by many as the most romantic of the great Newport houses.

"Makes your place look like a doll's house," Olivia teased, gazing up at the forty-room mansion, unable to conceive of living with the slightest degree of normality in such vastness.

She looked at Jamie now, astride the old bicycle, one foot on the ground, dark hair blowing a little in the wind, thought suddenly how noble he looked, and it was an odd thought for her to have, for God knew she'd never considered him quite that way before, and there was that pang again—*dammit*—and she'd believed she'd put that behind her, back in its box, and thoughts like that were no good at all, unless she wanted to lose one of her two best friends in the world.

"Peter and Carrie are planning to move into the west wing," Jamie said suddenly, his eyes black against the sunlight. "Michael told me while he was throwing steaks on the barbecue. He's awfully embarrassed—Louise is, too—but we all know it's Peter's house as much as his or mine, so there's not a lot anyone can do about it."

Olivia was silent for a moment, and then she said very quietly: "The hell with them both."

"I guess," Jamie said.

She looked at him sharply. "Don't tell me you've forgiven them."

He didn't answer right away, kept his eyes focused on Rosecliff for a few seconds more, and then he looked back at her. "No," he said. "But I'm starting to get used to it."

"Okay," Olivia said. "That's good. I guess."

"As good as it gets, I think."

She watched him for another moment, and a surge of emotion blew over her like an adrenaline rush.

"Let's race," she said suddenly.

"We can't," Jamie said. "The walk's too bumpy."

"You're getting soft on me."

One of those brief, painful images of his brother and his wife flashed across Jamie's mind.

"Wanna bet?" he said.

"Last one to The Breakers buys dinner tonight," Olivia said.

"Deal," Jamie said, and straightened out his wheels.

"On three," Olivia said. "You count."

Jamie smiled. "One—"

They both hunched over.

"Two—"

She was horsing around when it happened. They had both known before the start that racing on those cranky, archaic machines was absurd, and they were pumping the pedals as hard as they could and achieving little in the way of speed but laughing a good deal. Olivia's goal had been to get Jamie's mind off Peter and Carrie and to get her own off Jamie, and if they couldn't get a decent race going, she guessed she'd have to work harder, clown around a little, and so she stopped abruptly and climbed up on the low wall with her bike, and Jamie yelled at her not to be such a damned fool, that it was dangerous up there, but Olivia knew better—she *always* knew better—and she was off, and the wall looked wide enough so long as she kept a straight line, and she was pedaling furiously again, and Jamie, on the path itself, was fighting to keep up with her.

She went over a few hundred yards from The Breakers.

Jamie saw it happen, and yet it was as if he wasn't really seeing it. She veered suddenly to the left, corrected herself, and then her right foot seemed somehow to be stuck. He couldn't tell what had happened, if it was her sneaker or a lace, but she made a sound, gave a kind of low yell, a startled, warning kind of sound, and then she and the bicycle tipped slowly to the right and disappeared.

He'd seen it, but he couldn't believe it, *refused* to believe it. And then he heard her scream, and he screeched to a halt—it had seemed so slow, yet it had happened in just a few seconds—and his own bike crashed to the ground, and he heard yelling and did not quite grasp that it was his own voice yelling.

"Olivia!"

In his mind, he saw her as he would when he got to the edge of the wall and looked over, bloodied and unconscious, or broken, or—

He reached the edge and forced himself to look.

She was only eight or ten feet down on an outcrop of rain-smoothed rocks. She was quite still, facedown, her right leg drawn up and bent at the knee, the bicycle on top of her, and her left arm was thrown back over her head. She was not moving.

Jamie felt his heart literally stop.

"Olivia." It came out in a croak. He tried to clear his throat. "Olivia."

She still did not move. He could not see her face.

"Olivia!"

"Will—you—get—the—fuck—down—here."

Her voice was perfectly steady and quite calm, each word clearly separated, as if punctuated by dashes.

Jamie stared down at her, his heart pounding. "Are you okay?"

Her voice blew up to him again with the wind, its familiar, low huskiness as welcome to him as desert rain or manna from heaven or a sharp fingernail on a long-inaccessible itch.

"No, Jamie," Olivia said, "I am not okay." She paused. "I am not dead, nor do I seem to have broken anything much, but I am definitely not okay." She paused again. "Okay?" The question was acidic.

He smiled. "Okay."

"So are you coming down, or do we wait till I turn as rusty as this so-called bicycle?"

Carefully, forcing himself to stay slow, knowing that if he fell, too, he'd be no use to her at all, Jamie made his way down, using a drainage pipe for support, until he was beside her.

"Can I move the bike?" he asked, afraid he might hurt her.

"No, I really love having it on top of me," she answered.

"Your right sneaker's hooked on a spoke," he told her.

"Tell me about it," she said.

He started to extricate the lace, then stopped.

"Why have you stopped?" she asked.

"So you do want me to help you?"

"Yes, Jamie."

"Do you recall whose idea it was to go bike riding?"

"Mine, Jamie."

"And do you recall whose idea it was to have a race?"

"Mine."

"And do you recall who decided to be a wiseass and get up on the wall, even when someone else told her not to be such a damn fool?"

A moment or two passed. Somewhere above them on the pathway people walked and talked. Gulls wheeled and called over their heads.

"Jamie?"

"Yes, Olivia."

"Do you think you could please help me now?" Her voice was sweet now, compliant and gentle and utterly out of character. "I really would like to see if I can get back on my feet."

"I thought you said you weren't hurt." He was alarmed again. Quickly, he detached the lace and released the sneaker. "Where's the pain?" He lifted up the bicycle and set it over to their right.

Slowly, Olivia sat up. She flexed both arms, then both legs, one at a time, then she moved her head, tentatively, first to the right, then to the left.

"Nowhere." She smiled at him. "You looked really scared."

"I was," he said, sitting down beside her. "You have dirt on your face."

"Wipe it off, please," she said.

★　★　★

Like the fall itself, he didn't exactly know how it happened. He felt curiously disembodied, as if it were happening to another person. He went to wipe the dirt off her face, as she had bidden him, with his large white handkerchief, and then he saw that she had a scratch on her left cheek, saw that she was bleeding, and something deep inside him seemed to move, to come alive, something that he had not known— something he truly *believed* he had not known—was there. And instead of wiping her cheek, or telling her that she was bleeding, or getting her up on her feet and starting to get her back up onto the path, he kissed her. Not on the cheek or forehead or on her hair, the way he had done countless times in the past. On her lips. Right on her wide, soft, surprised mouth.

"Jamie," she said—nothing else—and kissed him straight back.

It was the most extraordinary kiss. All the first kisses he'd ever had until then had been either hungered for, pleasurably anticipated or, in less passionate encounters, bordering on obligatory. This one, flying into his life, into his body and soul, so abruptly, so entirely unpremeditatedly, seemed simply unavoidable. His mouth and Olivia's mouth were drawn irresistibly together. Their lips had to touch, had to kiss, they had to allow their mouths to open so that they could kiss more deeply; Jamie felt as if he might stop breathing, stop functioning, might literally curl up and *die* if he did not go on kissing that well-known, well-loved, oh-so-familiar mouth, and it wasn't really him kissing Olivia, it couldn't be, because that simply could not, would never happen. And yet their tongues were touching and exploring, and it felt like diving down, down, into some wondrous, fathomless, indescribable place, and Jamie heard a small sound and realized it was a moan, and he was not sure if it was his own or her moan.

And he stopped kissing her and drew back.

Olivia, who felt that perhaps she might have been struck by a bolt of genuine nonproverbial lightning, looked long and hard into his eyes.

She waited for him to speak, and when he did not, she knew, with an exquisite jolt of joy, that there was nothing to *be* said, and that he felt exactly the same as she did.

"Jamie," she said at last, and her voice was shakier than it had been right after the fall.

"Yes?"

"Let's go home."

They went back to the house hardly speaking. In the Arias drawing room, sitting beneath a sinuous, poetically lovely Gauguin original, they explained what had happened, went through the motions, let Louise fuss about how much worse it might have been, let her and Daisy clean Olivia up as well as they could given her refusal to take a bath and stay the night, and thanked them politely for finding her an unripped pair of Calvin Klein jeans and an utterly un-Olivia-like flowery silk blouse. They talked Michael out of calling the doctor and out of flying them back to Boston in either the Arias helicopter or the jet, and they bade them all farewell and got back into Jamie's car and drove back to Boston. Back to the apartment on Rowes Wharf.

Their conversation was minimal. They both knew that it was not over, that neither wanted it to be over. Jamie felt out of control, liked feeling that way because he was with Olivia, not with Carrie, and though he was aware that Olivia was taking control, there seemed to him to be no similarity at all between her and his wife. He was safe with Olivia. She was a little crazy, sometimes a lot crazy, but she cared for him as much as he did for her, always had, and so he let her take over, went on feeling as he had since the kiss. Slightly remote, slightly absurd, immensely excited, ready to do just about anything she asked him to. A normally responsible, conventional guy going AWOL.

Olivia knew exactly what she was doing—she'd have been a damned liar if she'd tried to deny it—yet in a sense she felt no more in control than Jamie. There was a nagging in her mind like a dull drumbeat, a warning that this was not wise, that it was, of course, not exactly dangerous because Jamie was Jamie, familiar and kind and safe, and Jamie would never hurt her, yet at the same time she knew they might both *be* hurt unless they stopped right there. Yet still she carried on regardless, encouraged him to open the bottle of Krug she'd put in the refrigerator three days before—they were both easy champagne drunks, always had been, just a glass seemed to go straight to its target, relaxing as a hit of sedative—and then she went right on into his bathroom and turned on the taps and threw about a third of a bottle of Guerlain foam bath into the water—she wondered, for an instant, why Jamie, a fast shower man, had such a thing in his bathroom and, more to the point who had given it to him, and a fierce and idiotic jealousy stabbed at her—and when it was full, she turned the taps off and went to fetch him and their champagne.

"Come on," she said after she'd downed half a glass, made him do the same, and refilled them both herself.

"Where?" he asked, dazed.

"Just come." She knew she had to act fast, in case her courage evaporated with the bubbles in the bath.

Jamie looked at the tub, turned around and saw, in awe and with immeasurable delight, that Olivia was unbuttoning Louise's blouse and unzipping the Calvin Klein jeans. She wore a pale blue, *broderie anglaise* brassiere and matching panties. Her body was slim and firm and smooth, and she had the most exquisitely perfect navel that he had ever seen.

"Did you fall off that cliff, or did I?" he asked, not knowing if the sudden wild pulsing inside his head was from the Krug or the sight of her.

"I think maybe we both did." She was a little breathless.

"Yes," was all he said, all he was capable of saying.

"Come on," she said again. "Before we change our minds."

"Have we made them up, then?" he asked softly.

"Oh, yes," Olivia said. She smiled. "I need a bath. Your family all said I should take a bath, so now I'm going to take one." She looked into his face. "You need one, too," she told him.

"Definitely," he agreed, and began, with fingers that had gone half numb, to unbuckle his belt.

"No sense in wasting water, after all," she said, and, taking off the brassiere and panties, stepped into the tub without another glance at him, lay back in the foamy, delicious water, gave a long sigh, and closed her eyes.

He was hard as a rock before he touched her.

"Do you mind if the rug gets wet?" she asked, not moving, eyes still shut.

"No." His voice was husky. "Not at all."

"Good."

It was a regular-size tub. He tried to settle in, facing her, his back against the cold steel of the taps. Still she didn't move, made no effort to make space for him, but her eyes were wide open now and she was watching him carefully. They were both long-legged, but the tub was large enough for her to be able to stretch out her legs while he had to bend his at the knees. His shins were level with her breasts. Her breasts were paler than the rest of her body, her nipples a dark peach color and erect. Jamie thought that he might, in a moment or two, have a heart attack.

"What now?" he asked.

"First," she said, "we have some more champagne."

"And then?"

"Then, I guess, we wash."

"Do I get to wash you?" he asked almost humbly.

"Well, I should hope so," she answered fervently, then added, as a polite afterthought, "If you like."

"Yes, please," he said, and reached for a bar of soap. It was Roger & Gallet sandalwood; he was glad it wasn't just Dove, which he often used. "Where would you like me to begin?"

"Sometimes," Olivia said, "I start with my feet, other times with my arms and shoulders and neck."

Her feet were surprisingly soft, their toenails painted the same shade of pink as her fingernails.

"For someone so active," Jamie said, contemplating the arch of the left foot, resisting the urge to tickle the sole, "you're not at all athletic looking." For the first time in many hours he thought of Carrie, who had gone to the gym like clockwork all through their marriage, and whose body had remained unquestionably splendid but had, he'd sometimes thought, feeling guilty for his sexism, seemed a little too hard, a little too unyielding. Nothing about Olivia's body, he reflected, soaping her ankle, was hard, except, of course, her nipples.

"Is this supposed to be therapy for me?" he asked her suddenly. "I mean, I don't mind, I don't mind at all, I'm not that crazy, but I'd like to know."

"Shush," she said. "Wash me and don't talk about it and don't think about it." She smiled at him. "We fell off a cliff, remember? Things happen after you fall off a cliff. The rules stop."

He kissed her then, dropped the soap into the water and made no effort to find it, and their bodies were touching now; he felt her breasts against his chest and if he had thought he was hard before, then he'd obviously never known what hard could be. He touched her left breast and felt her shudder, and with his other hand he reached down into the bubbles and parted her thighs a little way, though they were cramped between his own legs in the constraints of the tub, and he felt the soft curls of her pubic hair and looked down, blew away a little foam and saw it, with the most intense jolt of pleasure, like a small dark cloud, tendrils waving in the water like a mermaid's, and he felt it with his fingers and went a little further and heard her moan.

"Am I allowed to say that I don't really believe this is happening?" he whispered.

"You're allowed," she said. "Don't stop."

"I won't stop," he said, and stopped. "Are you sure it's okay?" he asked, with difficulty. "I mean, you can change your mind anytime if you want to."

"Are you nuts?" Olivia asked, huskier than usual, and her own right hand went down into the water and found him, encircled him.

"Jesus," he said. "Oh, sweet Jesus."

It began in earnest then. Everything went to hell, they were so hungry, so starved for each other. Their mouths became fused, and their bodies, and water cascaded over the sides of the tub onto the floor. They both wanted to touch each other everywhere, to feel, to know every part of the other's body, and it was every birthday and Christmas and, for Olivia, every Hanukkah, since time immemorial, and if this powerful, overwhelming need to have this man, this beloved, familiar man, inside her, to have him joined with her, was pure lust, or if it was, maybe, pure love, it didn't really matter, not now at least. It was what it was, and she only knew that she had never, in all her life, experienced anything more utterly, ineffably, joyously, perfectly right.

They had to get out of the tub, it was simply too small, and they knocked over the bottle of Krug, though it didn't matter—they were beyond champagne—and they grabbed at towels and half dried each other, but every new touch was inflaming, and the bathroom was snug and warm and they threw the towels down on the floor and pulled each other down. And Olivia had never been so ready, had never felt quite so monumentally wanton, and she flung her arms back over her head and opened her legs, and she saw Jamie hesitate, saw the question in his eyes—

"I'm on the pill," she answered.

"Thank Christ," he said—

And he entered her slowly, as slowly as he could bear, and he was bigger than she had imagined—though she hadn't realized till now that she *had* ever imagined—for such a slender man, with such beautiful hands. Oh, God they were beautiful, they were so clever and deft and giving, and they were on her now, everywhere, and so was his mouth, and he was moving inside her, and she was moving with him, and there was a molten place in her, and she thought she might erupt, knew she would—

"Oh, God," she said. "Oh, Jamie—"

And she did. They both did.

They both wept afterward too. Not for long, but lustily, in each other's arms, still on the pile of wet towels on the bathroom floor.

"Why are you crying?" Jamie asked her gently, kissing her tears.

"Why are you?" she asked back, licking his salty cheek.

"I guess," he said slowly, holding her tightly, "because today we fell off a cliff, and tomorrow we have to get back on real land."

"Not me," she said. "I get to fly."

"Oh, yes," he said, and held her even closer.

And now they both knew why they were crying.

Jamie awoke next morning to find Olivia already dressed and packed, sitting waiting for him in the living room.

"Why didn't you wake me?" he asked, seeing the time. "You know I'm taking you to Logan." He came over, bent down to kiss her. She accepted his lips but made no real response.

"I'd rather you didn't," she said. "Take me, I mean. I was going to wake you to say good-bye." She looked up into his face, saw confusion, guilt, and the start of misery in his eyes. "Don't look like that, Jamie."

"Like what?" He sat down beside her on the sofa. He was suddenly, uncomfortably aware of his nakedness beneath his white bathrobe. He tied the belt more tightly. He felt indescribably wretched.

"And don't feel that way, either," Olivia said.

"What way?"

"You're feeling guilty, aren't you?"

"Why should I feel guilty?"

"Not a single reason in the world. But you are." She paused briefly. "You think we acted on impulse, and you're right, we did, and that's me, isn't it? That's typical Olivia, leaping without looking, same way she fell off the damned cliff."

"Wonderful cliff," James said.

"Yes. I agree."

"Well, then."

"But you're not an impetuous man, Jamie, are you? At least you never have been, not like me, anyway. So now you're bound to start fretting and angsting all over the place, worrying about what I'm feeling, because we know you're not really over Carrie yet and so you're going to start thinking you've taken advantage of me."

"You ran the bath," Jamie said.

"I did. Quite. And I got you to open the champagne and get in the bath with me." Olivia smiled right into his dark eyes. "So you see, there really is no reason for you to look at last night as anything more or less than what it was."

"And what was it, Olivia?"

"Friendship," she answered.

"Uh-huh," he said, clearly unconvinced.

"It was, Jamie, darling. Friendship and true, true love—but only the kind of love we've always had for each other. And the rest of it was—"

He jumped right into her pause. "Yes? The rest of it was what?"

"A physical response to a buildup of tension," she said. "A wonderful response, and I'm not denying that we were very attracted to each other, but—"

"But?"

"But it was just one night." Olivia looked into his eyes again, then looked quickly away. "We both know that, Jamie, admit it."

Jamie shook his head. "I can't. I don't know it. I thought—"

"What did you think? That it was the start of something?" Olivia stood up, walked over to the alcove overlooking the harbor. "We are what we've always been. Best friends. You've been through hell lately, and we had a great week together, and I pushed you hard, made you do all kinds of things you wouldn't normally want to do."

Jamie got up, too, joined her by the window but kept a foot of space between them, didn't dare touch her, even brush against her. "I hope you're not suggesting that I didn't want to make love to you."

She smiled again. "No. Not that."

"That's something." He looked out over the harbor, toward Logan.

"It was beautiful," Olivia said. "It was good, better than good, for both of us, and I know I won't forget it." She took a breath. "But I don't think either of us should ever talk about it again, and I know we'll never do it again, and that's fine, too."

Jamie turned back to face her. "So we're just good friends, is that it? I mean, is that *it*? Last night never really happened?"

"I didn't say that."

"It's what you meant." He heard the tinge of bitterness in his voice and disliked himself for it. He knew, after all, what she was doing, that she was freeing him from an entanglement that she knew would only cause him more pain because she didn't want it.

"I guess," Olivia said. "In a way."

Jamie managed a smile. "You're right." At last, he reached out to touch her, lightly, gently, on the arm; it was safe now, the intimacy had gone, the danger had passed. "It is better this way."

"I wonder," Olivia said, with a brightness she did not feel, "what Annie would have to say to us if she knew."

"You don't think we should tell her."

"Maybe not."

Carrie's accusations and her malice came back into Jamie's mind. *Your own sick little affair with your two friends.* And her outrageous threats. *I'll drag them both through the dirt with you.*

"I guess you're right about that, too," he said.

They were both silent for a moment.

"If we're going," Jamie said, "we'd better go or you'll miss your flight."

"I told you," she said, "I don't want you taking me."

"I always take you."

"Not this time. I couldn't stand the airport farewell, not this time."

Jamie shook his head. "Me neither."

He called her a cab, pulled on some jeans and a shirt, and carried her bags downstairs to the lobby, where the doorman took them out to the waiting car. They embraced there, the way they always had, old, dear, trusted friends, and then they walked, arm in arm, out into the street. The traffic on Atlantic Avenue flowed past, thick and loud and fast; Olivia often remarked on the contrasting outlooks of the two faces of Jamie's building, the one inland unremittingly ugly, the other, the ocean, as calming and attractive as any city view could possibly be.

"I'll call you when I get home," she told him.

"You'd better," he said. "Anytime, even if you're delayed."

She got into the cab. "Just one more thing."

"What?" He crouched on the sidewalk.

"Only that if Carrie the Kvetch ever tried to cast any doubts about your lovemaking skills—and knowing Carrie I'll bet she did—then I am here to tell you that the woman's a fool as well as a liar."

At least, she thought, as the cab drew away, she'd left him smiling.

15

amie announced the opening of his own agency, JAA, that August. It had been a battle all the way, with Carrie—now married to Peter—blocking his plans wherever and whenever she could, and her new husband doing his darnedest to look the other way—which had greatly aggravated her—but a deal had finally been struck.

"I've left it all behind," Jamie told Olivia on the telephone. "All my clients, all my colleagues. I'm continuing to take care of my old accounts under the auspices of Beaumont-Arias—in which I'm still a silent partner—but in the meantime, I'm free to run my own ship with what Carrie calls a free hand."

"Sounds pretty accurate," Olivia commented wryly, "since it sounds as if you're going to be trying to function with one hand tied behind your back."

"Not really," Jamie said. "Sure, I've given up a lot, and Carrie is going to be holding a lot of the aces, but where new accounts are concerned, we're going to be rivals on the same turf, and I'll just have to see if I can still cut it. To be honest, I haven't felt so liberated or invigorated in years."

Three months later, word was out that James Arias's new agency was the place in Boston most likely to spawn original, product-selling, dollar-earning campaigns. Jamie's old skills at reaching into disparate worlds, his still-boyish capacity for excitement when a prospective client showed him a new product or service, his natural communication gifts, and, above all, his talent with words and pictures and images, had all soared back up to the surface the way a half-drowned diver might head through murky water back to sunlight. Word was out, and Carrie hated it.

When Maggie Carmichael and David Baum, Jamie's favorite old creative partnership, turned up on JAA's Boylston Street doorstep, his non-poaching agreement with Carrie forced him to resist the temptation to greet them with open arms.

"This wouldn't be poaching," Maggie pointed out over a cappuccino in the café next door to Jamie's office. "You know we left Beaumont-Arias five months back for Steinfeld-Nicholson in New York—"

"Where we were miserable as sin," David continued, "and pining for home."

"Except we both knew that home wasn't just Boston," Maggie went on, "and God forbid we should sound like we're brownnosing—"

"God forbid," David echoed.

"—but home to us is any agency you're running, Jamie."

"And with all due respect to Carrie Beaumont Arias Arias—"

"Or whatever you're meant to call a woman who marries a succession of brothers," Maggie chimed in.

"—she has no right to dictate to us where we work," David finished.

Jamie drank some more cappuccino. They looked at him.

"So?" Maggie said.

"So?" David said.

Jamie put down his cup.

"So let me talk to my lawyer."

"It's not exactly kosher," Bob Jacobson, his lawyer, told him.

"But would I be in breach of contract?" Jamie asked.

"Strictly speaking, no."

"But?"

"But we might be wise to think about the spirit of the agreement."

"The spirit of the agreement was to stop me taking away Beaumont-Arias employees—"

"And recently departed employees," Jacobson emphasized.

"Baum and Carmichael left five months ago. They went to New York, to another agency. Now they're back and they want to work for JAA." Jamie paused. "Can I hire them or not?"

"You might be inviting aggravation," the lawyer said.

"I'm used to aggravation from Carrie," Jamie replied.

"Then hire them."

There were no signs of retaliation for more than a month, and then, out of the blue, in the *Boston Daily News* of December 23—extracted, with due caution, in the next edition of *Advertising Life*—Carrie showed her claws again.

A man by the name of Silas Gilbert, whom Jamie recalled slightly as having worked unspectacularly in Beaumont-Arias's accounts department—gave an interview in which he talked about his personal impression of the dreadful years Mrs. Arias—a lady Gilbert said he both admired and respected—must have endured with her first husband, and how supportive and loyal she had remained to him in spite of her love for his brother.

Jamie read Gilbert's words in the *Daily News*, headlined in yellow, with swiftly mounting disbelief and rage.

> I heard them one day at the office. They were talking in the boardroom after some big meeting—I say talking, but really it got pretty heated and their voices were loud enough for anyone outside the room to hear.
>
> Mrs. Arias told Mr. Arias that once people knew the truth, no one would blame her for going to another man—not morally, anyhow—I remember she used that word, "morally." She asked him if he imagined she didn't know about the sick little affair he'd been having with his two friends. I could hardly believe my ears, but I'll tell you, I couldn't drag myself away—I mean, sure it's not nice to listen at keyholes, but it wasn't too hard to hear, and who wouldn't have stayed to listen, I ask you?
>
> I mean, a lady can only take so much, after all. Mrs. Arias knew her husband had been screwing around with two other women—

one of them married with kids, if you listen to gossip—and some kind of a junkie, too, apparently. I'd say Mrs. Arias was right. You could hardly blame her for leaving him for another man.

"How could you do this?" Jamie asked Carrie two days after *Advertising Life* had landed on his desk. He had been trying to confront her ever since he'd seen the piece in the *Daily News*, but she had been out of town until this morning, when he'd marched right into her office without giving Mark Reiss, her fresh-faced young P.A., a chance to buzz her first.

"How could I do what, James?" Carrie was sitting calmly at her desk, a single folder of papers in front of her. The rest of the surface was, as usual, gleamingly polished and almost bare, aside from one photograph of her with Peter on their wedding day. "And I'd appreciate it if you would not come bursting into my office without the courtesy of calling first."

Jamie slammed *Advertising Life* down on the desk. "I've known for years that you were a bitch, Carrie, but I honestly never dreamed you could sink this low."

She raised a beautifully plucked brow. "What can I have done to upset you so, James? Do tell me, please."

"How much did you pay Gilbert? I gather he left awhile back. Is he out of work? Did you take time searching for the right man for the job? How much *did* you pay him?"

"Wouldn't you prefer to sit down?" Carrie asked politely. "You look as if you need to."

"I intend to do my utmost to avoid ever having to sit down anywhere in your company again," Jamie said coldly. "Unless, of course, it's in a courtroom."

"Is that a threat?"

"Did you honestly imagine I'd let you get away with defaming a friend of mine?"

Carrie shook her head, her blue eyes wide with mocking innocence. "James, James, which friend can you be talking about?" She looked down at *Advertising Life*. "You surely can't be referring to that little interview with Silas Gilbert. What does that have to do with me?" She scarcely paused to draw breath. "And which friend of yours has been defamed by it? I've been longing to know—everyone's been longing to know—please do tell."

Jamie stared down at her, his expression pure disgust. "How do you sleep at night, Carrie?"

"Very well, thank you," she answered. "That is, of course, when your brother lets me." She smiled up at him quite serenely. "How are Olivia and Annie, by the way? I do miss hearing your little stories about them, you know."

"So you make them up yourself instead," Jamie said.

"Hardly," Carrie said dismissively. "It's so unnecessary when the truth is so much more fun."

"So you admit you were referring to Annie," Jamie said.

"You mean Silas Gilbert was referring to her, don't you?" Carrie paused. "Would you like me to admit that, James? Would you like Mr. Gilbert to name both your friends in another interview?"

"Do that, and you'll regret it for the rest of your life."

"Try bringing an action," Carrie countered, "and just see what I'll do."

"I want to sue for libel," he told Bob Jacobson, "and I want a court order to have her stopped from saying another word."

"I don't see how you can do either," the lawyer said, "since you tell me you and Carrie did have the conversation Gilbert's quoted—and the rest of it was gossip, which he admitted."

"But there's no way he or anyone could have heard us in the boardroom," Jamie said. "The walls are well insulated, the two doors are thick, and they were both closed. And neither of us was shouting. I'm telling you, Carrie put him up to this."

"I don't doubt it," Jacobson said, "but it'd be hard to prove—and pointless, too." He paused. "Bottom line, Jamie: You can't sue a man for telling the truth, and I repeat, you did have the conversation he says you did."

"It isn't the man I want to sue," Jamie said frustratedly. "Carrie paid for that story; we both know that."

"We'll never prove it, and even if we could, we still couldn't bring a case."

Jamie shook his head. "So she's allowed to call a friend of mine—and I stress a *friend*, Bob—a junkie and get away with it."

"The women weren't named, Jamie," Jacobson said gently. "Be grateful for that."

"Grateful?" Jamie repeated bitterly.

"From what you tell me, if you let the whole thing drop now, it's likely to die a not-too-ugly, natural death. If you try to fight Carrie, other people may get hurt."

Jamie knew Jacobson was right, that he had no choice but to sit back and grit his teeth and let it go. The attorney had made it plain enough; if he allowed this scurrilous but relatively minor piece of scandal-mongering to fade away, it was unlikely ever to permeate either Annie's or Olivia's European circles.

He thought about Olivia that evening at home, after his meeting with Jacobson, thought about her long and hard. He had seldom permitted himself either the luxury or the pain of thinking about what had happened between them the previous spring. He knew that it had meant nothing more to her than what she had told him. Friendship. Olivia had always been scrupulously, sometimes uncomfortably, honest. *Friendship and true, true love, but only the kind of love we've always had for each other.* He'd thought, with a leap of hope, that he'd seen something else in her eyes that morning, something more, but she'd been so adamant, and ever since then it had been business as usual between them. Friendship.

Bob Jacobson had not asked for the identity of the women Silas Gilbert had talked to the *Daily News* about, and Jamie had not volunteered their names. With nothing to be done, there would have been no purpose served. As it was, he could only hope and pray that no real harm had been done, especially to Annie. At least, thank God, he reflected, there were few, if any, people in Boston or in the agency business who knew about the close bond among the three of them.

A sudden chill went through him. What if Carrie had somehow learned about what had happened between Olivia and himself, if one of the family—Louise, or Daisy, perhaps, or even Michael—had talked about his bringing her to the Newport house? Michael would, after all, have seen no special reason not to mention that to Peter in passing, but

Jamie could imagine Peter and Carrie discussing it, remembered Peter's unpleasant innuendo when they'd met last January in F A O Schwarz, could easily envisage them building something out of nothing.

Except that it had not been nothing. And supposing, just supposing, Carrie had been having him watched. He poured himself a stiff drink and shook himself out of it. Nothing had happened until he and Olivia had got back to the apartment. No one could have seen them here. There were no bugs in his home, no hidden cameras; this wasn't some sick, paranoid movie. This was normal, not especially happy, Jamie Arias, doing precisely what he had just been mentally accusing his ex-wife and brother of doing, building something out of nothing.

He took his drink over to the window, took a swallow, and looked out over the harbor. There was, as Bob Jacobson had said, only one sensible course of action he could take. Carrie had thrown a nasty little jagged rock into the pool they both swam in. Now all Jamie could do was to stand on his dignity and wait for the ripples to disappear.

Olivia saw a lot of U.S. trade magazines and papers in the course of her working life, wherever she was, and she always scanned *Advertising Life* for any mention of JAA or Jamie himself. Reading the reprinting of the Silas Gilbert interview in the second week of January had her out of her chair and about halfway to the ceiling, spitting with fury.

She called Jamie.

"What are you doing about this?" she asked.

"Apparently, there's nothing I can do."

"What do you mean?" She was incredulous. "You have to sue, Jamie."

"I can't."

Olivia listened as he gave her Bob Jacobson's outlook and told her that, on reflection, he had to agree with the attorney. He sounded so calm, so *resigned*, even when he told her about his confrontation with Carrie, that Olivia felt like flying across the Atlantic to shake him.

"We *have* to do something," she said. "I mean, she's still making threats, Jamie—there's no telling what lies she could tell anytime she gets it into her head to start with you."

"Then I'll have to deal with that if it happens," Jamie said.

"But what about Annie?"

"What about her?" He was alarmed. "You haven't told her about this?"

"Not yet."

"You mustn't tell her, Olivia."

"Why not? Annie's pretty strong these days, and she and Edward are in great shape."

"Which is why I don't intend to rock the boat for them," Jamie insisted. "Or for you."

"For God's sake, Jamie." Olivia had never felt so exasperated with him. A realization struck her. "Are you concerned Carrie might know about us, about what happened after Newport? Because if you are, you can stop worrying—I don't give a damn what Carrie knows or says, okay?"

There was a brief silence.

"I don't want you to tell Annie about any of this," Jamie said at last.

"Don't you think she has a right to know?"

"She probably does," Jamie acknowledged, "but I honestly don't see there's anything to be gained by telling her, other than that Edward might go nuts and take Carrie on and for all that Edward's a smart guy, he doesn't know Carrie as well as I do."

"I can't stand the idea of Carrie getting away with it," Olivia said.

"How do you think I feel?" Jamie asked.

"I can imagine."

"Can you, really?"

"Of course," Olivia said more gently.

"Promise you won't tell Annie," he said again.

Olivia knew she wasn't going to change his mind.

"Okay," she said, giving what she felt was a reasonable portrayal of someone giving in gracefully.

"Promise me, Olivia."

Olivia crossed her fingers. "I promise."

And then she called Annie.

"I'm coming to see you," she said.

"How lovely," Annie said. "When?"

"Tomorrow."

"Couldn't you wait till the weekend?" Annie thought of her jam-packed calendar, full of study plans, arrangements for the children, and dinners with Edward.

"No," Olivia said.

"Oh. Okay."

"I have something you need to see," Olivia offered by way of explanation. "It's important." She paused. "But Annie, if you happen to talk to Jamie, don't tell him I called. If he finds out I'm coming to England, tell him you think I must be coming for a meeting with my father's foundation. Whatever you do, don't tell him about this conversation."

Annie was as outraged as Olivia had known she would be. It was the evening of the following day, and they were sitting at the kitchen table in Banbury Farm House, the clippings from *Advertising Life* and the *Boston Daily News* spread before them. Edward was in London; Sophie, William, and Liza were all in bed; Marie-Louise was out with her boyfriend—a cattle farmer who wanted to marry her—the two cats, Leo and Boots, were curled up asleep by the stove; and Bella, the golden retriever, was under the table, replete from the remains of the roast lamb she had just finished.

"I don't know what Edward's going to say," Annie said.

"Do you have to tell him?"

"Oh, yes," Annie said, definitely. "I don't let myself keep secrets these days. Too much trouble."

"You're right." Olivia remembered the awful, painful days and nights in Geneva with Gianni Dressler and his team, and then she thought about her own secret, her night with Jamie. She wished, sometimes, she had confided in Annie about that; it might have been a comfort. Too late now.

"At least we're not mentioned by name," Annie said.

"I wouldn't care if I was."

"I'm afraid I would," Annie said. "Very much."

"Of course you would. It's different for you, obviously."

Annie looked at the clippings again, at the photograph of Jamie with Carrie. "She really is a dangerous bitch, isn't she?"

"She sure is."

"Why did she do this now? Do you know?"

"Apparently she and Jamie had some kind of problem a month back, something to do with the agencies. He said he was expecting some kind of retaliation after that and he was only just starting to relax. He's mad as hell, of course—especially about you—but he believes there's nothing he can do about it because Carrie did once accuse him of having an affair with us both, and no one can prove this Gilbert character didn't overhear them."

Annie's eyes were very wide and blue. "But how could Carrie dream up such a thing? About *us*, for God's sake? I mean, forgetting the junkie reference, which is horrible enough—" Her cheeks were flushed with anger. It was one thing acknowledging her problems within the small therapy group she still regularly attended; this was quite another.

"I know," Olivia said, gently. "I know."

"I mean, it's *unthinkable*," Annie went on.

"Absolutely," Olivia agreed.

"Jamie's more like our brother—Carrie knows that."

"Carrie has a dirty mind." Olivia smoothed down both clippings on the table, using the flat palms of her hands. "Carrie has to be stopped."

Annie looked alarmed. "You really think there may be more?"

"Whether there is or not, I have no intention of letting her get away with this." Olivia paused. "You realize she's been using this accusation against Jamie all along, don't you? It has to be why he let her have the divorce all her own way."

"Did Jamie tell you that?"

"Not exactly. He didn't have to. Once he let slip that this sleazebag, Gilbert, could have heard them talking about us, I knew that Carrie must have been holding this over him."

"But there's nothing to *hold*," Annie said, anguished.

"You know Jamie," Olivia said. "He'd never take that kind of risk with us. He'd have been afraid of creating problems for you with Edward, for one thing."

"You're right. Of course you're right."

More appalled than ever, Annie stood up and walked over to the sink. She ran the cold tap for a moment, turned it on so full that the spray hit a spoon and spurted up at her. She turned it off again, forgetting why she'd run the water in the first place.

"My God, Livvy," she said. "What are we going to do about this?"

"Good," Olivia said, with some satisfaction.

"Good what?" Annie came back to the table and sat down again. "What's good? I don't see anything good."

"You agree we have to do something."

"Yes, of course." Annie was growing angrier by the minute and found, to her surprise, that the anger felt stimulating in a strong, positive way. "Yes, of course I agree we do. But what?"

Olivia smiled at her. "As a matter of fact, I have had an idea." She paused. "I made notes on the flight over. It's going to take a lot of working out, and we're going to need a little help. But I do seem to have a plan."

Annie smiled back. "Surprise, surprise," she said wryly. "Go on then," she added. "Tell me."

"Okay," Olivia said. "Here it is. We know certain things about Carrie, about what makes her run, don't we? We know that she's a selfish, narcissistic tyrant, that both success and her self-image are all-important to her, and that it follows that the best way to teach her a lesson would be to rip a good-size hole in that image."

"Go on," Annie said again, riveted.

"We know, too, that the lady is a whole lot more than just a giant ego. She's also megasmart, with eyes and ears everywhere. Which is why we need to plan this little revenge plot very, very carefully."

Annie frowned for the first time. "I take it we're only planning on teaching Carrie a lesson. We're not going to do her any real harm."

"Certainly not," Olivia said crisply. "But we are going to play dirty." She gave Annie one of her cool, challenging looks. "Wouldn't you say that Carrie deserves dirty?"

"Oh, yes," Annie said, thinking about Jamie, kind, easygoing, brilliant Jamie. "Oh, definitely yes."

"It's insane, and I still don't see how we can possibly pull it off," Annie said later.

"We can pull it off," Olivia said. "I know we can. It'll take a lot of work, and I'm going to need you with me a lot of the time, so we're going to have to talk to Edward—that is, of course, if you agree."

"I don't know," Annie said, and shook her head. "I mean, I can see that it really might be the perfect way to hit Carrie where it hurts. But I still don't quite understand why you've come up with something so—so extreme."

"What's to understand?" Olivia asked bluntly. "We both agreed she deserves dirty pool, didn't we? Don't we?"

"Definitely," Annie said. "That's not what I mean, Livvy." She looked intently at her friend. "I mean you've always been the most headstrong of us, the most daring, but you still lead a conventional, normal kind of life—you work hard, you play hard—you love life."

"Yes, I do," Olivia agreed.

"So how come you're willing to drop everything and run real risks with someone as nasty as Carrie? I mean, for heaven's sake, Livvy, if she finds you out"—Annie paused—"if she finds *us* out, she could make life hell."

Olivia shrugged. "I think it's worth the risk. For me, at least."

"But why? That's what I don't entirely understand." Annie was still perplexed. "I mean, is there something I don't know about? Has Carrie done something to you that you haven't told me?"

"No, of course not," Olivia said quickly. "Don't you think what she's done to Jamie in the past, and what she's threatening to do to us—to you, mostly—is enough?"

"Yes. I think." Annie was still unconvinced, still had the gnawing sense that Olivia was keeping something from her. "You realize how much money a plan like this could swallow up?"

"I have more money than I can easily spend," Olivia said steadily. "I'd like to spend some of it on giving Carrie what she deserves."

"Me, too," Annie said. "I guess it's not the money that bothers me."

"So what does?"

Annie shook her head again. "It's just so extreme."

"You said that already."

"I know." Annie paused. "So there's nothing else? Nothing I should know about?"

The Newport cliff flashed back into Olivia's mind and, following that, the way it always did, Jamie's bathroom, the two of them in the tub.

"Nothing," she said firmly, finally.

"Okay," Annie said.

"Okay, what?"

"Okay, I'm in."

"How come?" Olivia looked at her shrewdly. "I mean, if you think it's so wild, and so risky, which I guess it is."

"To help you help Jamie, of course," Annie said. "Our pact, partly. The fact that Carrie should be stopped in her tracks, and I agree that if we can pull it off, it would be a sensational way to stop her." She smiled. "A little because I'm so glad you think I'm strong enough again to join you in this." She paused. "Mostly because I can't conceive of deserting you—especially when I think you've flipped a little."

"But are you sure?" Olivia asked. "I don't want to force you into doing anything you don't want to, Annie."

"I'm sure," Annie said decisively. "But I'm still not quite sure about not telling Jamie. Doesn't he have a right to know?"

"No." Olivia shook her head definitely. "For one thing, knowing Jamie, he'd never agree to go along with it." She looked down at the notes she'd made, and her green eyes sparked at the thought of what was to come. "And for another, this whole thing is only going to work—really work—if Jamie doesn't know a damned thing about it."

Annie was silent for a while, and then she said, "How much of this do we have to tell Edward?"

"I thought you didn't like keeping secrets these days."

"I don't. And I can see that we have to give him some idea of what we're planning."

"Just not quite all of it," Olivia said.

Annie smiled ruefully. "No. Not quite. I mean, Edward wouldn't dream of trying to tell me I couldn't do something I really wanted to do, but he might try to talk me out of it, so don't you think it would be best to keep the details to ourselves?"

"Absolutely best," Olivia agreed. "As the old saying goes, what he doesn't know won't hurt him."

"So long as we don't get caught," Annie said.

16

The first approach arrived forty-two days later, on Monday, February 26, a letter in a gray envelope marked for Carrie's eyes only and brought directly into her office by her personal assistant. Carrie, on a call, indicated to Mark Reiss that he should leave the envelope on her blotter. It was another forty minutes before she opened it.

Dear Mrs. Arias,

I have been asked by the president of a Swiss corporation renowned in its field to approach you directly with regard to a dramatic breakthrough on their part which they will shortly be ready to share with the citizens of the United States of America.

Though I am not empowered, at this early stage, to disclose to you any further details, I have been authorized to assure you that the new product concerned will bring new confidence and renewed mental health to a large sector of the American nation, and vast, unprecedented revenue to its creators and those concerned with its introduction and distribution.

You will, I am certain, understand that something of such potential enormity will require exquisite handling for its launch into the public domain. In other words, Mrs. Arias, the perfect campaign. No other agencies are being approached at this point because of the necessity for maximum confidentiality, and your company has been selected for a number of reasons.

Beaumont-Arias is a compact agency, but substantial and

experienced enough to handle such a campaign. It encompasses the necessary talent in all required areas. It has, to our knowledge, no pre-existing accounts that might throw up an undesirable conflict of interests, and it has a chief executive who has already passed certain essential security checks.

I shall be in touch with you again in forty-eight hours. If you are interested in learning more about the product concerned, I would ask you to indicate accordingly at that time.

Sincerely yours,
G. Schnabel

Carrie read the letter twice, glanced at the letterhead—G. Schnabel, AG, and a post office box number in Bern, no actual address, no telephone or fax numbers—and laid it to one side. She pressed a key on her intercom.

"Mark, how was that letter delivered? The one marked my eyes only?"

"By messenger, Mrs. Arias."

"Which firm?"

"FedEx, Mrs. Arias."

She let the key snap up and gave the letter one more look.

"Bullshit," she said. Probably nothing, she decided, and even if one of the pharmaceutical majors had come up with the new Prozac or whatever, she was almost certain that every other chief executive of every other agency in the country had been sent the same letter.

The second letter arrived while Carrie was in a meeting. This time a telephone number was given. If Mrs. Arias was seriously interested in this unique opportunity, then Herr Schnabel would be available to speak to her between 9 A.M. and noon, eastern standard time.

Carrie made the call to the Bern number at five minutes to twelve.

"Herr Schnabel, please."

"Who is speaking, please?"

"Carrie Beaumont Arias." Carrie spoke reasonable French, but almost no German; there had seldom been a necessity to learn, since most Germans and Swiss had a fine command of English.

She was put through almost immediately.

"Mrs. Arias, this is Gerhard Schnabel speaking. I'm so glad to hear from you." His voice was pleasant, with the lilting quality of most Swiss-Germans.

"Your letters intrigued me," Carrie said. "A little cloak-and-dagger for my tastes, but I was prepared to make one call."

"And I thank you for that," Schnabel answered courteously.

"So what is this product?" Carrie looked at the new Cartier watch that Peter had given her for Christmas. She had a lunch meeting at half past. "I must tell you I have an appointment in fifteen minutes, so I can only give you two."

"Of course," Schnabel said. "Mrs. Arias, if you believe that your agency might be interested in preparing a presentation for my clients—"

"Who exactly are your clients, Herr Schnabel?"

"That I am not at liberty to tell you at this stage, Mrs. Arias."

"What are you at liberty to tell me?" Carrie was irritated.

"Very little, I'm afraid."

"Then why ask me to call?" Her irritation magnified.

"To establish a point of contact, firstly," Schnabel replied. "And to explain to you that my clients are adamant that there can be no direct meetings or even telephone conversations with them, and no in-depth details about their product can be discussed unless you have first signed a legally binding document to guarantee their confidentiality."

"This is absurd," Carrie snapped. "I'm a busy woman, and if your clients have done the research you claim they have, then they'll know my agency has handled a great many highly sensitive accounts."

"Mrs. Arias"—Schnabel sounded pacifying—"I can assure you they realize that, but nevertheless they are insistent that any agency who wishes to know more must first sign such a document."

"I thought Beaumont-Arias was the only agency they had approached."

"Until today, certainly." Schnabel paused. "If you indicate your willingness to discuss such a document with your attorneys, then that situation will remain unchanged."

Carrie drummed a perfect, newly wrapped deep red fingernail on her desktop. "I take it there would be no commitment implicit in signing such a document?"

"Of course not, Mrs. Arias," Schnabel assured her. "It is simply a vehicle for moving forward any possible negotiations—once the document is signed, you will be furnished with all the information available."

Carrie's mind hummed. Something told her that this might not, after all, turn out to be pure bullshit, and she had learned, through the years, to trust her instincts. *New confidence and renewed mental health to a large sector of the American nation.* Those words inclined her toward moving at least one step closer, since she could hardly have her people dream up the hottest campaign in history until she knew the whole story—and if, by any chance, this did turn out to be a dud or just another one of those sicko live-forever drugs, she could always either turn them down flat or sue their asses.

"Mrs. Arias?" Schnabel said softly.

"Get the papers to me. I'll have my attorneys check them over."

"They'll be with you tomorrow, Mrs. Arias," Schnabel said.

Carrie cut the call.

In the one-room office on Schänzlistrasse in Bern that Olivia had rented for the next month complete with telephones and fax machine, Olivia and Annie and Felix Pfäniger stared at one another with a kind of awe.

"She bought it," Olivia said. "She really bought it."

"My goodness, Felix," Annie said, "you were sensational."

Pfäniger shrugged modestly. "I'm an actor. If I can't manage a few lines in a simple telephone call, then I'm not much credit to my profession."

Olivia stood up from her chair, came over to where he sat at the desk, and bent to hug him. "Well, I'm with Annie—you were magnificent, Felix." She kissed him on his gold-highlighted hair. "Thank you, *Schätzli*."

"You're welcome." Pfäniger looked up at Olivia with undisguised adoration. They had met during her time in Geneva when her friend Diana Brünli had introduced them at a mutual friend's party, and he had fallen head over heels in love with her. They had gone out to dinner a few times, and Olivia had gone to Zurich, where Pfäniger was based, to see him perform at the Schauspielhaus, but Felix's lust for her had, to his great chagrin, been unrequited. Still, they had kept in touch, for Olivia always tried to maintain contact with the men she dated and liked, and since Olivia made a point of dating only men whom she did like, she had, over the years, assembled many good friends in many places.

"You do realize that this is just the beginning?" Olivia asked him. "Now that Carrie's taken the bait."

"If she signs the papers," Annie pointed out.

"She'll sign." Olivia was buoyant with confidence. "Even you thought they looked terrific, and you're the biggest worry wart here."

"What looks terrific to me," Annie said, "may not look so convincing to Carrie or her attorneys."

"Julius thinks they'll pass muster," Olivia said. She'd had another good friend, Julius Staheli, an ace corporate lawyer resident in Lausanne, draw up the confidentiality document.

Annie looked at her watch. It was a quarter past five. If she'd been home in Stone Bridge, she would have been giving afternoon tea to the children and helping Marie-Louise think ahead to dinner. "Shouldn't we call FedEx, Livvy? Confirm delivery?"

"Right away," Olivia agreed. "And don't let me forget to turn on the answering machine, just in case Carrie gets it into her head to call back."

Olivia thought she had it pretty much worked out, as far as it could be at this early stage. She'd talked Maria di Benetto, another freelance translator in Strasbourg, into taking over her engagements for the next few weeks, and had managed to assemble a considerable team of expert friends to join in what she had persuaded them all was a harmless, but hopefully effective exercise in late-twentieth-century monster slaying. Annie, impressed as hell by Olivia's array of friends and ex-lovers, all ready to play their specialist roles, called them "Segal's Standbys" and knew that, though she was still apprehensive about what might happen if and when Carrie found out what they were doing, she had never, in her entire life, had more fun.

Thirty-six hours after Carrie had signed the confidentiality agreement in the offices of Herbert, Morgan, and Bendell, her attorneys, Gerhard

Schnabel, a.k.a. Felix Pfäniger, arranged for her to be flown first class to Zurich.

"Do we have to waste all that money on first class?" Annie had asked Olivia. "Surely business would be good enough?"

"Carrie Beaumont Arias never flies any class other than first if it's available," Olivia answered firmly. "Try downgrading her, and we might easily lose her. Besides, I'd say it's money well spent."

"I just hate the idea of giving her pleasure," Annie sighed.

"Just think of it as a means to an end, Annie," Olivia reminded her. "A triumphant end."

A black stretch Mercedes picked Carrie up at Kloten and drove her directly to the Bellevue Palace in Bern, where a friend of Felix Pfäniger, a member of the Stadtheater, was waiting with Felix to play her role in one of the handsome Louis XV–style suites. Less than three hours later, Carrie was on her way back to Zurich, more galvanized than she had been for many years.

"Why are we meeting here?" Carrie had asked Gerhard Schnabel and Ruth Müller, an elegant, conservatively dressed woman in her mid-thirties, after Müller had introduced herself as a director of Lumitechnik AG, manufacturers of lasers.

"Partly for your convenience," Müller answered.

"But mostly because of security, Mrs. Arias," Schnabel added. "Lumitechnik is a subsidiary of a company with a factory near St. Gallen, but since some of their laser applications are for the weapons industry, the factory's address is unlisted and, of course, off-limits to visitors."

"Once the product has been launched," Müller went on, "and the full manufacturing process is underway, we will be glad to make arrangements for you to go to the factory."

"More secrecy," Carrie said, new irritation compounded by weariness.

"Perhaps, Mrs. Arias," Schnabel suggested, "you might like to take some lunch with us. There is an excellent grill room here in the hotel—"

"Just coffee, please," Carrie said crisply. "And some facts, if you don't mind." She paused. "I take it this product is not a weapon."

"Certainly not," Ruth Müller said. "Quite the opposite, as you will see."

Carrie settled back in an armchair rather too comfortable for her liking. She preferred a certain mild level of discomfort during important business meetings. Too much comfort could render one too relaxed, could dull one's critical powers. She had no great objection to having come thus far; first class Swissair, and a night to look forward to at the Baur-au-Lac in Zurich, the hotel of her personal choice, was no great penance. Carrie thought she deserved a vacation, had not taken one in some years, and had no intention of doing so, however much Peter tried to persuade her. By the time she got back to Boston and to the office, she would have been away for at least forty-eight hours—to Carrie that *was* a vacation. She had no objection to that, she reflected again, but any more delaying tactics by these people, and they would not see her for dust.

"Galvanized," she decided later that night, over filet mignon in her suite at the Baur-au-Lac, was the right word. Ruth Müller had done an excellent job of selling her the product merely by saying as little as possible and letting her judge the evidence for herself.

The product, as Carrie now knew, would—if it lived up to its promise—be a revelation in the practice of cosmetic surgery: a double-beamed laser developed for aesthetic applications by a Czechoslovakian scientist now working for Lumitechnik, with the power, precision, and delicacy to remove wrinkles and to heal the underlying skin so rapidly that, depending on the extent of the surgery, a patient could be returned to everyday life within days of treatment with scars already at a stage of healing normally expected several weeks or even months after more conventional surgery.

"There are a number of laser processes under development," Müller had explained to Carrie, "which will—as I'm sure you will discover for yourself when you conduct your research—at first glance, seem to offer the same end result—a resurfacing of the skin with rapid healing. When you examine those processes more closely, however, you will notice that initial improvement is normally promised within a few weeks, and that total recovery will take anything up to three months."

"But won't the lasers remove wrinkles by burning the skin?" Carrie was skeptical. "I can't imagine that burned flesh could very well heal in any less time."

"These lasers will resurface by vaporizing the water content of the surface skin, but so far as healing is concerned you are, of course, absolutely correct, Mrs. Arias," Müller had said. "Which is precisely what has made Lumitechnik so uniquely placed to revolutionize this whole area of surgery." She paused. "Frankly, once the men and women who are willing to endure having their faces literally peeled to appear more youthful learn about our laser, they will refuse to accept anything less."

"And the other processes will not reach the public for some years," Schnabel said with complacency.

"So what exactly is the invention?" Carrie persisted. "What makes your laser so different from the others?"

"You may have heard," Müller said, "of lasers being used to repair retinal tears. They can quite effectively seal small tears, or holes, if you prefer." She paused. "What we have done is to combine two separate lasers: one the more conventional, which, in the most simple terms, will remove the wrinkle; the other, called a *Heilunglaser*, which will heal the wound simultaneously."

"As if," Carrie said, trying to focus on an image, "a dentist were drilling and filling a cavity at the same time?"

"An almost perfect analogy," Müller agreed. "Removing the decay and drawing the healthy remains of the tooth together in one operation."

Schnabel smiled at Carrie. "Perhaps another application for the *Heilunglaser* in the future."

"I'll expect royalties," Carrie said.

"I imagine that patent has already been applied for," Müller said quickly.

"I was joking," Carrie said.

They took themselves so *seriously*, Carrie thought later. Lord knew she wasn't exactly famous for her humor, but Lumitechnik AG wasn't exactly planning on using this thing the Czech scientist had handed them on a plate for brain surgery. On the other hand, they were a thousand percent right when they said that with the right marketing approach, it would make billions and beat off everything else in the same marketplace. This was not perceived as being a treatment available to the masses. This would be a costly retail product, a package of equipment that would be supplied, together with training for its use, on demand to practitioners, and those practitioners would pay for the product only if their patients or clients were clamoring for it.

The marketing and advertising campaign, Ruth Müller had told Carrie, needed to be masterminded by an advertising wizard, someone who understood the pitfalls of hyping something that many might see as exploitative and exclusive, and Carrie, the manufacturers felt, was that wizard. And although Müller had explained that—with licensed testing procedures now officially ended and legal technicalities prohibiting any further use of the *Heilunglaser* until full production was underway—it would not be possible for Carrie to see the laser in action for herself, she was satisfied by the proof that had been laid before her: a folder of evidence—before-and-after photographs of two middle-aged women, dated and certified by a notary public, and, most convincing and reassuring of all, a letter of approval from the American Food and Drug Administration.

That night, as Carrie was climbing into her comfortable bed in Zurich, Annie, sharing a suite at the equally, perhaps even more comfortable, Schweizerhof in Bern, was getting an attack of the jitters.

"I wish you hadn't done that, Livvy."

"Done what?" Olivia was sitting curled up on the sofa, wearing a bathrobe and eating Lindt *truffes de jour*, content in the knowledge that the actors at the Bellevue Palace had done their job to perfection.

"A lot of things. Registered a dummy corporation, for one."

"We had to get Lumitechnik listed, Annie. You know Carrie would never do business without checking them out first." It had cost a small fortune in legal and accountancy fees, and Olivia now owed favors in Bern, Geneva, and Zurich, but she'd always known paying Carrie back would not be cheap.

"Mostly, I wish you hadn't faked that FDA letter."

"Why? It was easy." Gianni Dressler had got hold of a similar piece of FDA authentication, and Olivia had simply paid a small printing firm she had used in Geneva to use their state-of-the-art equipment to duplicate the letterhead and have their own letter printed in the same style as the original.

"It was forgery." Annie was pacing, running her right hand repeatedly through her blond hair.

"Surely not." Olivia went on calmly eating chocolate. "Not exactly, anyway. I didn't forge anyone's signature."

"Have you any idea what the jail sentence is for forgery these days?"

"No." Olivia looked up. "Have you?"

Back in Boston, Carrie's appetite began to grow, not only professionally for the marketing coup of a lifetime, but also on another, infinitely more private level. Carrie was still only in her mid-thirties, yet being the perfectionist she was, she had lately, despite all her strenuous, meticulous care and efforts, begun to notice some telltale flaws in her previously flawless skin, not noticeable, she was certain, to anyone else—not yet, at least. But they were there, those minute tracings and infinitesimal signs of slackening that promised betrayal, further down the line, of the immaculate beauty that had brought first James and then Peter Arias to their knees.

The temptation of being able to take no more than a handful of days away from the office and from her new husband and then to return renewed and sublimely confident that all was smooth again was almost too great to ignore. And if she played her hand well, Carrie realized that she would be uniquely placed to have the treatment before America knew about it, and no one else here would ever need to know; no one would ever suspect.

She called Ruth Müller at Lumitechnik and left an urgent message. Müller called back within the hour.

"What can I do for you, Mrs. Arias?"

"I want a consultation."

"Of course," Müller said steadily. "How may I help you?"

"You don't understand," Carrie said. "I want a consultation with a view to having the treatment for myself."

"For yourself?" Müller did not disguise her surprise. "To what end?"

"To the same end as all your millions of clients once the product hits the headlines," Carrie said. "I have some early lines, nothing major, but this seems an ideal opportunity to kill two birds with one stone—I get rid of my wrinkles, and I get the proof I need that this *Heilunglaser* really works."

"I thought you were satisfied with our evidence," Müller said.

"So far as it went," Carrie said.

Müller paused for thought. "I'm afraid, Mrs. Arias, that even if it were not legally impossible—as I explained to you previously—for the laser to be used again before production has officially begun, it would be both unethical and unwise for you to test it in this way."

"On the contrary," Carrie argued, "it's not only ethical but sound business practice. When an agency's asked to dream up a campaign for, say, a new brand of cookie, everyone concerned is encouraged to munch away on as many of those cookies as they can eat."

"This is not a cookie," Müller said gravely.

"No, it isn't," Carrie agreed. "For one thing, it's about twenty-five thousand dollars more expensive than a pack of cookies." She paused. "If I'm prepared to come back to Switzerland, and if I'm prepared to put my faith in your product, and if I'm prepared to pay anything for it—and I mean *anything*—then if you people refuse even to try to get over this license difficulty, I can only translate that into a lack of conviction in your own product."

Müller went silent for a long moment. "I will, of course, have to put your proposal to my colleagues," she said at last, rather stiffly.

"You do that." Carrie paused again. "I presume, Frau Müller, that you came to me because you figured I'd do the best possible job for you, which means, for one thing, that you must have done your homework pretty carefully when it came to checking me out."

"Naturally we did," Müller said.

"In which case," Carrie went on very coolly, "you must have found out that when I want something I either get it or I kick a lot of ass. That's a rather crude Americanism, Frau Müller, for which I apologize, but I'm sure you get the point."

"I believe I do."

"So when you speak to your colleagues at Lumitechnik, I would ask you to warn them that if they refuse to grant me this consultation, not only will I feel unable to allow Beaumont-Arias to proceed with

the campaign, but I will also see to it"—she sharpened her tone—
"without any way infringing the terms of our agreement, that no other
agency in the United States will touch you with a ten-foot pole."

"Holy shit," Olivia said in the office on Schänzlistrasse.

There were now two more telephone lines installed in the room,
one of them purporting to be Lumitechnik's main number, the other
Ruth Müller's direct line, and Olivia had employed a second actress to
play the double role of switchboard operator and Müller's secretary.

"We're finished," Annie said. She had gone home to Edward and
the children for a few days but, as luck would have it, had returned to
Bern just in time to listen in on Carrie's challenge.

"No, we're not," Olivia said.

"Don't be crazy." Annie had gone pale. "We have to stop now."

"No, we don't. There's no way we're going to stop now."

The actress playing Ruth Müller, wearing blue jeans and a baggy
pullover with patches at both elbows, shrugged her shoulders. "The
lady sounded as if she meant business," she said.

"Carrie always means business," Annie said. "Livvy, we have to
know when to stop. This is getting out of hand."

"I agree with you."

"Thank God."

"I mean, I agree we have to know when to stop, but we don't have
to stop yet. Carrie has no idea that this whole thing isn't kosher, so
there isn't any danger."

"Perhaps Olivia is right," the actress said to Annie. "I suppose the
worst thing that might happen if you don't agree to her terms is that
she pulls out."

"Since we can't agree to her terms," Annie pointed out, "that part
of it's obviously inevitable."

"Who says we can't?"

Annie and the actress stared at Olivia.

"You've flipped," Annie said flatly.

"Not necessarily," Olivia said.

Even in her wildest dreams, Olivia had to admit it had not occurred to
her that this highly intelligent, streetwise businesswoman would get so

suckered in by their invention that she would demand treatment for herself.

"You know," she said to Annie later over dinner at the Vieux Moulin, "this is almost enough to make me feel sorry for her—but only almost."

"It's certainly enough to make me feel incredibly guilty," Annie said, playing with her soup.

"You're such a softie, Annie Thomas."

"You're not so tough yourself," Annie said.

"Oh, yes, I am," Olivia said, and meant it. "I am when someone hurts a person I love." She looked intently at Annie. "Carrie's been hurting Jamie for years, and getting away with it, and now she's started lashing out at us, too. And we both know she hasn't finished yet—the moment Jamie tries to do the smallest thing she disagrees with, Carrie's going to use her ménage à trois invention, and then Jamie won't be the only one she hurts—you'll suffer, too, and Edward, and probably the children."

"I'm not sure she'd go that far."

"Why wouldn't she?" There was a harsh note in Olivia's voice. "She left Jamie for his own *brother*, Annie, and she left him without a trace of shame. What kind of a person does something like that?"

Annie said nothing.

"We can't just stop, you know," Olivia said. "If we did, and if Carrie found out that we were Lumitechnik before we'd got to the payback, then Jamie's life would be more hellish than before."

"And we'd be in jail," Annie said.

"She has to be taught a lesson," Olivia went on. "Okay, I have to agree that this looks as though it's getting a little more complicated, and maybe a little riskier than I thought—"

"A little," Annie said ironically.

"But it's nothing we can't handle."

"How, for God's sake?"

"Same way we handled the meeting at the Bellevue. With actors."

"Jesus." Annie, who still seldom drank, reached over for Olivia's glass and gulped down some burgundy.

"It's like you said," Olivia continued. "It's a question of knowing when to stop, and obviously there have to be limits on how much further we can take this thing."

"You mean you're not going to take a laser to Carrie yourself?" Annie asked sarcastically.

"Not quite," Olivia said thoughtfully.

"Not quite? Not *quite*?" Annie reached for Olivia's wineglass again.

"Get a grip," Olivia said. "I'm just trying to work this out in my mind, see how we can make sure we get to the perfect climax, the perfect payback."

"Without going to jail?"

"Certainly."

"I read somewhere that Swiss jails are terrible places."

"We're not going to go to jail, Annie."

"We will if Carrie finds out what we're up to."

"No, we won't, Annie."

"You're just making this up as you go along, aren't you, Livvy?"

Olivia looked across the table at Annie, saw that her panic was real.

"Do you want to go home, Annie? Do you want out of this?"

"No. Yes. I don't know."

"I'll understand if you do."

"But you're going on with it anyway."

"Yes."

Annie sighed. "Then I guess it looks like I'm as crazy as you."

Olivia went into overdrive. The computer and printer they'd had brought to their suite at the Schweizerhof grew hotter, the payments to the phony switchboard operator at the Schänzlistrasse office and to Federal Express grew larger as a compromise agreement was hammered out between Lumitechnik and Carrie. Olivia rejoiced; from all that Jamie had told them over the years, compromise and Carrie were about as incompatible as Jell-O and mustard, so that in itself was a small victory. Carrie was—Ruth Müller had persuaded her codirectors to agree—to be granted a consultation without delay, but licensing complexities aside, Lumitechnik felt that both Carrie and the corporation might be laying themselves open to accusations of corruption if she had exclusive access to the *Heilunglaser* prior to its official launch.

"They will contract, however," Schnabel told Carrie, "that you will be the first American citizen to undergo the new treatment, and that this will be paid for by Lumitechnik at whichever location you elect."

"I don't recall asking for a freebie," Carrie said brusquely.

"Of course not, Mrs. Arias," Schnabel answered swiftly. "This is merely a part of Lumitechnik's desire to take care of your concerns. I am authorized to tell you that, if convenient, you could plan your journey now, perhaps in order to prepare your colleagues for your brief absence. The treatment can be carried out anywhere in the United States, wherever you choose, and your confidentiality, of course, would be guaranteed."

"But you're telling me I can't do this until after the launch."

"I'm afraid that is so."

"And if I say that's not good enough?"

"Then, with great regret," Schnabel said courteously, "Lumitechnik will be compelled to take their business to another agency."

Carrie called Müller direct one hour later.

"I can come back to Switzerland this weekend for the consultation," she said. "I trust that would be in order."

"Perfectly," Müller agreed. "Let us know your flight requirements, and everything will be arranged."

"First Swissair of the day into Zurich," Carrie said, "and I want to return to Boston the same day, so I'd prefer to fly from Kloten to Bern."

"I see no problem with that," Müller said calmly. "The airport is just five or six miles south of the city, and the consultation should take no more than about two hours."

"I'll expect the tickets," Carrie said.

"You are unbelievable," Annie said to Olivia as they walked around the room in the handsome house in Neufeld, a suburb of Bern, that had been made ready for Carrie's consultation. The house belonged to a cousin of Diana Brünli who spent six months of each year in Canada and had agreed to its use in what Diana had called a "good cause" for one day.

"Why?" Olivia asked absently, checking over the leather-topped desk and steel trolley to see that everything was present and correct.

"All this." Annie shook her head. "It all looks so—authentic."

"I should hope it does."

"I didn't think you'd pull it off."

"We," Olivia corrected her. "And anyway, we haven't pulled it off yet."

"Did you have to remind me?" Annie's temporary burst of near confidence departed.

"Uh-huh." Olivia went on checking.

"What about him?"

"Who?"

"The actor—Felix's new friend."

"Professional Pfister, you mean." Olivia looked up and smiled.

The "professor"—at that time in the kitchen, perspiring and running through his lines and moves for the twentieth time with Felix Pfäniger and the actress who was to play the part of his assistant—was the kind of middle-aged actor who could make a fair living out of playing lawyers, judges, surgeons, and politicians. He had, Felix had told Olivia, done more than a little television, and was, therefore, less likely to overplay his role as the quiet, confident plastic surgeon than some theatrical actors. He had also been coached for several hours by a surgeon in Geneva, an acquaintance of Gianni Dressler's who had been misled into believing that the actor was preparing for a movie audition.

"He'll be fine," Olivia said.

"But we can't be sure," Annie said.

"We can't be sure of anything," Olivia agreed. She finished checking. "But he's been told to keep it simple. Gianni's friend says it's mostly down to basic logic."

Annie's eye caught the clock on the mantelpiece over the fireplace.

"Two hours," she said starkly. "She'll be here in two hours."

"We'll be ready for her," Olivia said.

"Felix is supposed to be meeting her at the airport."

"He will."

"But he's here, in the kitchen."

"Annie, it doesn't take two hours to get to the airport."

"But he has to get there and back—and he has to change—and the professor has to change, too—and the assistant—"

"Annie," Olivia said.

"Yes. What?"

"Stop."

Carrie was impressed by Professor Pfister, by his keen-eyed, gentle-fingered competence and by the thoroughness of his questioning and examination.

"My first question must be," Pfister had said almost as soon as she had sat down in his office, "why do you feel you need cosmetic surgery?"

"I have some lines," Carrie said. "I know they're minimal, but they're the beginning of bigger things, and I figure if I can get a head start—"

"You realize they won't be gone forever," the professor pointed out. "The *Heilunglaser* will remove your existing wrinkles but cannot prevent further lines forming in the fullness of time. We are, of course, resurfacing your skin, but the new surface will still be your own human skin."

"According to the people at Lumitechnik," Carrie said, "the effect should be good for a long time. I seem to recall a promise of years."

"In all likelihood, that should be accurate. I'm merely reminding you that it is not permanent." He shook his gray head. "I must tell you, Mrs. Arias, that I don't notice any significant wrinkling, or even creasing, on your face." He smiled, a gentle, twinkling smile. "You are, as I'm sure you realize, a very beautiful woman."

"Who wants to stay that way." Carrie smiled back at him.

"Very well. Let's take a closer look." He nodded to his assistant, who had until then stayed in the corner. "If you could help Mrs. Arias to remove all her makeup, please."

He agreed, after careful examination under a bright light through a magnifying glass, that the Lumitechnik laser would undoubtedly wipe away the tiny traces of aging that so concerned her. Working methodically alongside his quiet, efficient assistant, he had taken two cold-wax impressions of each section of her face, and then he had taken photographs from a number of angles and in different lights, asking Carrie alternately to smile, to scowl, to speak, to laugh, and just to sit in repose. And then he asked questions, more questions than she was able, later, to remember, some of which Carrie had anticipated—relating to her medical history, to general sensitivity, to allergies, to previous serious illnesses and problems with healing—and others relating to her personal life.

"Does your husband find you attractive?" Pfister asked, having established that Carrie was in her second marriage.

"He says he does."

"Do you notice him looking at other women, perhaps younger than yourself?"

Carrie frowned. "Is this relevant?"

"To your emotional state, yes."

"What does my emotional state have to do with the treatment?"

"Insofar as a patient in distress can sometimes take longer to heal, it is relevant, Mrs. Arias." Pfister paused. "Also, any physician of any integrity should be aware of his patient's needs and should also be certain that her expectations are reasonable."

"I don't expect you to turn me into a teenager," Carrie said briskly.

"Who would want to be a teenager again, Mrs. Arias?"

And she laughed.

Back home, wholly committed, she set to work, confident that no one, not in Boston, not in New York, not even in California, was better equipped to find the perfect way to sell this product to the ugly, the exquisite, and the tens of millions who fell someplace between those two poles and who could afford—barely, she supposed, in the majority of cases—to have it sold to them.

"We need your presentation in one month," Ruth Müller had told her.

Carrie had considered all her alternatives. She could put her two top creative teams on the Swiss account, remove them for ten days from the work they were currently engaged in, and force them to compete, to pit their wits against each other; she could choose just one team and pile all the pressure on them; or she could do what she had always been best at in the good old days, go it alone, at least with the early solo brainstorming.

"Why use two people to do the work of one?" she had once said to James when he'd been singing the praises of Baum and Carmichael, his pets.

"Two heads," he'd replied simply, aggravatingly.

It was funny, in an irritating kind of way, that the only other person Carrie had a curious desire to work with on this account, to share the excitement with and watch it stimulate his remarkable mind, was her ex-husband—though of course James and JAA would hear about this account over Carrie's dead body. Her new husband's world was shipping, the vast iron sea horses that rode the oceans and brought the Arias family their multimillions, yet Carrie knew that Peter didn't see even that in the same way that she did; Peter saw only figures, end-less reams of computerized numbers, and he saw very clearly what those numbers could buy. It was Michael Arias, Carrie realized, who had the passion for their family's industry that had wholly bypassed James—Peter was simply along for the ride. Carrie thought, sometimes, that maybe twice in a row she had picked the wrong Arias, thought that if she hadn't known that Michael was so irretrievably married to Louise, she might have made a play for him instead of Peter.

She decided to trust no one and shut herself into her office at Beaumont-Arias, had Mark Reiss divert all calls except those from Lumitechnik or Gerhard Schnabel to Mitzi Palgrave, her second-in-command, and began to work. Part of her brief was to create a brand name under which to market the *Heilunglaser*, but that had hit Carrie after her first visit to Bern. Light Years was both perfect and available—all she needed now was the right campaign to sell it. For ten days, she worked slavishly and entirely alone, more consumed by her task than she had been by anything else in as long as she could remember. She delegated the essential research to Mitzi Palgrave but explained nothing and undertook the more detailed work on her own, took no one into her confidence, not even Peter—*least* of all Peter, given her plans for undergoing the laser surgery herself; she had a second private fax line installed in her office, saw that every letter, every memorandum to Lumitechnik was sealed in its envelope before it left her hand, and directed Switzerland that each item for her continued to be marked strictly for her eyes only.

A kind of fever took her over. She slept little, ate only what she needed to keep going, saw only those people she had to see, and attended the minimum of meetings. She worked late into every night, letting her mind roam free, dragging ideas from the ether, some of them wild and foolish and useless except for the fresh thoughts that sprouted in the wake of their rejection.

She was dealing with a scientific invention with a medical application, but in realistic terms Carrie knew that she was dealing with the ultimate beauty product. Yet unlike so many of those miracle pots of night cream and moisturizers, this treatment was for *real*, and despite the fact that it would cost big bucks—what didn't, for goodness' sake?—it seemed downright criminal not to get the word through to the masses in the most appealing and effective way so that they could have their whack at going for it.

She couldn't book the ad spaces or billboards or TV prime-time slots or editorial feature spaces in *American Health* or *The Physician* or *Woman's Journal* or any of the other trade or consumer magazines or newspapers, not, at least, until she'd made her pitch and won the account, and that was a bitch because they'd be hard pressed to make it for what they'd alerted Carrie was their ideal launch date, June 1st. But they'd given her a month on top of the almost four weeks it had taken to get to that point, which indicated to Carrie that they believed in her and that she'd have to screw up pretty royally to make them hand it over to another agency.

Over at JAA on Boylston Street, Jamie had got wind that something was up with Carrie. People at Beaumont-Arias still talked to him, much to his ex-wife's chagrin, still let slip the odd morsel, always with a swift glance over their shoulder just in case, for everyone knew that Carrie was paranoid about Jamie and anything more than a passing nod in the street could be grounds for retaliation. But he heard snippets from time to time, and he knew right now that Carrie was locked into her office working on something big, and that Beaumont-Arias was, for all intents and purposes, grinding on almost without its leader. And

Jamie had to admit he was curious to know just what could have got her so steamed up, though even if it meant that JAA might have missed out on something important, at least while Carrie was so involved it meant she had no time to make mischief in his life.

He saw her just once during that period, in the offices of Herbert, Morgan, and Bendell, her attorneys, for the essential signing of some papers connected with their property settlement.

"I gather you're onto something big," he said to her afterward.

" 'Huge' would be a better word," she said. "Infinitely more exciting than anything you ever brought in."

"I'm glad," Jamie said, "for the company."

"You still think of it as your company, don't you, James?"

"It still bears my name."

"That is the one aspect of my marriage to Peter that I do regret," Carrie said with a smile filled with malice. "Still having to be named Arias."

"I guess you can't have everything," Jamie said wearily.

"I'm coming close, though," Carrie said.

Everyone Jamie knew seemed to be leading unusually crazed lives right now, come to think of it. He'd called Olivia several times in the past few weeks, but according to her office she was out of town; they didn't know where. He had wondered, with a brief, idiotic stab of jealousy, who she was with, and he'd called Annie, too, thinking they might be together, but she, too, was away, and Jamie missed them both, missed having them at the end of a telephone line to share stuff with, big or small.

Carrie had it worked out before the tenth day. It was simple and perhaps lacking in the uniqueness she had initially dreamed of bringing to the campaign, and yet she knew, in spite of that, that it was the perfect campaign, that it would make its point, reach its target—bottom line, the only line that mattered, it would sell the product wonderfully effectively.

Her artwork was rough and clumsy, the photographs she was using and the subjects contained in them could and would be vastly improved upon, but the concept was right. Three images. The first, a young girl's flawless, innocent face. The second, a teenager just into womanhood, skin still aglow with youth. The third, an older woman's silhouette, the face in shadow, no aging process to be seen, left to the imagination. And the copy:

You can go back in time
(and no one except your physician need ever know)
LIGHT YEARS

She brought in Mitzi Palgrave and Joe Moritzio, her art director, swore them both to secrecy on pain of never finding work again at any agency in any city, sold them the concept, brand name, and slogan and set them to work.

Two weeks later, three days inside the deadline, armed with a now perfectly formed campaign including the best logotype Moritzio had ever created for Beaumont-Arias or anyone else, Carrie was back in Switzerland, this time in a suite at the Dolder Grand Hotel in Zurich, making her presentation to Müller, Schnabel and a video camera.

"So that we may consult with my codirectors," Müller told Carrie.

"When may I expect your decision?" Carrie asked.

"Within one week," Müller said.

"I love it," Annie said the next day, when Olivia ran the tape for her. "God forgive me, but I think it's a fantastic campaign."

"Enough to make anyone look forward to old age," Olivia said.

"She sold me," Felix Pfäniger said, wryly fingering the laugh lines around his eyes. "I only wish Light Years existed—I'd be its first customer."

"After Carrie," Olivia reminded him.

"Poor Carrie." Annie sighed.

"Don't start, Annie," Olivia said.

"What now?" Felix asked.

"Now you tell her that Lumitechnik loved her pitch and the campaign is hers," Olivia said.

"And then?" Felix wanted to know. "You let her create the whole campaign or what?"

"We can't go quite that far, unfortunately," Olivia replied, "not because of any compassion for Carrie, but because we have to put a lid on the costs. The price of the print ad space alone would run into hundreds of thousands—we'd probably be talking millions for the whole package."

"So how much further are we taking it?" Annie asked.

"One more stage," Olivia answered. "Just one more."

Felix, back in his role as Schnabel, called Carrie within the week, as promised.

"Congratulations, Mrs. Arias."

Carrie felt the old shiver of success-related pleasure run through her. "Thank you, Herr Schnabel," she said, staying cool. "Beaumont-Arias looks forward to taking Light Years to the people."

"The name is perfect," Felix said. "Ruth Müller told me she found it almost a masterstroke."

"There's a great deal to be done," Carrie said, moving right along.

"Starting," Felix jumped in, "with a second presentation, this time for the practitioners—the physicians and surgeons and clinic directors who will be ordering the equipment for their patients and clients after the launch to the public in June."

"Is Lumitechnik sure that's a wise move?" Carrie was surprised. "The whole concept has been directed to the public; these professionals are bombarded month after month by pharmaceutical and equipment companies promising them new miracles—surely there's a danger in pitching at such a cynical audience?"

"You sound as if you don't believe in Light Years yourself, Mrs. Arias," Felix said rather coolly.

"Obviously that's not true, Herr Schnabel," Carrie countered, "or else I'd hardly be planning to have the laser used on my own face." She paused. "I'm simply doing my job by pointing out the risks."

"I understand perfectly," Felix said, his tone more conciliatory. "And I will, of course, pass your comments on to Lumitechnik. But I believe they are convinced that this approach will, in the worst-case scenario, pinpoint any weaknesses in the campaign"—he waited a beat—"and if, as seems to us far more likely, the opposite applies and they are enthusiastic, then the ordering, manufacturing, and delivery processes will be facilitated."

"So that Light Years could be available to patients on demand in their physicians' offices," Carrie said, warming to the notion.

"Precisely."

She prepared meticulously, keeping many arrangements in-house that would normally have been farmed out to professional conference organizers. Ruth Müller had informed her that the entire Lumitechnik team of experts would be in Boston for the presentation, scheduled for May 3rd, and that their responses to the medics' questions would, of course, need to be planned as a crucial part of the show. Schnabel would be taking care of Lumitechnik's travel arrangements, but so far as Müller was concerned, the rest of the event was in Carrie's hands.

She chose, of course, the Ritz-Carlton—the backdrop needed to be a class act—had Mitzi Palgrave put together an A-plus guest list of relevant medical and surgical movers and shakers across the country, and issued invitations to them and to both mainstream and specialist journalists telling them that one of the most important breakthroughs in aesthetic surgery since the skin graft was about to be announced.

"Carrie told Felix it's going to be a mix of dignity and razzmatazz," Olivia told Annie on the phone.

Annie had gone back to Stone Bridge, to Banbury Farm House and Edward and the children and a week or two of reflexology study and practice—a sampling of normality, as she'd put it, to keep her sane in the prelude to the grand finale. Annie dreaded the climax of what Olivia called payback time. She had nightmares about it, about Carrie having them arrested, about their lengthy, internationally publicized trial and their exile in some correctional institution. She thought, in her heart, that they probably deserved all the retribution that Carrie was going to sling at them, that even though Carrie was the bitch of the century, practical jokes were—had always been—reprehensible things, and that they had, quite simply, taken this one too far.

"It's a late-afternoon presentation," Olivia was telling her now, "with a champagne reception at five, and the presentation to be made at six, with the Lumitechnik team answering questions afterward."

"Except that they won't be there," Annie said, her stomach lurching.

"No, they won't. Just you and me."

"Quite," Annie said.

"I've told you before, you don't need to come if you'd rather not."

"You know I'd rather not," Annie said, "but I will be there."

"How much have you told Edward?" Olivia asked curiously. Edward had gone on being an angel, raising the odd eyebrow but little more when Annie had disappeared for days on end.

"Not as much as I should have."

"You're feeling horribly guilty, aren't you?" Olivia said sympathetically.

"Horribly," Annie agreed. "But I'll still be there."

Olivia hated to admit it, but she, too, was suffering intermittent acute pangs of shame, and she, too, was having the occasional nightmare. Not about going to jail, because she was just as confident as she had been all along that if they handled Carrie properly at the end of the affair, there was little risk of the law being brought in. She'd had one truly ghastly dream in which Carrie, presented with the truth, had taken a revolver and shot herself in the head, and another when she'd jumped through a window. But in the light of day, Olivia didn't think there was the remotest possibility that coldhearted Carrie would ever do such a thing. If she was going to shoot anyone, it would be Olivia. After all, that was more Carrie's style, and at least then, even if it was the last thing she did, Olivia would have to acknowledge that the woman had guts.

The trouble was, she knew Annie was right when she said they'd gone too far. She'd known it the instant Carrie had exposed her own vulnerability by asking for the treatment herself, and Olivia had seriously considered pulling out then, but she'd known that was impossible, had been aware that if you started playing games with someone as potentially dangerous as Carrie, you had to see it through to the bitter end.

Olivia had created this hoax telling herself that Carrie needed someone imaginative and bold to teach her the lesson she richly deserved, but she had a nasty feeling now that somewhere along the line she had come perilously close to being sadistic. She had always accepted, not altogether happily, that there was an unforgiving streak in her nature; she hoped now, with all her might, that she was not also cruel. The whole Lumitechnik creation had gone so much further than she had dreamed it would; it had become so complicated and so fascinating and so compellingly intricate that Olivia had almost begun to believe in it herself. And Carrie, poor Carrie—Olivia could hardly believe that she could think of her that way—had become utterly deluded, wholly and completely suckered in.

Jamie had once said to Olivia that she was the most honest person he had ever known. She wondered how he would feel about her if he knew what she had been doing, what she had been coercing Annie into helping her do.

She thought perhaps she'd rather not know.

17

Carrie had hoped that Peter would be with her that evening at the Ritz-Carlton, but he was in Athens with Michael on Arias Shipping business, had sent two dozen red roses to the suite she'd taken there for the night, with a card wishing her well, and so Carrie was all alone. She didn't particularly mind being alone, had always considered herself an entirely independent spirit, but she thought it might have been nice to have her husband in the wings while she took her bows. Though Peter was not really that type of husband; Peter didn't cater to her needs the way James had. James had certainly had his faults, and he, too, had been capable of great obstinacy, but he had unquestionably been a kind, generous and empathic partner, and if anyone in the world would have understood the mix of stage fright and excitement she was experiencing as she made her last-minute preparations for the biggest presentation of her career, it was James.

Schnabel had reported to Mitzi Palgrave that Lumitechnik's team of four experts were flying in from London with Ruth Müller and were due to arrive in Boston shortly before four, and Carrie had ordered two limousines to meet them at Logan and bring them to the hotel.

When the car company contacted Beaumont-Arias a little after four-thirty to inform them that the party had not arrived, Mark Reiss called the Ritz-Carlton and found Carrie still in her suite.

"I've tried checking with Swissair to see if they missed the flight,

Mrs. Arias," Reiss told her, "but I'm having trouble getting any information out of them. Should I call Lumitechnik?"

"I'll do that myself," Carrie said. "But tell the drivers to stay at Logan and check every incoming European flight—they may have changed their minds about London and be flying in from Zurich or Geneva or any damned place for all we know."

She called Lumitechnik. The number rang out, unanswered. It was, of course, after nine-thirty their time, but Carrie had spoken to Ruth Müller late in the evening on other occasions and there had always been a night service manning the telephones. She called Schnabel's number. It was unobtainable.

The first prickle of foreboding crept up her spine. She called Mark Reiss at the office.

"Anything?"

"Not yet, Mrs. Arias."

Carrie looked at her watch. It was a quarter to five. The guests would be assembling downstairs and she needed to go down.

"Make sure those drivers stay at the airport, Mark, and if you have any news at all, tell the hotel operator to find me wherever I am."

She put down the phone, took a few deep breaths. Time was still on her side, she told herself; there was more than an hour until the presentation was due to begin. But she'd designed the show around the Lumitechnik scientists, for Christ's sake, and though she was confident enough about her personal presentation of Light Years, there was no way on earth she was qualified to field the technical questions of almost two hundred physicians and surgeons.

"Don't panic," she said aloud. "No need to panic."

Snatching up the receiver again, she redialed Lumitechnik, then, on impulse, tried their facsimile number. Like Schnabel's line, there was just that long, unmistakable whine telling her it was unobtainable. She punched the number for the hotel operator.

"Operator, I need you to run an urgent check for faults on two numbers in Switzerland—and I mean urgent. This is an emergency."

"Of course, Mrs. Arias."

"Call me right back."

It seemed an eternity till the operator came back.

"Apparently both those lines have been disconnected, Mrs. Arias."

"They can't have been," Carrie said. "They're major business lines. I was talking on them yesterday. There must be a mistake."

"I don't believe so, ma'am," the operator said. "The Swiss supervisor was very definite. She said they'd been disconnected."

"Was she speaking English?" Carrie knew she was clutching at straws. "Maybe she told you there was a fault and you didn't understand her."

"She spoke very good English, Mrs. Arias." The woman paused. "Would you like me to have the lines checked again, ma'am?"

"Right away."

Carrie slammed down the receiver and checked her watch again. Two minutes past five. She had no choice but to go downstairs and to pray that the Lumitechnik no-show and the telephone failure were just coincidence, and that maybe the limo drivers had located the experts and were, even now, hustling them into their cars.

Fifty ghastly minutes later, with no word from Lumitechnik, with corroboration from Mark Reiss that the Swiss corporation and G. Schnabel AG both appeared to have suddenly vanished from the face of the earth, and with two hundred physicians, surgeons, and clinic directors draining their last drops of champagne and taking their seats for the main event, Carrie, having taken refuge back in her suite—ashen-faced and quivering with humiliation and fury—needed no further confirmation of the catastrophe that had befallen her.

It was her worst nightmare. She had been conned. She was the victim of a most elaborate, gold-plated hoax. She, Caroline Beaumont Arias—who prided herself on being one of the smartest, toughest, most impregnable women in the business—had been taken for a patsy, a sucker, an *imbecile*. Which, as it turned out, she clearly was.

She wanted, right there and then, to kill. She wanted to die.

But she did not know who to kill and she could not die, not just yet anyway, because there was an audience waiting and she had her image to preserve and she had to take care of that. And in almost any other crisis situation she could imagine, Carrie felt she might have been able to handle it herself, but this blow—this stunning betrayal—was so shocking, so physically and emotionally *painful* for her that she knew she could not walk onto that podium and face all those people.

"You'll have to tell them," she told Mitzi Palgrave on the house phone.

"Tell them what?" Palgrave sounded alarmed. "Mrs. Arias, what do I tell them?"

"Whatever you goddamned like, Mitzi." Carrie found she could not speak rationally. "Tell them Lumitechnik's plane got struck by lightning—tell them there's been an earthquake in Switzerland—tell them someone stole a laser and zapped the whole team of experts before they could get here. Tell them whatever the fuck you can think of."

"Better keep it simple, I think," Palgrave said gently, rising to the occasion, aware that for the moment, at least, her hard-ass boss was out of it. "I'll just tell them they've been unavoidably detained." She paused. "I'll say it's just a temporary glitch, but that unfortunately it means we've had to postpone the presentation."

"Fine." Carrie was still shaking. "Thank you, Mitzi."

Palgrave hesitated. "Are you okay, Mrs. Arias? Can I do something else for you? Call someone?"

"Nothing. Just get rid of those people."

She sat for a long, long time on the bathroom floor after she'd thrown up. She felt drained and exhausted, yet all the while her mind was racing, searching, seeking out her enemies. James was first up, but swiftly dismissed again—James would never, *could* never dream up anything like this, would not do such a thing to anyone, not even to her. And it wasn't as if she hadn't made a score of enemies on her path to success—who didn't when they were busy getting to the top of their chosen tree?

Whoever it was, Carrie thought bitterly as she rinsed her mouth and mechanically fixed her makeup, had to hate her one hell of a lot to want to put her through this. She looked into the mirror, looked into her angry, defeated eyes, and shook her head violently. She had seldom anticipated more from a campaign, but now there would be no fanfares, no Light Years to hype from coast to coast. No campaign, no fee, no commission. No magical, mythical instant laser surgery to wipe away her own early wrinkles.

She went into the bedroom and lay down on the bed. There were no words to describe what a fool she'd been. She'd wasted a fortune in time and money, she'd neglected valuable clients—*real* clients, god-dammit—and worst of all, worse than all the rest of it rolled into one, if the truth ever got out, if she failed to find a way to effectively silence Palgrave and Reiss and Moritzio (she thanked God, silently, briefly, that she'd kept the buildup so quiet, that she'd at least been so selective about whom she'd taken into her confidence), she would be laughed out of Boston, out of the whole advertising arena. Out of everything that had ever mattered to her.

Carrie began to weep, great wounding tears of rage and shame and misery, just lay there on the big bed and bawled as she had not done since childhood.

Until she heard, penetrating through the sound of her own raw sobs, the sharp rapping on the outer door of the suite.

"Go away."

The knocking went on.

"Go *away*."

It became louder, more insistent. Carrie lay there for another moment, trying to ignore it, but still it went on and she knew it might be Palgrave or someone more important, and at the end of this ghastly fiasco she might still have some kind of image left to preserve.

"Just a minute," she called, and got to her feet, ran back into the bathroom, splashed a little cold water on her face, offered a swift, sharp word of thanks for waterproof mascara, and, taking a deep, steadying breath, went to open the door.

And learned the truth.

Olivia and Annie stood on the threshold of the suite.

"You." Carrie almost spat the word.

"May we come in?" Olivia asked softly.

For a long moment, Carrie stared at her, right into Olivia's unwavering green eyes, and then she transferred her gaze to Annie, saw the apprehension and—damn her to hell—the pity on her face.

"By all means," she said.

They all walked into the sitting room.

"You'd better have a seat," Carrie said.

Annie looked at her. "Are you okay?"

"Why wouldn't I be?"

They sat, Annie rather gingerly on the edge of the sofa, Olivia in one of the armchairs, a black calfskin briefcase propped against her left leg. Olivia looked at Carrie's face, saw that she was ashen beneath her makeup and that she'd been weeping, and another brief but sharp pang of guilt stirred her uncomfortably.

"I rather think," Carrie said, "that I deserve a drink."

Slowly, keeping her movements smooth and careful, she went to the bar and fixed herself a vodka and tonic, then sat down in the armchair closest to her and took a long swallow.

"Now, then," she said, "can you give me one good reason why I should not call the police?"

"As a matter of fact—" Olivia pushed the guilt firmly away again—"I rather think I can."

Carrie looked at the briefcase. It was easy to imagine what it contained; if she had been running the scam, she would have done precisely the same as Segal. Her mind raced. Copies of her letters to Lumitechnik and Schnabel, of course, tapes of her phone calls, video recordings of her presentation, perhaps of her meetings, and certainly the photographs and wax impressions taken of her naked face at the "consultation" with Professor Pfister. The memory of that cold discomfort flooded her with fresh hatred and sharpened her wits.

"I take it," she said to Olivia, keeping her eyes on the case for another moment, "that this represents your graduation from hoaxer to blackmailer?"

"I wouldn't have put it quite like that," Olivia said.

"Oh, I would," Carrie said. She took another drink. "What," she asked, "do you plan to do with the evidence of my naïveté?"

"That depends," Olivia answered.

"Upon what?"

Annie, on the sofa, shifted nervously.

"You look very anxious, Annie, dear," Carrie said. "Perhaps you'd like a Valium?"

Some of Annie's shame melted away. "No, thank you."

"Maybe you're on something stronger these days?"

"Revenge," Annie answered, startling herself. "It's quite fulfilling."

"Yes," Carrie said. "I imagine it is."

Olivia wanted to get to the point. "What we do with the evidence, as you call it," she said, "depends on you, Carrie. There are a number of ways we could use it, and all of them would have the same end result."

"To make me a laughing stock," Carrie said, harshly. "I assume that was your goal."

"Not necessarily. Not if you agree to our terms. In which case, Annie and I will be happy to bury it all. All you'll have to worry about then will be your share of the costs and inventing a plausible explanation."

"My share?" Carrie's eyes darkened. "Have you the slightest notion of what this evening alone has cost?"

"Probably not quite as much as Annie and I have spent," Olivia said, good-naturedly. "Setting up Lumitechnik, all that first-class travel, the rooms at the Baur-au-Lac and the Dolder Grand. Such good taste, Carrie." She smiled. "Not that we'd have expected anything less of you."

Carrie drained her drink, stood up, still trembling, and went back to the bar and fixed herself another. "Who were all those people? Müller and Schnabel—the physician, his nurse?"

"Friends," Olivia said.

"You have interesting friends," Carrie commented, and returned to her chair. "You're very quiet," she said to Annie. "Perhaps you'd care to tell me about these terms of yours?"

"With pleasure." A curious new calm was flooding Annie now; she was almost beginning to believe that Olivia might be right, that maybe they were going to walk out of the Ritz-Carlton without handcuffs. "First," she said, and took a deep, cleansing breath, "a full retraction, together with an apology to Jamie for the libelous implications of Silas Gilbert's interview—"

"And not just one of those tiny pieces buried on page fifteen of the *Boston Daily News* or in the back of *Advertising Life*," Olivia came in. "It has to be substantial and clear in both publications."

"Together," Annie went on, warming up nicely, "with a whole new business deal with Jamie—legally signed and sealed, obviously—allowing him to move all his old accounts to JAA without delay or penalty—"

"Unless, of course," Olivia added, "any of them want to stay with you."

"How considerate of you," Carrie commented.

"And," Annie took back the reins, "you agree to hand over to JAA fifty percent of any profits that Beaumont-Arias has made from those clients and kept from Jamie since your split."

Carrie sat for several moments, her face expressionless, watching them both.

"Is that it?" she asked finally.

"Not quite," Olivia said.

"I thought not."

"You undertake never to make another poisonous innuendo that might tarnish Annie's good name."

"What about your name?" Carrie asked.

Olivia smiled again. "You're welcome to try, Carrie."

"What else?"

"Last, but most certainly not least," Olivia said, "you give your personal guarantee—prepared by our various attorneys and notarized—never to try to bring any action against us for this little charade."

Carrie's eyes were ice cold now. "Is that what you call it? Not fraud? Not forgery? Not blackmail?"

Annie's calm disappeared.

"I prefer charade," Olivia said.

Carrie took a long swallow from her glass and then set it down on the table beside her. "I never did enjoy party games," she said.

Time passed. The three women sat, silent now, alone with their thoughts.

Carrie asked one more abrupt question. "Was James involved with this?"

"Jamie doesn't know a thing about it," Olivia answered.

"I thought not," Carrie said. "Not his style."

They fell silent again. The telephone rang once, and Carrie moved swiftly to pick it up, spoke briefly and tersely, and listened to Mitzi Palgrave's report that the proceedings had wound up good-humoredly enough, thanks mostly to the champagne that had preceded the non-event. Carrie asked Mitzi to instruct the switchboard to hold all calls until otherwise directed, and hung up.

"So," Olivia said, at last. "What's it to be, Carrie? Do you come after us, or do we lay the whole mess to rest?"

Carrie sat back in her armchair and looked at them both.

"I could almost—*almost*—respect you for your skill," she said, "if you hadn't made a fool of me."

"No one has to know," Annie said.

"Some people know already."

"No, they don't," Olivia said. "They know that something's gone wrong, but they don't know what. Even the employees who've worked on the campaign don't ever have to know. You just tell them Lumitechnik's suffered a financial collapse and that you're going to sue. Tell them your lawyers are dealing with it and then get them back to work, hard and fast, as only you can, Carrie."

Another minute ticked by.

"Are you a gambler by nature, Olivia?" Carrie asked.

"Perhaps."

"Gambling with your own freedom and good name is one thing," Carrie said. "But surely you must have realized that Annie has far more to lose than you if I refuse to play the game your way."

Annie sat very still. "I took my own risks, Carrie."

"You're quite a brave woman, Annie. I'm rather surprised by that."

"Me, too," Annie said.

"Olivia, of course, knew she was taking a well-calculated risk," Carrie went on. "She gambled on the assumption that by bringing a prosecution, I would lay myself open to public ridicule and that, therefore, I would simply cave in to your demands."

"Was I wrong?" Olivia asked.

Annie held her breath.

Carrie lingered one more moment.

"Of course you were not wrong," she said.

She saw them to the door.

"Is there room for negotiation on the precise wording of the apology?" she asked. "I assume, for example, that Mr. Gilbert's contrition will suffice."

"I don't see why not," Olivia said.

"So long as it looks sincere," Annie added.

Carrie opened the door. "James is a fortunate man," she said.

"Thank you, Carrie," Olivia said.

Annie hesitated. "It was," she said softly, "a wonderful campaign."

A small, grudging, cold smile touched the corners of Carrie's mouth.

"It was an extraordinary product," she said.

Silas Gilbert's retraction appeared in both publications in the same week that Jamie learned from Bob Jacobson of Carrie's offer to renegotiate the terms of their business agreement in his favor.

Two days later, he telephoned Olivia in Strasbourg.

"What did you do?"

"Do?" Olivia, in her office, gritted her teeth and waited.

"Don't bother pussyfooting around, Olivia. Carrie told me that you and Annie are responsible for her change of heart."

"What change of heart?"

"Olivia, cut it out. There's no point—Carrie's told me."

"What exactly has she told you?" Olivia picked her cordless phone off its base and began to spin her chair, as she often did when she was in good spirits. It was going to be all right; she could tell. At worst, Jamie was going to get on his high horse and say he didn't need help and that she shouldn't have got involved and she *certainly* shouldn't have dragged Annie into it.

"She hasn't really told me anything," Jamie said, "except that if I want to know what's been going on, I should ask you."

"You can ask," Olivia said brightly. She spun the chair twice to the right.

"So I'm asking."

"Doesn't mean I'm going to answer." Now twice to the left.

"Do you want me to ask Annie?"

"You can try." Olivia stopped spinning, feeling a little dizzy. She and Annie had come to an agreement that it really was best if Jamie never learned exactly what they had done.

"Olivia, this isn't fair and it isn't right. I didn't ask you to get involved."

She grinned to herself. "You know me."

"And as for Annie—you promised you wouldn't tell her about the Gilbert interview."

"I crossed my fingers, so my promise didn't count."

"Olivia, it's not funny."

"Tell me something, Jamie. Are things better or worse for you now than they were before?"

"Better, goddammit, but that's not the point."

"Maybe you should make it the point," Olivia said gently.

Jamie paused. "Are you going to tell me how you did it or not?"

"Not," Olivia said. "Never. Nor will Annie. And Edward only knows we were up to something, no more than that."

"Oh, Olivia," Jamie said.

"Oh, Jamie, stop." Some of the brightness went out of her. "I admit I took a few risks that I probably shouldn't have—with other people, too, not just myself, and I don't feel too good about that. But no one really got hurt, thank God—Carrie's pride took quite a tumble, and you may not believe this, but I came close to feeling bad about that, too." She gripped the phone more tightly. "But I'm not going to tell you any more than that, Jamie, and it did pay off in the end, so please, please don't spoil a happy ending by worrying too much about how we got to it."

Jamie was silent for a long moment.

"Tell me just one more thing," he said at last.

"If I can."

"Why did you do it?"

"You know why," Olivia said.

"Tell me anyway. Please, Olivia."

It was Olivia's turn to be silent. A parade of thoughts and hopes and longings swung through her mind, all of them leading back to those hours in Newport and Boston. Perhaps, after all, Jamie had not forgotten, had not wiped it out. Perhaps he was waiting, hoping for her to say something now, to give him a sign.

No, she told herself. *Not now. Probably not ever.*

"Olivia?" Jamie's voice urged her on. "Tell me why you did it."

"You know why we did it," Olivia said. "You, me, and Annie. Our pact."

"Was that the only reason?"

She thought she heard a yearning in his voice, but she wasn't sure, could not be sure. "Of course not," she answered softly. "We both love you, Jamie."

"Oh," he said.

OLIVIA'S BOX

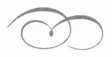

18

On November 6, 1938, a young Jew from Hanover studying in Paris named Hirsch Grynszpan, enraged by news he had received concerning the inhumane treatment of his family by the Nazis, went to the German embassy in Paris and shot an official named Ernst vom Rath.

Two days later, on November 8, Georg Brauner came to our house for what was to be his final visit. Of the few paintings that still remained in the cellar, he chose just two: a Hodler and a Redon. On most previous occasions, Brauner had conducted what he still euphemistically termed "business" in a manner so leisurely that I know it had driven my mother almost wild with the effort of having to suppress her outrage. He would go, with Papa, down into the cellars and make his selection; he would refuse every offer of help from me, claiming that only my father could be entrusted with the handling of the precious paintings. Then he would stand back and watch as Papa fetched and climbed a ladder and struggled to bring down the works from the racks in which they—together with the one hundred and thirty other paintings already stolen by Brauner—had previously been so meticulously and lovingly stored, and then he would observe as my father carefully wrapped the works and made them ready for transport.

On this occasion, however, Brauner was plainly in a great hurry, allowing me to assist my father, chivying us down to the cellar, urging us repeatedly to move faster, to be certain not to damage the two paintings but to work more rapidly nonetheless. As my mother stood, fists clenched, waiting at the top of the cellar steps, listening to Brauner's commands, hearing our breathless efforts to comply, I think we all knew, without being told, that the end of the Georg Brauner episode was near. And though a part of us rejoiced at the prospect of never seeing him again, I think that the greater part was aware that our troubles had barely begun.

"A word, before I leave," Brauner said upstairs in the hall.

"Of course," Emanuel said, still fighting to catch his breath. Hedi, anxious for his health, had wanted to snatch the Redon out of his arms as he had struggled up the cellar steps in front of Anton, who was carrying the Hodler, but Emanuel had been too proud, too obstinate—things were bad enough, bad enough, without allowing his wife to schlepp for a thief.

"In the salon, if you please," Brauner told them.

Hedi, straight-backed, head held high, refusing to show her apprehension, led the way into the room in which Brauner had so often made an irritating point of taking a drink before leaving, his manner always so damnably cordial, as if he actually believed they might enjoy his presence in their home.

"A schnapps for you?" Emanuel asked wearily.

"No," Brauner said, as Anton, thin and tall and strikingly like his mother, closed the door. "No more schnapps."

They waited. Brauner did not sit, as he always had, perfectly relaxed, legs elegantly crossed, taking his time. His suit was as exquisitely tailored as ever, his shoes as finely made and highly polished, yet he was, indisputably, ill at ease.

"This is the last time I shall come to this house," Brauner said. He spoke softly, as if he feared that someone outside the room might be listening to their conversation. "But I leave you with some important news. Important, at least, for you." He paused. "You know, of course, about the shooting in Paris."

"We do," Emanuel said, his stomach tightening painfully.

"I have learned from certain of my contacts," Brauner went on, still speaking quietly, "that reprisals against Jews all over Germany are imminent."

"Here, too, in Baden-Baden?" Anton asked quickly.

"Here, too." Brauner regarded them all with his sharp, dark eyes. "I have managed to obtain assurances that, so long as you all remain here, inside your home, you and your family will be safe."

There was a brief silence. Emanuel had become very pale.

"Where else could we go, Herr Brauner?" Hedi's question was wry. "Since our travel documents have still to materialize."

Brauner gave her a small, curt nod. "Your papers, Frau Rothenburg, should very soon be with you."

"Are you sure?" Anton asked.

"Unfortunately," Hedi added, "we've heard that many times before."

"But the situation now is changed," Brauner told her, "because our business dealings have come to an end."

"Have they?" Emanuel asked.

"Alas, yes," Brauner said, "since the cupboard, so to speak, is almost bare." He paused. "It has been," he added smoothly, "I know, a disappointing period for you all, but when times are difficult we must all look after our own. I'm sure you agree."

Neither Emanuel nor Hedi nor Anton spoke.

"The time has come," Brauner went on, "for me to fulfill my side of our bargain, and this I intend to do. You will not hear from me again, but your papers will come, and they will come soon."

"That's very good news." A little of Emanuel's tension left him.

"If it's true," Anton said.

"Anton, please," Emanuel said.

"I understand your son's skepticism," Brauner said, "but I assure you all that what I tell you is, to the best of my knowledge, the truth."

"And the reprisals?" Emanuel asked cautiously.

"Imminent, as I said." Brauner moved closer to the door, preparing to leave. "Do as I tell you, Herr Rothenburg. Stay here, with your family, in this house, until it's all over, and nothing will happen to you." He paused. "They may come, there may be some small trouble—a little damage, perhaps—but I'm promised it will be purely for show."

"Can you guarantee that?" Hedi asked him.

"I can only tell you what I have been promised, Frau Rothen-burg," Brauner replied. "I have no reason to doubt it."

My mother did doubt it, with every fiber of her being. She told us, after Brauner had gone, that she did not believe that their visas and other necessary documents would materialize now any more than they had in the past; neither did she have any real faith in Brauner's assurances of safety. Papa argued with her: Brauner had seemed to him so frank. In stressing that the situation was different now because the cellars were almost empty, Brauner was admitting that he had blocked their departure so long as he had still needed their cooperation. Why should he not admit it, Mama asked ironically, since there was no action they could take against him? She, for one, could not believe in the word of a thief.

"What would you have me do?" my father asked her.

"There is nothing to be done," she answered flatly. "We must stay, as he told us, and we must wait, and then—"

"Then?" Papa asked.

"Then we'll learn the truth," she said.

And I said nothing at all.

We waited all through the rest of that day and night, and on through the next, long day. It was Leo Landau's birthday, and I wanted to go next door to visit him, but Papa would not permit it. I felt restless and irritable; Lili became argumentative; Trude became tearful. Perhaps, Mama suggested gently to our father, we might all go to the Landaus' for a little while, but Papa stood firm. Brauner's instructions had been clear and, given no better alternative, we would all remain in the house. And if my mother's instincts warned her that if there was to be trouble of some kind in the area there might be greater wisdom in dividing the family, she clearly had neither the heart nor the will to argue the point with him.

I know now that as the night of November 9—Kristall-nacht—unfolded, Jewish neighborhoods all across Germany were facing a wave of unprecedented wanton destruction and violence, but for our family it began quietly, with an uneasy calm, our house remaining, as Georg Brauner had promised, untouched.

Shortly before eleven, after Maria, our housekeeper, had gone to her own home for the night and with Lili and Trude already asleep in their rooms and Mama, too, getting ready for bed, I looked at my father.

"Shall we go to bed, Papa? Try to sleep?"

His smile was so strained, I can still see it now.

"We can try," he said.

As we had done the previous evening, after Brauner's departure, we took the two Danes and made a last patrol together, checking the locks on every door, going from room to room ensuring that each window was properly closed, that each curtain was securely drawn.

Outside, to the front and sides and rear of the house, all seemed silent, all seemed peaceful.

We, too, went to bed.

Emanuel dreamt that his father was beside him, standing close, his prayer shawl wrapped around his shoulders, a skullcap on his head, and he knew, even in his dream, that it was Yom Kippur, and the more devout among them were rocking back and forth, lost in their prayers, but his father was standing quite straight and he was looking down at Emanuel, his son, and his face was filled with pride and his eyes glowed.

"You can leave soon," he said very softly, so that no one else would hear. "You and Hedi and the children, you can come to us now."

"But we don't have our papers," Emanuel said to his father.

And his father smiled down at him. "You don't need papers," he said, and he put his strong left arm around his son's shoulders. "Your mother will be so happy to see you again, so happy."

The cold woke him. Against his right temple.

He opened his eyes. He was lying on his side and Hedi was close beside him, her warmth pressing into him, her left arm around his shoulder. For one more infinitesimal instant he thought that the cold had been a part of the dream, and then he became aware that it was still there.

Cold steel.

Emanuel blinked, once. He heard the movement from behind him. And he knew that the steel was a gun.

He began to pray.

Please, dear Lord, don't let her wake.

The man said just two words.

"Die, Jew."

Emanuel saw Hedi's eyelids flutter, felt her body stir. Quickly, he slid his right arm about her.

Please, God, Creator of the universe, save our children.

I heard nothing. Not any of the sounds that our dogs must have made before they were silenced. Nor the shots. Nor the spilling of the gasoline, or the rasp of the matches being lit.

Lili, Trude, and I slept on, right through the murder of our parents, through the burning of our house around us. Gretel Landau, Leo's mother, woke just after one o'clock and went to her window, saw the light from the flames, and roused her husband, Samuel, who threw on his dressing gown and ran downstairs and out of the house, feet bare, ran across the lawns and through the gate that linked their land with ours. His voice, as he screamed out our names, over and over again, was my awakening, tore me, choking from the smoke, first to my bedroom door, where the flames forced me back, and then to my window, where I watched, bewildered and terrified, as Landau found a ladder and put it up and helped me safely down.

Next morning, on November 10, I have heard that all the Jewish men in Baden-Baden were marched through the streets to the synagogue and ordered to read aloud extracts from *Mein Kampf.* Neither Samuel Landau nor I were among them, for we were already on our way to the recently opened concentration camp at Buchenwald.

I had seen the fire destroy the house, incinerating the bodies of my parents and my sisters, as well as the pitiful remnants of my father's once great art collection. I am certain there will have been no postmortems, no investigation.

Neither into the shootings, nor the fire.

Nor into the man known as Georg Brauner.

Two months have passed since they brought us here, and I know now that I am very ill. They separated me from Samuel Landau on our arrival, and I can only pray that he has fared better than I. I have eaten nothing at all for more than a week, and I am coughing blood. My lungs have been bad since the beginning—I think that the smoke must have damaged them, made it harder for me to fight.

I found this little notebook on my first afternoon in the camp. I stepped on it in a patch of muddy earth, and almost overlooked it. Paper is like gold dust here. I have written down our story as well as I could manage, and I keep the book carefully hidden. Before the end comes, I hope to pass it on to someone stronger than myself.

I would like someone outside this place to know the truth.

Otherwise, what hope is there?

FOR OLIVIA

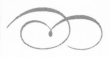

19

*O*livia was the only person either Annie or Jamie knew who liked moving. Most people—normal people—agreed that moving was hell, not exactly up there, as some statistics claimed, with bereavement and divorce, but certainly something to be endured with gritted teeth and overdraft.

Olivia said that moving was fun. She said that every move she had made—excepting the leaving of her parents' house in 1976—had seemed to her a joyous leap into unknown territory.

"It's all adventure," she told Jamie and Annie when they visited her for the last time in Strasbourg in August of 1994, as she was preparing to uproot herself again for a spell in Brussels. "It's finding another set of walls and turning them into home—it's making new friends and working out where to buy great food and which restaurants to go to—"

"And which language to speak on the way to work," Jamie said, scrubbing potatoes in Olivia's kitchen. They were all wearing T-shirts, jeans, and aprons—they'd eaten out for the last six nights, so this evening Annie and Jamie had agreed to stay home, cook pot-au-feu, and help Olivia with some of her packing.

"French and Flemish this time." Olivia lifted the lid of her big casserole to inhale the aroma of beef, chicken, pork, and herbs.

"Flemish is almost Dutch, isn't it?" Annie asked.

"Just about," Olivia answered. "And Brussels is a bilingual city—every street has a French and a Flemish name." She spooned out some broth and held out the spoon to Jamie. "Taste, please."

Jamie tasted. "Gorgeous. How soon can we eat?"

"When you've boiled those potatoes."

"I'd hate it," Annie said.

"What?" Olivia said.

"Moving to another country."

"You did it and survived," Olivia pointed out.

"Not exactly easily," Annie said.

"Would you do it again," Olivia asked, "if Edward wanted to?"

"I can't imagine Edward ever wanting to leave England," Jamie said, lighting the gas under the pan of potatoes.

"Thank God," Annie said.

"What about you, Jamie?" Olivia asked. "Would you think of relocating again?"

"I might," Jamie said. "For a good enough reason."

"A woman," Annie said. "You went to Boston for Carrie."

"It wasn't exactly alien territory for me," Jamie said, "with my family home almost around the corner."

"Funny," Olivia said, sitting down at her table, "but I've never seen the Newport house as your home at all."

"But it is, in a way," Jamie said.

"I know," Olivia said, "but it still doesn't feel like it to me."

One of the things Olivia loved about moving was the excuse it gave her to delve into what she called her family trunk—the vastest of the handsome, solid pieces of dark green leather luggage Arthur Segal had bought from Swaine Adeney & Briggs in Piccadilly soon after the family had moved to London, and into which Olivia had placed many of his and Emily's possessions when she'd closed down the house in Hampstead. Moving was an appropriate time to rummage through old belongings and clear away some of the detritus, the accumulated nonsense that she always seemed to hold on to for no good reason, like matchbooks and theater programs and Christmas store catalogs.

Every time she moved, Olivia told Jamie and Annie as they sat around her dining table and ate the pot-au-feu, she seemed to find something new in that old trunk. When she'd moved from New York to Geneva, she'd found an old dictaphone of Arthur's with a previously unnoticed tape still inside; Olivia still remembered the excitement of scrabbling around for the right battery to make the old machine work, and the pure joy, when it did still play back, of being able to hear her father's voice again, dictating to his secretary.

"And then, when I left Geneva, it happened again," she said, pouring more wine for them all. "I'd often seen this old camera of my mother's, but for some reason I still can't understand, it seems I'd never checked to see if there was film inside—maybe because Mom was always so busy working, I didn't really remember her taking pictures. But there was this film, and I was so upset because I thought it wouldn't develop—"

"Surely it didn't," Jamie said, "after so many years?"

"Oh, yes, it did," Annie said. "Livvy showed the pictures to me just after she moved here, didn't you?"

"Wonderful, happy pictures," Olivia said. "I'll show you later, Jamie—Mom and Dad away together somewhere—it looks like France, but it's all countryside and there were no signposts or other clues, so I could never be quite sure."

"So what are we going to find this time?" Jamie asked.

Olivia shook her head. "I'm going to assume there's nothing new left to find—that way I won't be too disappointed." She stood up, started clearing dishes from the table. "Not that I mind either way—it's fun just looking at the same old stuff again."

They dragged the trunk together into the middle of the spare-room floor and began, and there were all the wonderful old familiar items: the report cards, the rolled-up diplomas, the bulky shortwave radio Olivia remembered Arthur tuning into late at night to listen to news reports from distant places; diaries, letters galore of gratitude to Arthur from international charities, photographs—endless piles of black-and-white and color snapshots never stuck into albums—and her parents' love letters, tied up with ribbon by Olivia after she'd first found them back in 1976 and never, she'd promised silently, to be read by anyone else again.

"What's in here?" Annie asked.

Olivia looked at the old pigskin briefcase with the broken lock and remembered, suddenly, sitting on the floor in her father's study in their house in Hampstead picking that lock with the blade of a small kitchen knife. And she remembered, too, what she had found in the case. A strange, starkly worded little note from Carlos Arias to Arthur, written shortly before their deaths. *Shock and dismay,* that was it, Olivia recalled, seeing the note again in her memory, remembering that it had been handwritten and that it had jarred her, disconcerted her a little. She remembered too, now, that she had mentioned it to Annie and asked if she should show it to Jamie, but that Annie had thought it better she didn't, and so Olivia had put it back in the case.

"Livvy?" Annie was looking at her questioningly.

"What's up?" Jamie asked her.

Olivia took the case from Annie and opened it up.

"I just remembered something that was in here," she said, looking for it.

It was there, folded up, as she had left it all those years before.

"What is it?" Annie asked.

Olivia unfolded it and read it again.

Dear Arthur,

Deeply shocked and dismayed to learn that your suspicions are not, after all, unfounded.

We must meet soon.

Carlos Arias

"I'd forgotten this," she said to Jamie. "I found it while I was clearing out the London house, and then I put it away and forgot about it." She held it out to him. "I didn't understand it then, and I told Annie about it and she thought it might upset you, so I put it away."

Jamie read it, frowning, then shook his head. "It doesn't mean anything to me. I wonder what it was about?"

Annie leaned across, read it, and remembered. "It could have been about anything," she said. "Something really trivial."

"The words don't make it sound trivial to me," Olivia said. "They didn't to me then either, Jamie. I'm sorry. Maybe I should have shown it to you at the time."

"I can't see that it would have meant more to me then than it does now." Jamie paused. "And I think Annie was probably right—it might have upset me."

"What surprised me most was that I didn't remember our fathers talking to each other that often," Olivia said. "I mean, there were the occasional charity affairs and American School stuff, but I wasn't aware of much more than that, were you?"

"Not really." Jamie thought for a moment. "Maybe they were doing some business."

"What kind of business?" Annie asked. "Shipping and art don't seem to go hand in hand."

He shrugged. "Don't know."

"Ask Michael," Olivia suggested.

"What for?" Jamie asked.

"He might know if they were involved in any kind of deal."

"More than eighteen years ago?" Jamie said.

"I think you should both leave it alone," Annie said warmly.

"Why?" Olivia asked, surprised.

"Because you're not going to find anything out," Annie answered. "And because it seems a very private note. It sounded to me back then—and it still does—as if Jamie's dad was really upset about something." She paused. "And whatever it was, neither he nor your father probably got to do too much more about it. So what's the point in dwelling on it?"

"Curiosity," Olivia said.

"You're way too big on curiosity, Livvy," Annie told her.

"I know, I know, and it killed the cat," Olivia said.

" 'A man should live if only to satisfy his curiosity.' Yiddish proverb." Jamie grinned.

"How come you're quoting Yiddish proverbs?" Annie wanted to know.

He shrugged. "It just popped out."

"New Jewish girlfriend?" Annie asked.

"Not this month," Jamie said.

Olivia said nothing.

The day after Olivia's move that September into the Amigo—a luxurious hotel built in the fifties on the site of an old Brussels prison, which she had decided to make her base while she hunted for her new home and office—Jamie phoned from Boston to check on her.

"How're things?"

"The usual at this stage." Olivia was sitting on the bedroom floor surrounded by suitcases. "This is where I always discover that I've put the really important stuff that I need right away in the boxes that have gone into storage. So far, I have all my saucepans and no underwear."

"Good thing it's summer," Jamie said.

"Good excuse to go shopping, too."

"Speaking of boxes," Jamie said, "I mentioned my father's note to Michael one day last week. It didn't mean any more to him than it did to us."

"Did he know if they'd ever done any business?" Olivia asked.

"No, he didn't. He thought it sounded a little strange, too—he asked if you'd found any more correspondence. I said I assumed you hadn't."

"I never came across any more," Olivia said. "But then I don't think I really looked."

"That's what I thought."

"I have a whole cabinet jammed with my parents' papers. I could take a look if you'd like me to."

"I don't see the point," Jamie said. "Like Annie said, it's all so long ago."

"Then I think I'll focus on buying underwear instead," Olivia said. "I'm dying to go shopping anyway."

"Olivia," Jamie said.

"Yes?"

"Stop talking about underwear."

"What do you have against underwear, Jamie?"

"Nothing at all."

"So why can't I talk about it?"

"Olivia," Jamie said again.

"What?"

"Go shopping."

It was extraordinary, Olivia reflected, after putting down the receiver, how even after so many years, just the merest, tiniest *scrap* of a hint that Jamie might, after all, remember—perhaps even sometimes think about—what had gone on between them that one single night in

Boston, was enough to inflame her every nerve-ending. It was more than extraordinary, she decided, still sitting on the floor. It was far worse than that; it was both depressing and pitiful.

Unless, of course, Jamie really did remember. Unless, of course, he, too, still felt something more than friendship for her.

But if that was the case, that would mean they were both fools, outsize idiots for having done nothing about it. And, alas, neither of them was a fool.

"Only one thing to do," Olivia said aloud, and got to her feet.

Like the man had said.

"Go shopping."

She met Bernard Martens three weeks later. It was a dull, cool October afternoon when she strolled into Martens Antiques just off the rue des Sablons, partly to take a closer look at the treasures inside, partly to get out of the rain. Within half an hour, she had fallen in love with a Georgian silver teakettle, and Bernard, the proprietor of the store, had fallen head-over-heels in love with her. He was fifty-seven years old and a widower with grown-up children and five grandchildren, living in solitary splendor in a great house outside the city near Foret de Soignes with only his full complement of household staff to keep him company. Bernard was the oldest man Olivia had ever had a relationship with, but he was in such wonderful shape, was such an attractive man, such a great companion with his marvelous blend of intellect and earthy humor, that she could hardly imagine herself ever again being satisfied by a younger man.

Except, perhaps, Jamie. If Olivia was honest with herself, there was no longer any perhaps about it. She had not meant to, certainly hadn't *wanted* to, fall in love with her best male friend, and she knew that she'd done and said all the right—all the *sensible* things—after that night in Boston, about it having been pure friendship and nothing more. But the truth was that she had not really meant a word of what she'd said, had known that right away. Yet she was still sure it had been the right thing to say to Jamie, who'd only just begun to recover after being put through the wringer by Carrie.

"How is Carrie?" Olivia asked him from time to time, trying to be casual, wanting to find out if his ex was still keeping to her side of the bargain more than four years after she and Annie had brought her into line.

"I don't hear much from her," Jamie usually answered, and Olivia said that was good, wasn't it? And then she would ask—also casually—about other women, and Jamie would mention the occasional name and sometimes tell her a little more but there was never anything serious going on. And Olivia—shame on her—would experience, in spite of herself, an instant of almost overpowering relief, and it was so wrong of her because Jamie deserved someone wonderful, someone loyal and generous who would respect him and be faithful. Someone, she supposed, a little like Annie. Nothing like her.

It was Bernard Martens who helped Olivia find her apartment in rue Charles Hanssens near the corner of rue Ernest Allard and almost a stone's throw from his own store. It was a rare find in the exclusive, artistic, entirely cobbled Sablon area: an exquisitely renovated, beautifully furnished home on the ground floor of a narrow old house belonging to a wealthy diamond merchant from Antwerp. The three apartments above had attractive small balconies, but Olivia's pride and joy was her tiny, private, white-walled backyard, which she swiftly turned into a cobbled garden with big earthenware pots planted with flowers from the market in Grand Place and La Palmeraie in rue Ernest Allard.

"And I've found an office in the place du Grand Sablon," she told Annie on the phone in the second week of November. "I can hardly believe my luck—it's just one room, and it's really small, so I'll have to keep it tidy—"

"That's impossible," Annie said.

"I know, I know"—Olivia, as Annie and Jamie both knew, had inherited Arthur Segal's knack of untidying a room the moment she entered it—"but in this case I'll just have to try."

"So you can walk to work?"

"In minutes, Annie—and it's just so gorgeous around here—it really is the nicest part of the city by far."

"And Bernard's store must be practically next door, too, mustn't it?"

"Yes, it is, though he's not there that much."

There was a smile in Annie's voice. "He sounds like such a nice man, Livvy."

"Yes, he is," Olivia said. "But don't start reading too much into that—I've met a lot of nice men, as you know."

"Are you happy, Olivia?" Bernard asked her one evening in December as they were finishing dinner at La Maison du Cygne, one of his favorite restaurants. "Is life in Brussels enough for you?"

She looked at him in surprise, replete as she was with fine food and champagne and the pleasure of overlooking what really had to be, at night, one of the most enchantingly illuminated great squares in Europe. "Can't you tell that I'm happy, Bernard? Brussels has been so good to me."

"But is it enough?"

She understood then what it was he meant. "For now or for always?" she asked.

"You tell me."

"I seldom think about always," Olivia said.

"Do you think you could try, just for once?"

Olivia regarded him for a moment. He was a quite wonderful-looking man, with his perfectly groomed silvering hair and his merry, kind blue eyes, and his firm, straight mouth. He was also extraordinarily good to her, so decent and gentle and generous. He deserved honesty.

"I think," she said, "for now." She paused. "*Ça va?*"

He gave a tiny shrug, but his smile, if a touch wistful, was all warmth.

"*Pas bien,*" he said, "*mais ça va.*"

He was a clever man, far too intuitive not to be aware that emotionally theirs was an uneven relationship, that although Olivia was immensely fond of him, she was not in love with him. And because he was also a fair-minded man, he had no wish to tie her to him any more tightly than she might be comfortable with. That, Martens knew, would be the swiftest way to lose Olivia Segal, and while he knew, just as surely, that the day would dawn when that would happen, he had every intention of postponing the evil moment for as long as possible.

Which was one of the reasons he had helped her to find her apartment. Martens would have infinitely preferred Olivia to come to live in his house, but even if it had not been much too early in their relationship, he was far too wise not to recognize her need for space and privacy and, most of all, independence. As it was, because she had a home in which she felt more comfortable and at ease than she had felt anywhere since her parents' house in London, and because Bernard Martens was perfectly willing to spoil her with love and affection, yet knew when to stand back and let her breathe, Olivia felt better able to respond to him, both physically and emotionally.

"Which is why," she told Annie in another of their telephone chats, "the time we spend together is just so great."

"I must say," Annie commented, "I've seldom heard you sound quite so comfortable with any man."

"Comfortable?" Olivia hated the sound of that. "I don't think comfortable is the word at all."

"Settled then," Annie suggested.

"Hardly settled either. We're too busy, for one thing."

"You've always been busy, Livvy," Annie pointed out, "always the most active of us. It just sounds different with Bernard—you do different things—all those concerts, the opera, the ballet, the gallery openings—those are settled, comfortable kinds of things, whether you like it or not."

"Grown-up things, you mean." Olivia was wry.

"Well, yes." Annie paused. "Is that such a bad thing?"

"For a thirty-something-year-old woman?"

"Well, yes," Annie said again.

"I guess not," Olivia said, but she was not entirely sure that she meant it.

Life in Brussels did suit her wonderfully well, at least for the time being. Being the restless spirit she was, Olivia did not truthfully imagine for a moment that she would be able to consider settling there forever, but for now her daily life was pretty close to sublime. As there had been in Geneva and Strasbourg, there were a vast number of translation agencies in Brussels, but because Olivia's preference was to deal with artists, novelists, and media people in general, and because she was relaxed about tailoring her fees to her clients' means—often working for several weeks at a heavily cut rate because she liked and respected one of these talented, but tight-budgeted individuals—the Segal Translation Agency's books were generally filled with interesting bookings.

With Bernard, Olivia wandered farther afield, and when she was in a shopping frame of mind, she visited the chic and seriously expensive boutiques on avenue Louise, but she seldom tired of the Sablon district. She loved to browse through the weekend market stalls in front of the church in Grand Sablon, and she liked wandering along the cobbled lanes near her home, delving into the less traditional of the antique shops and galleries. She delighted in buying delicacies at Confiserie Wittamer and then—on one of those sunny, energizing winter days that she had always enjoyed—sitting on a bench to eat them near the goldfish pool in the lovely statued garden of the place du Petit Sablon, listening to the pealing bells of Notre-Dame du Sablon. She looked forward to lazing at tiny tables in one of the street cafés when spring and summer came, reading or watching the tourists go by, and in the meantime, on rainy days, she was content to sit inside the cafés and brasseries or at one of the long communal tables at Le Pain Quotidien, eating slices of their wonderful brown bread spread with brie and walnuts.

Nineteen ninety-five began auspiciously enough, with Olivia staying for three weeks in Gstaad in a marvelous chalet with Bernard and two other couples, all old friends of his and all entertaining and relaxing to be with; yet she felt almost relieved to be back in her own apartment after the trip because, she supposed, it had been just a little too comfortable, a little too much like being half of a permanent partnership. She bought a small blue Renault a week after their return to Brussels, partly so that she could drive herself when the fancy took her out into the Belgian countryside, but partly, if she was honest—with herself if not with Bernard—because it made her feel more independent, less hemmed in, when it came to staying at his house. She worked hard through February and March, interpreting for and generally helping out an Australian television crew on location in Brussels; and then in early April she went to England for Edward Thomas's fiftieth-birthday celebration before accompanying Jamie back home to Boston, where they spent five lovely days together, sailing in the *Joie de Vivre* and just hanging out. Jamie wanted Olivia to stay in his apartment, but she preferred, these days, to stay close by at the Boston Harbor Hotel, had done so ever since that night in 1989, though that was so long ago, and she was almost sure that while she had not and never would forget it, Jamie must have by now.

Bernard flew to New York to meet her at the end of that trip, and they had a few days of shopping and buying at antique auctions, and it was always quite a struggle persuading him not to spend a fortune on her. Olivia was happy enough to let him buy her the occasional gift—they both enjoyed surprising each other and neither was short of a few dollars—but she had to draw the line, otherwise Bernard might have gone wild at Harry Winston or Tiffany's, and that didn't seem right, somehow, given that Olivia had no more intention of moving in with him than she ever had.

They flew back to Brussels on April 22. Olivia, who had parked her car at Zaventem Airport, dropped Bernard off at his house and then drove back to rue Charles Hanssens alone.

The cool breeze brushed her face, stopping her in her tracks, as soon as she stepped inside the apartment. Slowly, fully alert, she bent to pick up her two suitcases from the doorstep and set them down on the parquet floor of the entrance hall. She listened for a moment for strange, alien sounds and then, hearing nothing, closed the front door.

"Hello?" she said, her voice low and tentative, not knowing what she would do if someone answered.

No one did.

The breeze was unmistakable. Somewhere, a window was open and Olivia knew she had closed and locked everything before the journey. She was many impractical things—untidy, impulsive, sometimes irresponsible—but when it came to securing her home before a trip abroad, even before going to work, she was pretty methodical.

"Shit," she said softly.

The right thing, she supposed—the smart thing—to do would be to go to a neighbor, but she and the people who lived to the left and right of her had exchanged little more than a passing nod, usually when she was in a tearing hurry to get somewhere, and she knew that the two upper flats in her own house had not been leased.

Another puff of wind blew her short hair, coming through the narrow hall from the kitchen and garden room. The garden door, Olivia thought, with a chill.

She took a few paces forward. The door to the sitting room was ajar. Taking a deep breath, she opened it fully and stepped inside.

"Oh, shit," she said again.

They had turned the whole room and its contents upside down. Lamps, tables, and chairs lay fractured like so many fatal accident victims on the rug. Books, some of them with their spines broken, were strewn everywhere, as if they had been hurled around. Her lovely mid-Victorian mahogany writing table lay on its side, its drawers several feet away, their contents scattered around. The handsome mahogany dresser that had been included in the apartment's inventory had clearly been rifled, all its doors open and the ornaments that had stood on its exposed shelves smashed. Yet still, Olivia supposed, standing looking at it, even at that awful, depressing, angering moment, it might have been worse—they might have taken an ax to it or urinated all over the place, and they had done neither.

"The whole place is such a mess," she told Bernard three hours later on the telephone while the police were still dusting for prints. "We figure they must have done it about a week ago, because they got in through the garden door and the carpet close by is pretty wet, and apparently it rained really heavily around then and it's been dry ever since."

"But you're all right?" He was anxious. "I wish you'd called me straight away."

"There's nothing you could have done, Bernard. I'm fine," she said. "Furious, but resigned. I guess it's the price you pay for living in any city these days, especially if you're lucky enough to have a little garden like mine."

"Maybe you should move to another place."

"Like yours, I suppose?" Olivia smiled.

"Sounds like a good idea to me," Bernard said lightly.

"I think, for the moment," Olivia said, "I'll get a stronger set of locks."

"Ah well"—he took the rebuff in stride—"at least I can come round now to help you."

"There's still not much you could do, Bernard. The police need me to compile lists of everything that's missing, and someone's going to call from the insurance company, and they're sending people to fix the glass and the locks, so I'm going to have my hands pretty full."

"Just for company, then," Bernard said, "if you refuse actual help."

"The place is crawling with company, Bernard." Olivia paused. "Tomorrow," she said. "Tomorrow I'll accept all the help you're willing to give me."

"And tonight?"

"Tonight," she answered ruefully, "I expect I'll crash."

"Have you an idea yet what they've taken?"

"The silver teakettle, for one thing. Remember it?"

"It brought us together," Bernard said warmly. "I'm not likely to forget."

"And my silver menorah." She paused. "And my mother's jade horse."

"The Ming? I'm so sorry, Olivia. I know how much you loved that."

For the first time since she'd discovered the break-in, Olivia felt angry tears pricking at her eyes. "She never cared much for possessions, you know, but she really loved that horse. I remember she used to touch it very lightly with her fingertips and say it made her feel she was connecting with the past."

"I can understand that kind of feeling."

"I expect you can."

He waited a moment. "Don't you think you might be nervous alone tonight, *chérie*?"

"I don't think so, Bernard." Olivia paused. "But if I am, can I call you?"

"Anytime. I mean it, anytime at all. I'm always here for you, Olivia."

"I know you are."

★   ★   ★

Cleaning up seemed to take Olivia forever. Every drawer of every wardrobe, desk, and night table had been turned upside down by the thieves. The contents of the three personal filing cabinets in her study had been strewn over the floor. Her own briefcase and a handbag she had left behind before her trip to Britain and the United States had been tipped out, too—even the refrigerator had been ransacked. One of the police officers had told Olivia that the burglars had, more than likely, been searching for cash.

"In the refrigerator?" She raised an eyebrow.

"You would be surprised," the policeman had told her, "where some people keep their money."

"Though in many cases," his fellow officer had said, "intruders simply get excitement from rampaging through their victims' homes."

"I like a mess as much as the next person," Olivia remarked drily, "but I can't say it's ever turned me on."

They had been selective, had taken mostly easily portable antiques like the teakettle and recumbent jade horse, three lovely silvered bronze art deco dancers, a late-eighteenth-century French mantel clock, and a pair of Flemish tapestry-covered cushions; and they had taken, too, the solid silver Victorian frame that had housed Olivia's favorite picture of her parents, though the photograph itself was thankfully still there, just torn a little at one corner, Arthur and Emily standing, arms entwined, smiling out at her. And that seemed symbolic to Olivia, a reminder, if she needed one, that no one had been hurt and nothing truly irreplaceable had been lost, and so it was simply a case of gritting her teeth and riding out the aggravation.

Three days later, Olivia's office in place du Grand Sablon was broken into. These were, of course, thieves of a different bent, their target her computer, photocopier, and fax machine, but once again the greatest source of irritation was the wreckage they left behind, as well as the chaos and inconvenience and the apologies to clients that Olivia had to make while items were replaced and lost work was redone. But still, Olivia said to Bernard at the end of another day's cleaning up, it was just an office, not the place in which you slept or ate breakfast or made love.

"It must be catching," Jamie said on the phone from Boston a few days later. "I've just had a break-in at the apartment, along with three of my neighbors."

"Did they take much?" Olivia asked.

"The usual—TV, video recorder, hi-fi. Nothing I really care about—guess they didn't think much of my taste. Peter and Carrie had a break-in at the Beacon Hill house last month, and I gather they lost a whole lot more."

"Who told you about it? Michael?"

"Carrie told me herself, actually." There was a smile in Jamie's voice. "I saw her at a party last week and she was quite civil. I mean, things have been pretty straight between us for a long time now, but last week I'd almost say she was hovering on the edge of warm." He paused. "Maybe it's true what they say about time and old wounds."

"Maybe it's just because she has different wounds to rub salt in."

Jamie had told Olivia awhile back that Carrie's second Arias union was foundering, but that cousin Michael, his Catholic faith by now grievously offended, was pulling rank within the company and pretty much ordering Peter to fix his marriage or have him to reckon with.

"Is there any more news on that front?" Olivia asked.

"Not that I know of," Jamie said.

"Are they still living together?"

"Some of the time."

Olivia detected reluctance in his tone. "Jamie, tell me you're not still carrying a torch for Carrie."

Jamie laughed. "Not even a match. Why do you ask that?"

"Because you manage to sound almost guilty for just discussing her problems, and I know it can't be because you feel bad for Peter."

"I don't, not really. But just because my marriage didn't work out doesn't mean I don't want it to work out for them either."

"God, Jamie," Olivia said with feeling, "if it were me, I'd be jumping up and down with the *justice* of it. They deserve to be miserable—they deserve each other."

"I can't disagree with you there," Jamie said readily.

"That's something, I guess."

★   ★   ★

A fortnight later, on a Sunday afternoon, Olivia decided to stay home and try to restore some order. Untidiness was one thing, but the ugliness left by her intruders had been something else entirely, obliging her to set to cleaning up with unprecedented vigor; yet still, the pressure of work during the last two weeks meant that the lovely apartment had still not fully recovered.

Filing. Lord, she hated filing more than anything, did just about *everything* before she got around to that—even cleaned her new cat's litter tray in preference. Bernard had given her little Cleo, her gorgeous, independent, free-spirited tortoiseshell kitten, a few days after the burglary.

"I'd prefer to give you a dog," he said. "A big one to make you feel safe, but I know it's not possible for you."

"It wouldn't be fair," she'd agreed, "leaving it alone so much."

"But little Cleopatra"—he had handed the little complaining creature over to her in its wicker basket—"will occupy herself while you are out."

Many men, Olivia knew, would have sulked after her rejection on the night of the break-in, but Bernard instead had managed to turn the aftermath of the burglary into a pleasure, for he did, of course, have a store full of gorgeous antiques as well as a wealth of marvelous contacts. And Olivia had loved the new excuse to spend hours on end in galleries and shops, replacing what she had lost—though nothing she or Bernard bought proved as much sheer fun as Cleo. The kitten had, as he had predicted, certainly learned to occupy herself during Olivia's absences, had studiously ignored the scratch post and basket that Bernard had bought for her, and had swiftly taken to exercising her claws on the Persian rugs and armchairs, and to sleeping on Olivia's bed, preferably, when Olivia was not home, on her pillow.

"You're not helping, Cleo," she told the kitten now as she came flying from the hall into the study, making a riotous dive into a pile of alphabetically sorted letters. "You're not helping at all."

The kitten took off again, and the papers flew.

Olivia groaned.

"Chocolate cake," she said. "I need chocolate cake."

She had bought a handsome slice the previous afternoon at Wittamer, and now she settled herself comfortably on the sofa in the sitting room and prepared to enjoy it.

Within a minute of taking her first taste, Cleo bounced onto her lap.

"No way," Olivia said.

The kitten stared at the cake.

"Cats don't eat cake," Olivia told her.

Cleo went on staring, her black pupils huge.

They went halves, Olivia eating the cake part, Cleo taking the cream, purring loudly. They had just finished when the telephone rang. It was Bernard.

"I'm bored," he said. "Are you finished with your work yet?"

"I've hardly begun."

"Come out to play," Bernard said.

"I can't," Olivia said. "I'd love to, but I can't."

"Tonight?"

"Maybe. If I've done enough."

"Shall I come and help you?"

"I've already had more help than I can cope with," Olivia told him, "from your cat."

"She's not my cat," Bernard said.

"She is when she's bad," Olivia said.

"Like children," Bernard commented.

"I wouldn't know," Olivia said, and put the phone down.

It rang again.

"How're you doing?" Jamie's voice asked.

"Trying to file papers and tidy up."

"Oh, God."

"You said it."

"I'd say I wish I could be there to help you, but you'd know I was lying."

"I would," Olivia said.

"So you don't want to take time out to talk to me," Jamie said.

"I'd love to," Olivia said. She thought about the mess of filing that Cleo had made even worse. "But I can't."

"Call me when you're through," Jamie said.

"If I ever get through."

★   ★   ★

Olivia was back in the study, the door firmly closed against Cleo, restacking the papers on the floor, when she thought, for no particular reason, of Carlos Arias's note. It occurred to her suddenly that she couldn't recall noticing the old pigskin case either at the time of the break-in or since.

She went into the spare room and hunted through the wardrobes, and there it was, on the floor at the back of one, probably, she thought, where she'd left it. She took it out and opened it, leafed idly through the small wad of old papers still inside, but the note was not there.

It irked her. She was certain she'd put it back into the case right after she and Jamie and Annie had talked about it. And she had not, she was just as sure, taken it out since. She sat down on the spare bed and tried to remember if, perhaps, the case and its contents had been strewn around the place with the rest of her belongings—she'd cleared away so much, had done much of the work almost automatically. Which meant that Carlos's note could be in any number of places in the apartment.

Olivia knew it was of no real importance and that she ought to leave it, to return to the job she was supposed to be doing, but she'd always been like this when something bothered her, like a dog with a bone, especially when she had lost something.

She went back to the study, opened one of the filing cabinets she had been meaning to sort through, and looked under the section marked A–D. There was one letter from Carlos Arias's secretary in connection with a forthcoming event at the American School, but no note. She put the file back, closed the cabinet, and went to her bedroom, where Cleo had gone to sleep on the bed. There was a chest at the foot of it, the kind of box in which most people stored blankets but in which Olivia kept her own personal store of memorabilia, including her great hoard of letters from Annie and Jamie.

She stared distractedly down into the chest.

"Why?" she asked Cleo. "Why does it matter?"

The kitten went on sleeping.

Olivia considered calling Bernard, telling him to come over and take her away from all this, but the urge to find the note remained strong.

She began to search. She looked for a long, long time, regularly sidetracked by the correspondence with her two friends. She found one letter that Annie had written her from England about a year before her confession to her drug dependency, another, much older, sent from San Francisco during the late autumn after the helicopter crash, and a third that had been written during a school vacation long before the accident. Annie had sounded so different in that early letter, not just because she'd been so much younger, but mostly, Olivia realized, because she'd still had safety and normality—she'd still had her parents—and reading between the lines of those and some of the other letters, it seemed clearer to Olivia than it ever had before how much more damage the tragedy had done to Annie Aldrich than to either Jamie or herself. Except, she suspected—idle again for a moment, watching Cleo, who was now awake and lavishly washing on the bedspread—that Jamie might not have put up with Carrie and all that pain for so long if he had not lost his father so early. If Carlos had lived, Jamie would not have needed to go through life agonizing about whether or not he might be letting down his father. If Carlos had been there, they could have thrashed out their differences as they went along, the way most fathers and sons did.

She went on searching. The kitten came to the edge of the bed and wiggled her behind intensely and rapidly before diving headlong into the chest, and for a time Olivia played with her, tossed envelopes into the air to watch her bat at them or try to catch them, and then she went on searching for a while longer, but she did not find the note.

"If it wasn't important," Bernard said to her later over dinner, after Olivia had abandoned both the search and her attempts to tidy up, "why are you so concerned to find it?"

"I'm not sure," Olivia said.

Bernard waited for more. "Some intuition, perhaps?" he asked. He set great store by women's intuition.

"Perhaps." Olivia paused. "That note always got to me, even when I first found it. Its tone was—disturbing, I guess. Or maybe it was just a symbol of so much unfinished business." She stopped again. "But I think what's bugging me now, more than anything, is that I can't seem to think of anything else that's missing that wasn't valuable."

"But would you know?" Bernard asked. "How could you tell?"

Olivia smiled at him. "Are you referring to my untidiness?"

"I love your untidiness, Olivia," he said. "It's a part of you."

"You're right, of course." She went straight on, avoiding, as she always did, any allusion by Bernard to his love for her. "There's no way I can be sure of what's missing or not, but what I do know is that every single item I have looked for—my bank books, old check stubs, my birth certificate, other old letters that I particularly remembered—you name them, I've found them."

"But not this note."

"No." Olivia shook her head. "And I know I should just drop it, forget about it, but what's happening instead is that I'm back where I was when I first found it nineteen years ago—I am disturbed by what Carlos wrote, and I'm still really curious to know what it was about."

"Your father's foundation is based in London, isn't it?" Bernard asked, referring to the Arthur Segal Foundation, which owned and administered her father's art collection, as well as continuing to look after Arthur's favorite charities in the manner he had wished. "Perhaps they have kept his personal correspondence on file? After all, he and Arias might have exchanged a number of letters."

"I never thought of the foundation," Olivia said.

"It's a possibility, surely?"

Olivia nodded slowly. "But isn't it a little over the top to go bothering people in London?"

"A little," Bernard agreed.

"I should drop it, shouldn't I?"

"Perhaps," Bernard said. "Perhaps not."

"You're a big help."

"You don't need my help, Olivia."

"I'll drop it," she said.

"Whatever you think," he said.

She waited until eleven o'clock the next day to make the call. She had gone to bed the previous night, at her apartment, intending not to do this, meaning to forget the note, to bury the foolish, annoying niggle that had drawn her back, again and again, to wondering why that insignificant piece of paper had vanished when everything else seemed to be present and correct, and why it mattered to her. Olivia seldom lost anything. She mislaid things all the time because of her dreadful untidiness, but she rarely lost them for long because what she lacked in method she made up for in instinct and accuracy in memory. If, in a moment of absentmindedness, for example, she had placed an invoice in her dressing-table drawer instead of on her desk, Olivia had only to command herself to think things through for a few moments, to retrace her steps or actions, and she would go to the dressing table. This, she realized, was one of the things bothering her about Carlos Arias's lost note. She knew that she had last seen it during Jamie and Annie's last visit to Strasbourg, she knew that she had replaced it in the pigskin case, and she knew, just as certainly, that because the burglars' mess had offended her in an entirely different way from her own personal disorder, she had taken considerable care when she had tidied up after the break-in. She would, she was almost positive, have been conscious of finding that note in the wreckage, and she would, consequently, remember where she had put it if she had found it.

She had determined, nevertheless, before going to sleep, not to telephone the Arthur Segal Foundation. Olivia thought that perhaps she thrived on real drama, but the intuition to which Bernard had alluded smacked of melodrama, which she despised, and so she had decided not to indulge it in herself. On waking, however, Carlos's note had been the first thing to come into her mind, and drinking her first cup of coffee it had come again, and strolling over to the office it had drifted in and out, and then, sitting behind her desk sorting out administrative tasks, it had gone away, quite satisfactorily, for two whole hours.

And then, there it was again.

She asked to speak to Jerry Rosenkrantz, a New Yorker and one of the foundation's older directors, a man who had known Arthur personally and with whom Olivia had had a few dealings in the past. Rosenkrantz was in Israel, his English secretary said, then asked if there was anything she could do to help. Only, Olivia said, if she could gain access to her father's old personal correspondence files.

"Goodness," the secretary said.

"It's probably an impossible thing to ask, isn't it?" Olivia said.

"Well, no, not really—not ordinarily, anyway," the other woman answered. "But we're still in such a frightful mess after the burglary."

Olivia sat up straighter. The tiny hairs on the back of her neck prickled.

"You've had a burglary? At the foundation?"

"Goodness, yes," the secretary answered. "It was a couple of weeks ago now, but I can't begin to tell you what a shambles they left us in—papers absolutely everywhere."

"What did they steal?" Olivia asked.

"Office equipment, mostly—computers, you know the kind of thing."

"I do," Olivia said. "The same thing happened to me just around the same time."

"Then you'll understand—the mess, honestly. I can't imagine why they have to do all that, throw stuff all over the place, instead of just unplugging the computers and walking out with them."

"They did exactly the same to me," Olivia said sympathetically. "The police say they do it for kicks."

"Charming," the secretary said. "But that's why if you were going to ask me if I could find something in Mr. Segal's old files, it really would be easier said than done."

Olivia's neck prickled again. "Did they wreck those, too?"

"Oh, yes, goodness, yes."

"Was anything taken from the files?"

"I wouldn't know," the secretary answered. "I don't suppose so, but then again, I don't suppose we'd be able to tell. No one would, apart from—"

"Apart from my father," Olivia said.

"Well, yes. Quite. I'm sorry."

Olivia replaced the receiver in its cradle. Her home, then her office, then Jamie's home, too. And now the foundation. The coincidences were becoming bizarre.

She picked up the telephone again and called Banbury Farm House, longing suddenly to speak to Annie, but she was out, according to Sally Breecher, the Thomases' housekeeper, an amiable, attractive local woman who had taken them on when Marie-Louise had married her cattle farmer.

"Is everything all right?" Olivia asked Sally.

"Everything's fine, thank you," Sally answered solidly.

"No problems at all? I haven't talked to Annie for a bit."

"Nothing," Sally said, "touch wood. Not since the burglary."

Olivia's blood temperature dropped a few degrees.

"You've had burglars?"

"Afraid so," Sally said. "Awful mess, but not too much taken—nothing too sentimental, anyway—and no one hurt, which is all that matters, when all's said and done, isn't it?"

"Of course," Olivia said.

"I'll tell Annie you've telephoned. I'm sure she'll phone you back later."

"If she has time," Olivia said.

She was glad, on reflection, that Annie had been out, for she might not have been able to conceal her reaction from her and then she'd have had to explain what had been going on and she wasn't ready to do that. Annie was okay these days—better than okay—but all Olivia's instincts were warning her that something seriously weird and possibly sinister was going on, and Annie didn't need to know that, not yet, anyway. But what? *What?*

She worked on a script translation through the morning, ate a sandwich at her desk, then ploughed on, glad to be focusing her concentration, as she needed to, on ensuring that her translation was accurate in words, nuance, and spirit. At seven, she walked home, fed Cleo, changed into one of her little black dresses, and drove herself to place de Brouckère, where she was needed to interpret at a lavish cocktail reception and dinner at the Metropole Hotel for a Texan film producer who spent much of the evening enthusing about her long silk-stockinged legs instead of paying attention to her translations.

It was after one when she got home again. Her message light was flashing, showing three calls. Bernard, telling her she could ring back even if it was very late; Annie, sorry to have missed her and she'd call again tomorrow; and Jamie, saying nothing in particular but sending his love.

Olivia kicked off her high heels, unzipped her dress, poured herself a large glass of fresh-squeezed orange juice, and sank onto the couch in the living room. Cleo, snoozing in an armchair, twitched her ears but didn't otherwise acknowledge her homecoming.

"Hi, Cleo," Olivia said. "Don't bother getting up."

She drank some juice and switched on the television, watched the headlines on Sky News, and turned it off again.

She'd switched off the other thing for almost thirteen hours, but tired as she was, there was no way she was going to be able to drop into bed and sleep if she hadn't at least tried to confront her thoughts first.

She reassembled the facts. Not much. Five burglaries inside the space of a week or two. Her home, her office. Jamie's apartment. The Arthur Segal Foundation's offices. And Annie's house.

She remembered Jamie saying there'd been a rash of robberies in Boston, so it was crazy to discount the possibility that his break-in was mere coincidence. That they were *all* coincidences.

"But I don't really believe that, do I?" she asked Cleo, still out for the count, her soft kitten stomach moving rapidly with her swift kitten breathing. "No, I don't."

She drank the rest of her orange juice and rested the glass on her left silk-stockinged knee.

If this was not a coincidence, that meant that she and Jamie and Annie had all been targeted. But by whom? Carrie Arias came to mind first as the only common enemy Olivia had ever been aware they shared.

She shook her head. "No way, Cleo." No motive, not anymore, and anyway, Jamie said Carrie and Peter's house had been burglarized, too, as part of the Boston rash. Or were they targets, too, along with the three friends? That made no sense at all that she could think of, and besides, Jamie had said their robbery had happened a month before.

So where was the sense in thinking that Annie and Jamie and she were linked in this thing? Setting her glass down on the rug, Olivia stood up and walked restlessly over to the window, pulled one curtain a little way to the right, and peeked through the curtains into the street.

If all three of them were somehow unwittingly involved in something—whatever the hell it might be—then the connection had either to be through their special friendship or, perhaps, through their parents. And what did their parents have in common? Not much really, aside from the fact that they had all been United States citizens who had gone to live in London and their kids had all gone to the American School. Nothing much else, except for a few school events and spin-off parties and maybe the odd business connection and a number of charitable events organized by Arthur. And a single, discomfitingly worded note from Carlos Arias, now vanished.

And, of course, their final, fatal helicopter ride.

Olivia let the curtain drop back as a sharp, almost jagged shiver passed through her.

"Don't be silly," she said out loud, briskly.

It was impossible. It had been an accident. Everyone had said so. There had been a full investigation; the pilot had been exonerated. Mechanical failure.

"Don't get crazy," she said, and went to bed.

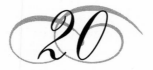

"*What's wrong with you, Olivia?*" *Bernard asked a few evenings later as* they dined on turbot and langoustines at L'Ecailler.

"Nothing's wrong with me."

"You're not yourself."

"I'm sorry."

"I don't need an apology," Bernard said gently. "I would simply like to share your problem."

"Who says I have a problem?"

"Your eyes. Your mouth. Your demeanor."

Olivia smiled. "What kind of a problem does my demeanor say I have?"

"Apparently a secret kind."

"It's misleading you," Olivia said lightheartedly.

"So you have no problem?"

"None," she answered firmly. "My turbot's delicious, my companion's delightful, if a little paranoid about my demeanor." She looked into Bernard's face, saw that his concern was real. "I'm sorry," she said again. "I know I may have seemed a little preoccupied for the last few days, but actually I think I'm just a bit tired."

"You're very seldom tired, Olivia," Bernard commented.

Her chin went up. "It can happen, even to me."

"And that's all it is? Fatigue."

"That's all."

"Nothing to do with the note you lost."

"No," she said. "Nothing to do with that. I've decided to forget that it ever existed."

"So you didn't call your father's foundation."

"No," Olivia said.

It troubled her long into that night. She had lied to Bernard for the first time, and she wasn't even quite certain why. Olivia prided herself on her honesty, had more often, through most of her life, been guilty of being too honest, too blunt. She could fib with the best of them, had, of course, created the most enormous lie when she'd invented the Light Years laser, but she thought she could still truthfully say that in general she abhorred dishonesty.

"So why," she asked Cleo, who lay snugly on the duvet close to her feet, "did I tell Bernard that I hadn't made that call? And why haven't I told him about all the other burglaries? Why am I shutting him out?"

Because if she couldn't talk to Jamie or Annie about it, came the answer, then she could hardly talk to an outsider.

Outsider. She gave a small shudder of shame, for she knew there had to be something badly wrong with their relationship if, after all these months and all that they'd shared, she was still thinking of her lover as an outsider.

"Which is probably why I'm sleeping here alone with a cat," she said, and added quickly: "No offense meant."

Unable to sleep two nights later, she called Jamie in Boston.

"What's up?" he asked.

"Why should anything be up?"

"Because it's four o'clock in the morning in Brussels."

"I couldn't sleep."

"You always sleep," Jamie said.

"No, I don't."

"Yes, you do; you've told me enough times."

"Well, I can't sleep tonight," Olivia said.

"And that's why you're calling me."

"Do you mind?"

"Of course I don't mind." Jamie paused. "What's wrong?"

Olivia sat up in her bed and held the phone more tightly. "I'm worried about something, Jamie."

"What?" Anxiety sharpened his voice. "What's the matter? Are you sick?"

"No, nothing like that."

"So what is it?"

She told him about the five burglaries and his father's missing note.

"You didn't take it with you after Strasbourg, did you?" she asked him as an afterthought.

"No, I didn't."

"I didn't think you did."

"Anyway, you said you knew you'd put it away," Jamie said.

"I did. I just thought maybe—I'm not infallible." She paused. "So what do you think? Am I overreacting or what?"

"I'd say so."

"You think it's all a great big coincidence," Olivia said.

Jamie thought about it. "What I think is that I'd take a bet that if you ran a survey of the homes in Annie's kind of neighborhood, as well as your own, at least a third—maybe a fifth—of them would have been robbed in the past few months. It's normal to be burgled these days— heck, it's almost insulting to be left out."

"Don't tell me it's normal for three best friends living in three different countries all to be burgled in the same couple of weeks."

"No, that's not normal," Jamie said. "That's coincidence."

"What about the note?"

"What *about* the note?"

"That's a coincidence, too?" Olivia asked ironically.

"I can't see the slightest connection with the burglaries," Jamie said. "It's just a little piece of paper that's gone missing."

"That's all."

"I think so, yes."

"Okay," Olivia said.

"You're really rattled, aren't you?" Jamie was surprised. Olivia was hardly ever, almost never, rattled.

"Yes, I am."

"Will it make you feel any easier if I ask Michael to check through my dad's personal files for a copy? I think they're all at the New York office."

"Would Michael be willing to spare the time?"

"I don't imagine he'll do it himself." Jamie paused. "I guess it's reasonable to assume that if my father wrote to yours, there might be a copy on file."

"It was handwritten," Olivia said. "He might not have made a copy."

"Then there might still be something from your dad. It'd be worth checking anyway, if it's going to help put your mind at rest."

"I think it might."

Michael Arias called Jamie back just over a week later.

"I had my secretary check the files herself."

"And?"

"Nothing at all. She told me she looked through every conceivable section, but the only thing she found relating to Olivia's father were a few letters connected either with Segal's charities or your old school."

"Nothing more personal?"

"Absolutely not." Michael paused. "Why's Olivia getting herself so steamed up about this, do you know?"

Jamie told him about the burglaries.

"So what do they have to do with your father's note?" Michael asked.

"Not a thing, so far as I'm concerned, but Olivia's got some kind of gut feeling about it."

"I've never had the impression she was the fanciful type."

"She isn't," Jamie said.

"Maybe the break-in at her place freaked her out a little?"

"She's never been easily freaked out either," Jamie said.

"Oh, well," Michael said. "Tell her from me I think she's working herself up over nothing."

"Michael says he thinks you're working yourself up over nothing," Jamie reported back to Olivia.

"And is that what you think, too?"

"I think," Jamie said, "that it's too unlike you to do something like that, for me to say I think it. If you follow me."

"Not easily, but yes," Olivia said.

"So that's that," Jamie said.

"I guess."

"But you're still not certain."

"No." She paused. "I don't suppose you asked Michael if they'd had a break-in at Arias Shipping."

"I did, as a matter of fact, and the answer is no. No burglaries at head office or at Newport." He waited a moment. "So really that does have to be that, doesn't it?"

"I guess," Olivia said again.

"Are you okay?" Jamie asked. "Should I fly over, maybe spend some time with you?"

"I'd love nothing more," Olivia answered. "But not if it's because you think I'm flipping out."

"I don't think that, Olivia."

"Good," she said. "Then feel free to fly over anytime."

"I can't, not for a couple of weeks anyhow. Too much work."

"That's great."

"Yes."

"How's Carrie's agency doing?"

"Doing fine."

"No bad stuff happening between you?"

"Not for a long, long time."

"That's good," Olivia said.

"Are you sure you're okay?" Jamie asked.

"Peachy," Olivia said.

There was one avenue left to explore. If there was any validity to the creeping paranoia—as much as she disliked it, there was no other word for it—that had begun to plague Olivia after the burglaries, if there was any truth to her uneasy theory that all their parents might be linked in the affair, then, having had Carlos Arias's old files checked and having attempted to do the same at the Arthur Segal Foundation, it followed that she should pay Franklin Aldrich's archives the same attention.

The Aldriches hailed from California, but Franklin's still flourishing law firm had three offices: one in London, one in San Francisco, and its head office in New York. Olivia made some calls and managed to locate Richard Tyson, one of Franklin's partners and the man who had helped Annie after the accident by removing her father's papers from their mews house to the London office.

She came directly to the point. She was aware, she told Tyson, that Franklin had, during their time in Britain, handled some aspects of her own father's legal work, but she was uncertain if he had ever taken care of Carlos Arias's affairs.

Remembering Arthur Segal quite well and knowing Olivia to be a close friend of Annie's, Tyson was courteous, though brisk.

"I can tell you," he said, "with reasonable certainty, that Mr. Arias was never a client of Mr. Aldrich's, and that I personally can't recall any particular connection between the two gentlemen. But as to Mr. Aldrich's private papers, they were moved, years ago, to the archives in our New York office."

"I see," Olivia said.

"I'm sure you won't need me to point out to you, Ms. Segal, that such private papers are precisely that, private, and for family's eyes only." Tyson paused. "If Mr. Aldrich's daughter needs access to her father's archives, that could, of course, be arranged."

"I'll pass that on," Olivia said, knowing that she would not do that.

She knew, too, when she ended the call, that that was that. There was no place left to look. Jamie and Michael were probably right. She had been working herself up over nothing. It was time to curb her too vivid imagination, time to forget the note.

Coincidences, clearly, did happen.

One week later, on Friday, June 2, Bernard took Olivia to a concert at the Conservatoire Royal and then to Vincent for dinner. They walked together, as they had several times before, through the kitchens to their table, admired the old tiled murals, and then Olivia ordered T-bone steak and Bernard ordered fish, but when the food arrived, Olivia noticed that he was picking at his.

"Are you sick?" she inquired, concerned.

"No," he answered. "I'm well."

"Then what's the matter?"

Bernard smiled.

"What's funny?"

"Our role reversal," he said. "For some weeks, it seemed I was always asking you to explain what was wrong."

"Yes," she said. "I know. I'm sorry."

Bernard laid down his knife and fork. "I'm not hungry, I'm afraid."

"But you're always hungry." Olivia grew more anxious.

"Not when I'm upset."

She said nothing, waited for him to go on.

"I'm going to take a trip," he said. "To the Far East."

"When?"

"Soon. A week or two."

"Sounds exciting." Her own appetite a little diminished, Olivia cut another slice of steak, ate it, and laid down her own knife and fork. "Where exactly?"

"Tokyo, Taipei, Hong Kong, perhaps Bangkok."

Olivia's eyes brightened. "That's wonderful—you never mentioned you were planning it. Will you be buying or selling or both?"

"Both, I imagine. But mostly looking, experiencing." Bernard paused. "I had hoped that when I made such a trip you might travel with me, share it with me." He looked at her for a long moment, his blue eyes searching, almost piercing. "I've hoped for other things, too, Olivia, as you know."

"I do," she said softly.

"I've tried very hard to stay inside the parameters you laid down for us," Bernard went on. "To play what you call our 'relationship' your way."

"I know you have." Olivia knew now, thought she knew, what was coming, steeled herself for it.

"I thought I didn't mind too much, but I realize now that I was lying to myself." Bernard drank a little of his Sancerre. "I told myself how fortunate I was to have this young, beautiful, vibrant woman in my life; this woman who enriched me so, yet was so anxious never to crowd me, who was content to be my friend and my lover, without wishing for any more commitment." He drank a little more. "Whenever I found myself thinking of more, wishing that we were living together, longing for us to be married, I told myself to stop. No,

Bernard, I told myself—you're a fool. Every man you know would leap at the chance to have such a woman, yet to keep his freedom."

"But you didn't want your freedom," Olivia said.

"No, I did not. I do not." Bernard paused. "But still, I think, I believe, I could have gone on that way, even with those differences between us. If you had just been willing to commit your heart a little further."

"I care for you a great deal, Bernard."

"I know you do," he said. "But not enough to share your troubles with me."

"Oh," Olivia said. She didn't know what else to say.

"You've lately been so distracted, Olivia, and I've never complained, or not too much—"

"You've been wonderful."

"I have not been wonderful at all, but I longed for you—more than you can imagine—to come to me, to confide in me, to depend on me. To *use* me."

"But there hasn't been anything to confide in you about," Olivia tried to explain. "Or nothing real anyway."

"Real enough for you to be distracted," Bernard said.

"Yes. That's true."

"Real enough, I imagine, for you to confide in Jamie or Annie."

Olivia felt her cheeks grow warm. "I haven't talked to Annie about it."

"But Jamie."

"Briefly, yes." She felt defensive. "But he thought there was no problem, and that was the end of it." She paused. "There really was nothing for me *to* share with you, Bernard."

"Olivia." Bernard reached out across the table and took her hand lightly. "You are an honest woman."

"I hope so. On the whole."

"Then be honest now, for both our sakes."

"All right."

"You are fond of me, I know that." He went straight on, giving her no chance to speak. "But I love you. And that, for me, means that I want—that I need—to share my life with you. My small doubts and anxieties as well as my bigger fears or troubles. *Tu comprends?*"

"Of course."

"In order for us to go on, in whichever way we choose—you choose—you would need to feel the same way about that. About sharing." He paused. "Can you do that, Olivia?"

She waited a moment or two before answering.

"I don't know," she said.

Bernard nodded. "Voilà." He took his hand away and returned it to the stem of his wineglass. His eyes were deeply sad.

"What do you want to do?" Olivia asked gently.

"What I think I must do," he answered carefully, "is to travel to the Far East alone. Don't you agree?"

"I suppose I do," she said. "With regret."

"I believe that," Bernard said.

"How long will you be gone?"

"A month, maybe a little longer. The business here is perfectly run without me—better, I think, sometimes."

"And afterwards?" Olivia asked.

"Afterwards," Bernard said quietly, "I will come home to Brussels, to my large, too empty house, to my business, to my friends. To my life."

"Will you—?" Olivia took a sip of her red wine to moisten her lips. "Will you be willing to count me among your friends, do you think?"

"After a time," Bernard said. "If you wish it."

"I value your friendship, more than I can say."

Bernard's smile was wan.

"You have a great many friends, Olivia."

The weeks passed. Bernard left Brussels for Tokyo. Annie and Jamie came for a long weekend. Olivia caught a cold, which she passed on to several of a troupe of visiting dancers from Toronto for whom she had been interpreting. Cleo graduated from catnip-impregnated toy mice to the real thing when a small gray mouse found its way from the cellar beneath the house into Olivia's apartment. At least Olivia assumed it had come from the cellar, which she had never seen. There was a door, solid, locked, and keyless, in the wood-paneled hall that the real estate broker who had first shown the apartment to Olivia and Bernard had dismissed as of no relevance, since the disused cellar that lay beyond the door did not form part of the property Olivia was planning to lease.

"Good kitten," Olivia, who did not care for mice, told Cleo as she crouched, purring loudly, over her prey. "Excellent almost-cat."

She got over her cold and launched herself into her next assignment, which was to help a Welsh crime novelist named Ian Jones with his research in Brussels and Antwerp. Jones was middle-aged, craggy, lively, intelligent, and amusing, but he drank too much Belgian beer and made no bones about his latest ambition, which was to get Olivia into bed. Olivia, who was well practiced in the art of diplomatic rejection, spent almost as much time avoiding Jones's beery kisses and smacking his wandering hands as she did translating old editions of *Le Soir* and helping him track down and comprehend the books he needed in FNAC and other book shops, and by the time he returned to Cardiff she was glad to see the back of him.

Olivia missed Bernard. That is, she missed his companionship, their conversations and intimate dinners, but asking herself if she felt bereft without him, she had to answer honestly that she did not. There was a gap in her life into which Bernard had slotted rather comfortably—she remembered Annie, some months ago, using that same word when describing their relationship, and she remembered thinking then that "comfortable" was for armchairs or beds or big, old sloppy sweaters, not for relationships, certainly not for lovers—but it was a gap that would be, for her at least, all too easily refilled once Bernard returned from the Far East and became—she hoped—resigned to being no more than her friend. They would see each other once in a while, would attend the occasional gallery opening together, would have lunch, would value each other's friendship greatly but feel no need for anything more profound.

July came, the city grew warm—Bernard, back home, made brief contact but, alas, nothing more—and with the summer weather came a slackening of Brussels' pace as some offices, restaurants, and stores began to close for their summer vacation. Olivia, who had feared that by August, like Paris, the city might seem almost entirely dead, found, to her pleasure, that she enjoyed this slowing down, liked the softer, sleepier atmosphere. Her own business calendar was filling up for the autumn, and she brought home piles of brochures and maps and travel books in order to contemplate a real holiday for herself. Something adventurous, she thought, something decidedly *un*comfortable—white-water canoeing, maybe, or an African safari—or maybe just something rare and fascinating like a visit to Russia or China or to India, where she longed to go.

She had almost forgotten the note and the burglaries when she came in to her apartment on July 19 and listened to the message on her machine asking her to call Jerry Rosenkrantz at the Arthur Segal Foundation in London.

She telephoned first chance next morning from her office.

"Olivia, how are you?" Rosenkrantz always sounded breathless. He smoked two packs of cigarettes a day and every head cold he ever had turned into bronchitis, but nothing and no one had ever persuaded him to quit.

"Fine, thank you, Jerry. How about you?"

"Pretty good, can't complain." Rosenkrantz paused. "Heard you called a few weeks back when I was in Israel. My secretary said you were hunting for something in your dad's old files."

"That's right," Olivia said. "But you'd just had your robbery—"

"And the place was pretty much a shambles," Rosenkrantz finished for her. "Thing is, we've gotten it all back together now, which was one reason for calling you."

"That's kind of you—"

"But the main reason is that I've just come across something that might interest you. Seems your father rented a safe-deposit box in London awhile before his death, but because he rented it through the foundation it never came up when his estate was being prepared for probate." Rosenkrantz coughed twice, then cleared his throat. "Seems we've been paying for the box ever since by direct debit, and no one thought to ask me about it."

"It's been nearly twenty years, Jerry." Olivia was disbelieving.

"Tell me about it." He coughed again and wheezed. "Thing is, no one at the foundation seems to have a key to the box, and I wondered if you either knew about it or if you'd maybe ever come across some keys you hadn't been able to account for."

"I don't know." Olivia's mind flew to the big leather trunk in her spare room at home. Keys. She had seen a bunch somewhere, sometime. "Listen, Jerry, I didn't know anything about the box—"

"I presumed you didn't."

"But I'd certainly like to take a look around for the key."

"You think there's a chance you might find it?"

"I have a zillion things of my parents'—it's a good excuse for another rummage through."

"You sound like your dad," Rosenkrantz said warmly. "He was always a hoarder, I seem to remember."

"Like father, like daughter," Olivia said.

She picked up a container of fresh pasta and ready-made sauce on her way home, together with a carton of cans of the only brand of cat food that Cleo seemed willing to eat and a pack of microwavable French fried potatoes—Cleo was predictable in that she'd virtually kill for fresh fish, but Olivia had learned over the past few months that her little cat also had a passion for French fries.

"Hi, Cleo," she called as she came through the front door.

There was no response.

"Come and greet me," Olivia threatened, "or I'll get a dog."

The tortoiseshell was curled up beside the fruit bowl on the kitchen table. Olivia swept her off onto the floor, chastised her, then, feeling guilty, tried to pet her, but the cat stalked off into the hall.

"You'll be back," Olivia said, "if I make you fries."

Olivia fed Cleo, cooked her own pasta, heated the clam sauce she'd bought, and opened a half bottle of wine, and then she sat at the kitchen table and ate her dinner reading *Le Soir*.

She was perfectly conscious of putting off the moment when she would finally drag out the trunk and start searching for the key. It was her reason—or her reasons—for all the delaying tactics that she wasn't quite clear about. She would, she supposed, be disappointed if she failed to find the key, but rather more than that, she found herself reluctant to open herself up again to all that edginess and confusion if she did find it. And then there was something else besides, a curious feeling, connected, she imagined, to what might be inside that safe-deposit box. A feeling no more logical than any of the others she had experienced since the coincidences had begun. Olivia thought, perhaps, that it was fear, but it was hard to be certain because she so seldom knew real fear, was one of those people who just happened to be blessed with a natural absence of the commonplace, everyday kinds of fear that others appeared to suffer from. Some people seemed afraid of so many things, most of them outside their control and mostly starting out with "What would happen if . . . ?" What would happen if they had left the gas turned on and the house blew up? What would happen if they came down with the flu the week they'd booked their vacation? What if they went to New York and got mugged? What if they went to San Francisco and got caught in an earthquake?

Olivia remembered how many of Annie's problems had been hypothetical, mostly groundless fears concerning Edward's reaction if he found out that she, like most people, had feet of clay. And how Jamie had always—still did, perhaps—fret over what Carlos might have felt about him had he lived. Olivia knew how to be scared of real things, had experienced, many times, the adrenaline-pounding chill of taking one too many risks on a ski slope, or hang gliding too close to a mountain, or taking a corner too fast on the road and going into a skid. But she'd never been prey to those pointless anxieties; there were enough real things in the world to be afraid of, she thought, *real* diseases and wars and famines and accidents.

Which was why she couldn't understand, and did not like, what she was thinking now. That if she found the key and went to London and opened her father's old safe-deposit box, she might, somehow, live to regret it.

The bunch of keys was there, in the green leather trunk. Four keys on a tarnished silver ring. Three of them perfectly ordinary, one made to open a British front door, one smaller, probably the key to a filing cabinet, one the kind of key made to fit a padlock. And the fourth, silver-colored, flat and slim, with a number engraved on it.

That feeling struck Olivia again. Like a small, hard fist against her stomach. Part excitement. Part apprehension.

Cleo was sitting in the doorway watching her intently. Olivia took a deep breath, detached the flat key from the ring, tossed the other keys back into the trunk, shut the lid, and stood up.

"Looks like I'm going to London," she said.

★ ★ ★

She went five days later on July 25, a Tuesday, traveling on the breakfast Eurostar, the best way now, she felt, to get quickly into the heart of London. She parked her Renault in the underground car park at the SNCB building, walked over to the check-in, and strolled on board with nothing but the huge Hermès shoulder bag that Bernard had bought her for Christmas—into which she had tossed her passport, credit cards, some sterling currency, a tiny bottle of First perfume, and the latest John Grisham—and sat in a state of suspended calm comfort while the train carried her smoothly through the pretty, undulating Belgian countryside toward England.

At least, she thought, leaning back between chapters, she hadn't had to decide whether to see Annie or not, or to tell her what was going on, for she and Edward had left for New York three days earlier and would not be back for a fortnight. It was more years than Olivia could remember since she had come to Britain without seeing, or even talking to, Annie.

"Is something up with you?" Annie had asked her the previous week.

"Nothing," Olivia had answered, knowing she could get away with that because Annie was so unlike her, was too discreet by nature and upbringing to pry or push. Annie would always be there for Olivia, just as Jamie would, but unlike Olivia, she would never thrust herself forward, would wait to be asked and would then do anything, *anything*, for her.

"Are you sure you're okay?" Annie had persisted that time because, though she was discreet, she was also too intuitive not to know when Olivia was keeping something from her.

I'll have to tell her, Olivia thought now as the announcement was made that the train was about to enter the Channel Tunnel, and some of the passengers turned their faces to the windows to watch the sunlight of France funnel down with breathtaking speed to the size of a penlight and then disappear into darkness. *If, that is, there's anything to tell.*

She had arranged to meet Jerry Rosenkrantz—who had ascertained that as a foundation director, he would need to sign if Olivia was to be allowed access to her father's box—at the Britannia Safe Deposit in

Leadenhall Street in the City shortly after eleven o'clock. She had not seen Jerry for years, was a little startled at how old he looked, still as immaculately dressed as she remembered him, and with a fine head of white hair, but his increased frailty made Olivia realize, with a mix of emotions, how old Arthur would now have been had he lived.

"Mind if I smoke?" Jerry asked while they waited in the general seating area for papers to be brought out to them.

"If I smoked," Olivia said, her Eurostar tranquillity long since gone, "I'd want one, too."

"Why?" Jerry glanced at her, surprised.

She shrugged. "Just wondering what I'm going to find."

"I shouldn't expect too much," Jerry cautioned her. "Probably just some fusty old legal papers. Or maybe nothing at all—some people hold on to these things for just the odd eventuality."

"I know they do," Olivia said, trying to settle down.

"You okay?"

"Fine, Jerry."

She went alone, with a uniformed man, past a great, heavy vault door into a cavernous room with wall upon wall of locked steel safes of varying sizes. Her father's safe was large, much larger than Olivia had anticipated, about the size of a small suitcase.

"You put your key into the left-hand lock, madam," the man told her, "and I put the master key into the other lock." They turned their keys simultaneously, and the hinged gray door opened.

There was a box inside. Quite large, made of heavy cream-colored card, its lid sealed down with brown sticky tape.

"Would you like one of our rooms, madam?" the uniformed man asked.

"Please."

He walked ahead of her, carrying the box carefully in his arms, took her to a small room, not much bigger than a cubicle, with a wooden table and a plastic chair. He set the box down on the table and stepped out of the room.

"The door will be locked, madam. You just press that buzzer when you've finished."

"I will," Olivia said. "Thank you."

The door closed.

She looked down at the lid. There was nothing written on it or on the sides of the box, no identification, no hints as to what lay within.

Olivia sat down on the plastic chair. It was uncomfortable, and there was a slight smell of dampness in the room. She folded her hands in her lap and stared at the box for a moment longer. She knew, without opening it, that this was it, that she had found what she had been, half unknowingly, seeking ever since the first burglary at her apartment almost three months before.

The fear came back, the same sickly, unfamiliar chill.

She unfolded her hands.

"Okay, Dad," she said softly, almost on a sigh. "Here goes nothing."

And leaning forward, she peeled off the old, half-perished tape.

And opened the box.

OLIVIA'S BOX

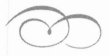

he box contained a foolscap-size, stoutly filled manila envelope and two packages wrapped in brown paper and tied with string. The first package, when Olivia opened it, appeared to contain copies of correspondence: letters and notes between her father and Carlos Arias, and a third man named Paul Walter Osterman. The second contained documents, sworn statements and photographs, several old monochrome pictures, of a man, woman, and three children, all of them attractive, finely dressed and happy-looking, a family of strangers. And two of another man, black-haired, dark-eyed, elegant, and—though Olivia was certain she had never laid eyes on him before—disturbingly familiar.

She turned the photographs over. The family shots all bore the same words on the back, written in blue ink by hand. *The Family Rothenburg: Emanuel, Hedi, Anton, Lili, and Trude.* She turned over one of the pictures of the other man. *Georg Brauner,* the handwriting identified him. *Also known as Juan Luis Arias.*

The chill passed through Olivia again, gripped her briefly, seemed almost to paralyze her. There it was. The final proof that the crazy instincts and events that had driven her to this point had been neither coincidental nor symptoms of paranoia. She didn't know what she had expected. Some long-buried sin, perhaps. An explanation. But this was going to be bad for Jamie; she was certain of that now. Whatever she was about to face was likely to affect him deeply in some dark, possibly dangerous way, and the thought of bringing pain to Jamie, of all people, was almost unbearable.

She thought of stopping, felt a great desire to do so, to go no further, simply to stuff the papers back into the box and leave. But the manila envelope lay on the table, still sealed. By her father. Olivia knew she could not ignore it.

She opened it. There was a typewritten letter inside and a small, badly stained, very old brownish-colored notebook, its covers worn down and frayed, the handwriting within tidy but urgent on the early pages, growing wilder, perhaps weaker, as it went on, changing from faded ink to pencil and then back again to another shade of ink. The letter, addressed to Arthur Segal from Paul Osterman of Philadelphia, Pennsylvania, and dated April 13, 1976, fell into two clearly separated sections, with directions for the first part to be read prior to reading the notebook and the second, much longer, section to follow.

Olivia began to read.

You will wonder, my dear, unfortunate Mr. Segal, why I have chosen you, of all men, to share Anton Rothenburg's story with. It is a dark, evil, sickening tale, and it concerns you not at all, not directly at least. Yet I do choose you, for a number of reasons. Partly because of your acknowledged love of fine art. Partly because of your well-documented contributions to the Wiesenthal Center in Vienna. Partly because of your dealings with the late Max Wildenbruch of New York City. But most of all, because of your acquaintance with Carlos Miguel Arias.

I have borne the weight of this tale alone since 1952, and in almost a quarter of a century I have gathered a fair amount of evidence. Enough, yet not enough. And all of it too late. Too late to help. But I believe, with all my heart, that the story of the Family Rothenburg of Baden-Baden must live on, no matter what. I am a sick man now, nearing the end of my life, and so, as young Anton did so many years ago, it's time for me to pass my burden to another man.

It's your misfortune, Mr. Segal, that I have chosen you.

Olivia turned her attention, as directed, to the notebook. She had no idea how long she read. Time seemed simply to cease to exist as she read the tale of Emanuel and Hedi Rothenburg and their three children, from the day in 1932 when the man calling himself Georg Brauner had first come to call on them, to the night of November 9, 1938, Kristallnacht, when all the Rothenburgs, except for Anton, had been murdered.

She paused for a few moments then, composed herself sufficiently to press the buzzer and summon the uniformed man, and to ask him to tell Jerry Rosenkrantz to leave, not to wait for her. And then she returned to the second part of Paul Osterman's letter.

It is true that none of the family survived, that Anton Rothenburg died, just over two months after the others, in Buchenwald. But he did, as he had hoped to, live just long enough to tell their tale and pass the notebook to a fellow inmate in the concentration camp. And it was that Holocaust survivor who passed it all on to me in the autumn of 1952 during one long, rather drunken night in the bar of an Amsterdam hotel.

We were two strangers, both businessmen traveling alone, both lovers of art, both Jews. As I said before, at the beginning of my letter, I had heard—we had all heard—so many terrible stories of those nightmare years, and yet this particular one seized my imagination, my heart, so profoundly, so savagely, that I knew immediately that it would remain with me until my dying moment.

I was consumed that night by a curiously wild compulsion to discover the true identity of Georg Brauner, and by an equally passionate yearning for justice. The first, at least, was not so difficult to achieve. Brauner believed that by arranging the deaths of the Rothenburgs, the chief witnesses to his crimes in Baden-Baden, he had eradicated every significant shred of evidence. No one, after all, in Nazi Germany of 1938 was going to query the end of another handful of Jews.

But the disappearance of a great painting by a famous artist is harder to conceal forever. Emanuel Rothenburg's collection of Symbolist art was recorded and reported by the Nazis as having burned to ashes in the Kristallnacht fire. Georg Brauner was a man of property, a man—not, in that at least, unlike Rothenburg—who took great pride in the art he owned and stole.

I guessed, from all I had learned, that if I waited long enough, at least one of those paintings would emerge into the light. I employed scouts to cover all the major art centers in the world. (Not such a vast undertaking and certainly no penance for a lover of paintings, to scour catalogs in museums and galleries and auction houses, waiting for one work from the Rothenburg list to emerge.)

I thought, once, in early 1956, that I was on the right trail when I received word that one of Emanuel's Hodlers had recently been donated to the Kunsthaus in Zurich. But it turned out to be one of the nine paintings that Georg Brauner, covering his tracks perfectly, had allowed to reach Max Wildenbruch in New York. One of the paintings, Mr. Segal, that Wildenbruch had sold to you after the war.

Nothing else, not a trace, not a whisper, came to light for another five years. Until I read for myself a report in the *Herald Tribune* that a Paul Gauguin work, long buried in a private collection, had been loaned to the Museum of Fine Arts in Boston. I had a hunch (more than a hunch, really) even before I read the painting's title, *La Rêveuse—The Dreamer*—that, at last, I was on my way.

I flew to Boston less than a week later, went directly to the museum, wanting, needing quite passionately—as if foolishly, egotistically, perhaps, I might in some way be keeping faith with Emanuel Rothenburg by just standing before the painting, *his* painting—to see it for myself. I had expected that this would be only a beginning, that the plaque beside the Gauguin might tell me, enigmatically, that the work was on loan from an unnamed source, but the small, polished plaque told me all I wanted to know.

Paul Gauguin - La Rêveuse
On loan from the Juan Luis Arias Private Collection.

It was a wonderful painting, a thing of great beauty. I understood, standing before it, how a person might ache for the privilege of owning such a work of art. But nothing, no part of me, thank God—not even the tiniest, darkest fragment of my mind—was, or is to this day, able to comprehend how a man might have conspired to destroy not just one person, but an entire family, for that privilege.

In the small locked room in the depths of the Britannia Safe Deposit, Olivia leaned back against the small hard plastic chair and closed her eyes.

She was thinking about the painting, about the Gauguin. She was seeing it again in her mind, as she had seen it the last time, in the drawing room of the Arias mansion in Newport when Jamie had brought her back there after her fall, back in that strange, briefly remarkable spring of 1989. She remembered looking up at *La Rêveuse* while Louise and Daisy Arias fussed about her, remembered its sinuous beauty, remembered registering, even in the midst of that abruptly, crazily awakened desire—no, lust—for Jamie, how much Arthur would have loved the work.

And she was thinking about the painting now partly because she wanted, desperately, not to think about Jamie, because thinking about Jamie, right now, in the depths of this ugly, monstrous tale, was unbearable.

Go on, she told herself. *Get to the end. The sooner you reach the end, the sooner you can get up off this chair and leave this room and get back up into the light and air.*

She opened her eyes, leaned forward again, and went on reading.

I remained in Boston for a time, gathering what information I could about the Arias family of Newport, Rhode Island. In general terms, it was not difficult, listed as they were, still are, in *Who's Who* and various other registers.

Juan Luis Arias and his younger brother, Carlos Miguel, were the second generation of the Arias family of Bilbao to be citizens of the United States, Juan Luis the First having immigrated during the period of unrest and anarchy that had swept much of Spain after the First World War. The Ariases were an old family of shipbuilders, high-born, wealthy, and proud, both of their ancestry and their considerable achievements in America. It was

Juan Luis the First, a man with a liberal heart and conscience that blended intriguingly with his vast ambition, who determined to gain the most solid foothold possible in his new country, who fell in love with and, against great odds, bought the Newport mansion, who must have used every ounce of his innate good breeding and charm to gain acceptance for himself and his family in this old-moneyed enclave of giants with names like Vanderbilt and Astor.

I considered, at this point, employing a private detective to investigate the second Juan Luis Arias and, more particularly, his art collection, but I chose instead to employ a local researcher. The facts she gleaned for me were sparse, but devastatingly clear evidence (clear enough, at least, to me) of his guilt. Like many proud, arrogant men, Arias—a widower with one son—simply could not bear to conceal his trophies for the whole of his life. He had striven too hard, too ruthlessly, to accumulate his treasures. Now, presumably, he ached to show them off. Until 1960, there was no public record to be found of the Juan Luis Arias Private Collection, and then suddenly mentions of it began to creep into specialist journals, catalogs, and newspapers. Though my researcher found no comprehensive documented list of the works forming the collection, she did find details of twenty-seven of the Symbolist paintings that had once been owned by Emanuel Rothenburg.

I left Boston for a while, returned to my home in Philadelphia, trying to prepare myself, to steel myself to confront the man I was by now certain had been Georg Brauner. I spent many restless, feverish nights tossing and turning, finding myself suddenly afraid of the prospect. I was a businessman, an ordinary, run-of-the-mill American Jew with a small company, a wife, and one son. How, in God's name, I asked myself over and over again, was I to confront a man of vast wealth and influence and to accuse him of conspiring with the Nazis to steal and to commit murder?

I thought, for a while, as I had thought many times before during the preceding eight or so years, that perhaps I should hand the case over to Simon Wiesenthal or one of the experienced Israeli Nazi hunters, but I found that even after so much time I still could not let go. Emanuel Rothenburg and his loved ones had become, in some illogical, ghostly fashion, my family, *my* responsibility. To a man like Wiesenthal, the Rothenburg story might have been just one more horror, one more crime, to add to the list, but it had become everything to me. I was, I suppose, obsessed.

I lived my own life, going about my business, trying to feign normality with my wife (who knew something, of course, of my quandary, though not—for which I am grateful—the full extent of my absorption) and our child, for three months.

And then I returned to Boston, where I learned, within twenty-four hours of my arrival, that I had come back too late.

Juan Luis Arias the Second had died.

Olivia paused, aware suddenly that she had, in her suspense, been digging the fingernails of her left hand so deep into her palm that one of the nails, a little sharper than the others, had drawn a tiny crescent of blood.

She stood up, pushed the chair back, almost knocked it over, and reached out to steady it. Her breathing was rapid and shallow, her pulse rate felt as fast as if she'd been running, and she was both warm and cold at the same time. Jamie came into her mind again, and forcibly she ejected him. And then, in his place, was Arthur. Her gentle, philanthropic, beauty-loving father. If she felt this way now, so many years later, two generations past the evil, if she felt this degree of horror and revulsion and rage and outrage, how must Arthur—always, she remembered, so contented with his lot, so grateful that his own father had escaped in time from Nazism—have felt receiving this out of a clear blue sky? This burden, as Paul Osterman had so accurately described it, this challenge from a long-dead family.

Olivia drew the chair back to the table and sat down again. The letter, she saw, was nearing its end, most of the pages stacked to the left of the table, only a few more remaining to be read.

I was at a loss. It might have been one thing to try to tackle the man himself, but I still had no more than circumstantial evidence and intuition. For all I knew, Arias could have come by those twenty-seven Symbolist paintings legitimately, perhaps from the real Georg Brauner. How could I approach the man's grieving relatives, not knowing whether one, or more, or perhaps all of them had been guilty of complicity? I had evidence but, as yet, I had no absolute proof, which meant that yet again I had to wait, had to find a way to get that proof.

I had to wait much longer than I had anticipated. Back in Philadelphia, my son was sick, my wife distraught, her emotional state not helped by my repeated absences from home. Priorities were brought home to me, and there could be no question that the needs of my own family—my own, thank God, *living* family— had to come before the memory and honor of people I had never known. It was more than a year before my son's health had improved sufficiently for me to consider the Rothenburgs again, and then, alas, I realized, too late, that my marriage was in deep trouble.

It was 1964 before I felt free to turn back to Georg Brauner. Juan Luis Arias had been dead for three years. There was, at least, no question that I might be intruding on fresh grief. I took a gamble. I instructed an art dealer in Boston to approach the Arias family, saying that he had a buyer for one of the paintings in their collection. I named a work from Emanuel's list by Gustave Moreau, *Nymphe Dansante*, which had not appeared on the list compiled by my researcher of exhibited paintings from the Juan Luis Arias Private Collection. The dealer, I directed, was to ascertain that *Nymphe Dansante* was in the possession of the Ariases and was then to make an attempt both to authenticate the painting and to establish provenance. It took time, of course. Everything connected with Brauner and the Rothenburgs took time; I had long since become resigned to that. But in all respects my gamble, or rather my hunch, paid off. The Moreau painting was in the Arias collection, and my dealer was as satisfied of its authenticity as he could reasonably be, but with regard to provenance, he had not even managed to ascertain the work's previous owner let alone its origins.

Every lingering doubt dispelled, I tried to make an appointment to see Juan Luis's younger brother, Carlos Miguel Arias, now the head of the family and shipping company, but was given no choice but to make do with Juan Luis's son, Michael. The Newport mansion was not, I was politely informed, open to visitors, and so we met in the Manhattan offices of Arias Shipping on a Monday morning in May. Michael Arias was only twenty-one years old, but I found him a smooth, articulate, mature man for his age. His uncle, he explained, with immaculate courtesy, was away in Europe but had empowered his nephew to speak for him on the subject of the Moreau, which, Michael told me immediately, the family was not eager to part with.

Deeply disappointed by Carlos Arias's absence and uncomfortable having to speak to Juan Luis's own son (knowing in any case that it was immensely unlikely that the young man might know anything of use to me), I set about my business regardless, asking about the painting's history. Michael told me that he knew only that his late father, in common with many private collectors, had accumulated his collection over a great many years. I asked if there was a record of when and where and from whom his uncle had obtained any of the other works—*La Rêveuse*, for example, the Gauguin that had, for a time, been lent to the Boston Museum of Fine Arts. Michael paused for a moment and then replied that the family's admiration had always been for the paintings themselves and for his father's remarkable overall achievement in gathering them under one umbrella. Whether *Nymphe Dansante*, for example, had previously been owned by an old lady in Marseilles or by a museum in Guatemala, had never been of the slightest interest to any of them.

That was when I posed the question I most wanted to ask. It was an unwise question, clumsily put, and yet I found that I had to ask it.

"I don't suppose you happen to know," I asked the young man, "whether your father spent much time in Germany between 1932 and 1938?"

Michael Arias frowned, a small furrowing of his smooth, handsome young brow. "How could I know?" he asked me in return. "Given that I hadn't even been born."

"Your uncle would probably know," I said.

"He might," the young man said. The frown grew a little deeper. "Why is that of interest to you?"

"I think," I said carefully, "your father may have had some dealings with an old friend of mine who lived in Germany at that time."

"Who was that?"

I took a breath. "A man named Emanuel Rothenburg," I said.

Arias shook his head. "The name means nothing to me, I'm afraid."

"He was an art collector, too," I said. "He lived in Baden-Baden."

Again the young man shook his dark head. "I'm sorry," he said.

"Perhaps you could ask your uncle?"

"I could." Michael Arias paused. "It seems important to you."

"It is," I said.

"More important, apparently," Arias said slowly, "than buying the Moreau."

"But didn't you imply," I answered with a small shrug, "that your family doesn't want to sell the painting?"

"Yes," the young man said. "I did imply that."

That was the end of the meeting. He had remained courteous throughout, and he was, of course, as I've already said, far too young for me to have expected him to know much about his father's prewar activities. I can't even claim to have sensed that he knew more than he was saying. Yet a wall had gone up from the instant I had begun asking questions about Juan Luis Arias, and I had a picture in my mind of that dark young man telephoning his uncle in Europe as soon as I'd left his office, reporting my curious questions. Whether or not Juan Luis's son or other relatives knew about his crimes, it was obvious to me that this was the kind of family that protected its own, and that a stranger asking personal questions about any family member was decidedly unwelcome.

I found out exactly *how* unwelcome less than a month later when, back home, I received a letter from a Boston firm of lawyers warning me that any further intrusion into the private affairs of the family of Juan Luis Arias would be responded to by legal means. It was the clearest evidence I'd had to date that I was right about Georg Brauner, but it still left me no closer to proving it.

While taking care to steer clear of the family, I have assembled more through the years. Photographs of the Rothenburgs, found in a Jewish library in Baden-Württemberg, and of Juan Luis Arias, alias Georg Brauner, retrieved from the picture library of the *Boston Daily News*. Signed documents attesting to Emanuel's prewar ownership of many of the works now in Juan Luis's private collection. Character "references" obtained by a private investigator from men and women who knew both men during that wartime period, demonstrating the substantial differences between Juan Luis and his younger brother, Carlos. It's clear from the descriptions that Juan Luis was the more powerful man, invariably charming but also vain and prideful, while Carlos was strong but gentle and more liberal in his opinions, like their father, Juan Luis the First. There's an account from a female acquaintance, a lady from New York who prefers to be unnamed, detailing an encounter she had experienced with both brothers at a party in Manhattan in 1936. The lady says that at that party Juan Luis Arias drank a great deal and disclosed to her not only his sympathy with but also his immense admiration for Adolf Hitler. She also says that his younger brother, Carlos, displayed both shock and the most intense embarrassment at Juan Luis's statements.

I send you all these things, Mr. Segal: the photographs and statements and the information about the paintings that once belonged, without doubt, to Emanuel Rothenburg and then came into the hands of Juan Luis Arias. I send them to you because where I have failed, perhaps you, who are personally acquainted with Carlos Arias—who can unquestionably reach the man I was never permitted to speak to—may find a way to make use of them. And I say to you now, in the hope that it may ease your mind at least a little, that in spite of the family's strenuous efforts to keep me from peering more closely into their private history, in all these many years I have found no trace of evidence of any direct involvement by Carlos Miguel Arias in his brother's crimes.

I have asked myself so often since that chance encounter in 1952 why the fate of the Rothenburgs gripped my heart so fiercely, so relentlessly. I have no profound answer to pass on. Perhaps it was because the stranger's descriptions of Emanuel Rothenburg reminded me so much of my own father. Or perhaps it was simply because the evil perpetrated by Georg Brauner or Juan Luis Arias—a man in no possible way compelled by his environment or his masters to do as he did, a man who could so easily just have stayed away, could have left the Jews alone, could have gone on with his own comfortable, successful life in his own world—seemed in its way so much more evil than anything I had ever come across before.

I asked the stranger in the Amsterdam bar why he had not gone forward to the authorities after Buchenwald to give evidence against Brauner, and he explained that he had been too physically and emotionally scarred by his own wartime experiences, too afraid, too weary to face another ordeal. Yet Anton Rothenburg's story, and the young dying man's longing for the truth to reach a world beyond Buchenwald, had affected him deeply, and he suggested to me that perhaps if I had the strength and the will, I might try to accomplish what he was too weak to do.

I remember thinking when I fell at last into bed that night that the sudden, violent urge for justice, created perhaps by a surfeit of whiskey, would probably have left me by next morning. But it did not leave me. To this day, it is still with me.

And now, perhaps Arthur Segal, it is with you.

For a long while, after she had finished reading Paul Osterman's letter, Olivia sat in the little room and stared at the pages and at Anton Rothenburg's notebook and at the photographs that Osterman had so painstakingly gleaned of the Jewish art collector and some of his priceless treasures; and at all the other signed declarations and documents that still, in spite of Osterman's conviction, added up to insufficient evidence of Juan Luis's guilt.

A rapping on the door jolted her.

"Are you all right in there, madam?" It was the courteous voice of the Britannia Safe Deposit's manager.

Olivia looked at her watch and saw, startled, that she had been in the cubicle for more than three hours.

"I'm fine, thank you," she answered.

"Could I get you something? Some coffee, perhaps?"

"No, thank you," she said. "No coffee."

"Sorry to have disturbed you, then," he said.

"I'm sorry to be taking so long," Olivia said.

"Take as long as you like, madam."

Olivia heard him walk away, and then she turned her attention to the package of correspondence, and here, at last, were copies of every letter that her father had sent to Carlos Arias between April and June of 1976, and the replies he had received. And there was a small cassette tape, too, and Olivia guessed that it might be a recording of a conversation between the two men. And the tone of all Carlos's letters and notes was the same as in the first one Olivia had found in the pigskin case, the one that had disappeared after the break-in: Jamie's father had been, as Osterman had believed, innocent of any complicity.

Carlos wrote in one letter:

I knew nothing of the existence of Georg Brauner. But I did know that my brother often traveled to Europe and, in particular, to Germany during those prewar years, and that he returned after many of these trips with magnificent additions for his art collection. Including, alas, the Symbolist paintings that you have listed. Juan Luis explained to me, when I asked how he had obtained them, that because of the ever growing atmosphere of fear and uncertainty in Europe, works were becoming widely available that otherwise would have remained forever out of reach. People, Juan told me—Jews especially—needed funds more than they needed paintings, and when I suggested to him that this sounded to me like exploitation, his response seemed frank enough. He was, perhaps, he agreed, taking some advantage of a bad situation, but I ought to understand how infinitely preferable it was for the Jews to sell their treasures to a family like ours in a free country, rather than to see them ultimately confiscated without compensation.

I did not, in all honesty, either understand or agree with my brother, but Juan Luis was the head of our family, and it was not my place to question him. Respect and family loyalty were everything to us, you know. But I tell you now that if I had had even the smallest inkling of the evil that my brother was perpetrating, all the family loyalty in the world could not have kept me either silent or quiescent.

I am, my dear Arthur, horrified, and deeply ashamed. There are matters that must be dealt with and addressed. I wish with all my heart to make such amends as may be possible, though nothing, I realize only too painfully, can ever make up for the loss of an entire family.

We must, as you suggest, meet soon.

And there, Olivia realized, in her hand, was the final proof that Paul Osterman had sought for so many years. He had chosen her father for all the reasons he had given: his love of art and his dealings with Max Wildenbruch and the Hodler that had once belonged to Emanuel Rothenburg and that now hung in the Zurich Kunsthaus; his established wish to help—albeit previously only in financial terms—anti-Nazi causes; but chiefly because Arthur Segal would be able to reach the ear of Carlos Arias.

Osterman had tried, but had been restrained by law from doing so. Olivia's father had got through to Carlos, and it seemed clear to her from his letters that Carlos had been thinking of ways to make restitution of sorts, but then both men had died in the crash.

Too drained to think further, Olivia packed the contents of the box into her big Hermès bag, apologized to the Britannia manager for having taken so much time, and made a swift telephone call to Jerry Rosenkrantz to thank him for his help, to tell him that the papers in the safe-deposit had been of a private nature, and to explain that she would not now have time to come to the foundation's offices for a drink as he had suggested, because she would be returning directly to Brussels.

She emerged into Leadenhall Street, momentarily confused by the

City of London hubbub, found an empty taxi, and headed for Water-loo Station. Perhaps, she considered, she ought to have abandoned her train reservation and gone to a hotel to rest for the night, but she was too shaken by what she had read, so hugely weighed down by the burden she suddenly realized she had now taken from her father's shoulders that she could hardly seem to think straight, found she did not really want to think at all. She just wanted, needed, to be back in her own home, where she could be by herself until she was ready to think again, to plan the next step of this dreadful voyage back into the past, to be rational again, *normal* again.

She boarded the Eurostar at five o'clock, allowed herself just one glass of white wine before the dinner she knew she would be unable to eat. She wished now that she had not parked her car at the Gare du Midi, wished she could have simply fallen into the back of a cab, preferably too drunk to remember Anton Rothenburg's notebook or Paul Osterman's letter. But the Hermès bag on the empty first-class seat opposite her was a tangible reminder—if she needed one—that she had a duty now to her father and to Carlos Arias, and to the long-dead art collector and his family.

And, she was beginning to realize—though it was, of course, too bizarre, too *hideous* to contemplate—to Emily, her mother, and to Grace and Franklin Aldrich and to the pilot of their helicopter whose name, God forgive her, she could not at that second recall.

For Osterman had been prevented from getting too close, after his single meeting with Michael Arias. And Arthur had deemed it pru-dent to lock the box into a vault. And Carlos had written that there were "matters to be dealt with and addressed." And he and her father must have been making plans, must have been working out what step to take next.

Before death had stopped them.

She didn't notice the dark-haired man in the black leather jacket in the next compartment who sat, with tinted glasses covering his eyes, read-ing the *Daily Express*. She had not noticed him earlier that morning, either, on the journey from Brussels to London, or, later—a lifetime later—when she had come out of the safe-deposit into Leadenhall

Street and he had followed her, had watched her climb into her cab and had hailed another behind her.

And she did not notice him when she left the train shortly before ten o'clock and headed, still wearily, still half numb, toward the SNCB building and the underground car park.

It happened too fast, much too fast for her to have time to react, to do anything, even to see anything. There was only the sound of a car abruptly, aggressively picking up speed, and then a blinding glare of headlights, forcing her free hand up to shield her eyes, and then a screeching of tires.

And the awful, ugly noise that was the fender of the car hitting her.

And after that, nothing at all.

FOR OLIVIA

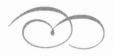

22

She came to in the emergency room of the Saint-Pierre Hospital. They were kind to her, gave her something to ease the pain, and told her that she'd had quite a miraculous escape, that her left arm was fractured but otherwise her injuries were minor, mostly small cuts and bruises.

"First," one of the doctors, young and harried and tired looking, said to her, "we'll get your arm set in plaster, and then we'll get you to a room for one night's observation, and then, if all's well, you can probably go home in the morning."

Olivia looked dizzily up at him. "The car didn't stop, did it?"

"No, mademoiselle," he said. "The police will speak with you soon."

"Good," she said.

He touched her right arm gently and shook his head. "*Vraiment*, mademoiselle, you have been very, very lucky."

Olivia believed him, just as she'd almost believed the nurse who'd mentioned miracles, for there was not a single, solitary doubt left in her mind that whoever had been driving that car had intended to kill her.

She knew, too, even before she asked, that the Hermès bag was gone.

"It was a deliberate hit-and-run," she told the two officers from the gendarmerie who came to see her while she waited for her arm to be set.

"The driver failed to stop," one of them said. "Probably he panicked."

"Or she," the other officer said.

"You say you didn't see the driver, mademoiselle?"

"I didn't see anything," Olivia said, "except the headlights. I couldn't even tell you what kind of car it was."

"They may report the accident later," the first man said. "It sometimes happens that way."

"It won't this time," Olivia said fuzzily. "And it wasn't an accident."

"Why do you say that, Miss Segal?" he asked, frowning.

She closed her eyes for a moment. "It's a very long story."

"Perhaps you should rest, mademoiselle."

She opened them again. "What are you doing to find the car?"

"There's not too much we can do," the second officer said with a hint of a shrug, "without any description."

"You're sure there's nothing you can remember?" the first man asked.

"It was dark," Olivia said very softly. "It happened too fast." She paused. "No one else saw it happen?"

"No one has come forward, alas," he answered. "Not yet, at least."

"Maybe later," the second man said.

They began to turn away.

"I need to tell you," Olivia said, "about the bag."

"You told us, Miss Segal," the first officer said patiently. "It's missing."

"Stolen," she said.

"It's possible," he said. "An opportunist, passing by after the accident—"

"It was stolen by the driver," Olivia said. "Or by an accomplice."

The two policemen glanced at each other quickly.

"You should rest, mademoiselle," the first man said again.

"But I need to tell you," she said. "I have to explain."

"Not tonight," he said soothingly.

"*Ecoutez, mademoiselle,*" the other man said more firmly. "You told us yourself that you've made two long journeys today, and you admit that you were very tired and perhaps a little careless, and you drank some wine on the journey from London—"

"One glass," Olivia said as firmly as she could, but the drugs and the pain were making her feel sick, making it hard for her to be assertive, to be herself. "And it wasn't an accident."

"You may be right, Miss Segal," the second man said. "But we still won't achieve anything more tonight, so we're going to leave you now and let you get some rest."

"How can I rest," Olivia asked him, "when someone's trying to kill me?"

"You'll rest when they operate on your arm," the first man said, smiling.

The second officer looked down at her seriously for an instant. "Why are you so sure that it was deliberate?"

"I told you, it's a long, long, awful story," she said, wearily. "And it's pretty wild—and maybe I wouldn't believe me either if I were you—but it goes all the way back to war crimes in Germany, and if I'm right, then whoever tried to have me killed did the same thing to another six people nearly twenty years ago."

She knew, as soon as the words were out, that she'd made a mistake. She'd had their attention—skeptical, but on the job nevertheless—until she'd said those two things, "war crimes" and "another six people," but now she'd lost them, and she knew they'd written her off as suffering from shock or concussion or having an overactive imagination or maybe having her period. Or perhaps, looking at their faces, they thought that she was just downright crazy.

In a private room for the night, she slept for a little over two hours, then woke again at around four o'clock, still groggy but with the sudden, urgent realization that what she needed now, more than anything, was to speak to Jamie. He would listen to her, he would believe her—she would *make* him believe her—but more important than that, she needed to make him understand that once he, too, knew the truth about Juan Luis, he might be in just as much danger as she was. It occurred to her, briefly—while she was struggling with her freshly plastered, startlingly heavy left arm and fumbling with the telephone, telling the operator that she needed to call overseas and she needed to do it now, whatever the time was—that Jamie might be better off being left in the dark, but that thought was swiftly dismissed. He had to know; Carlos would want him to know. It was his right to know.

He wasn't at home, his machine was picking up, and suddenly Olivia remembered Jamie telling her that he was going to be spending a few days at the Arias house in Newport because Louise was throwing a birthday party for Michael.

She put the phone down and, struggling not to fall asleep, started to hunt around for her address book, but it had, of course, been in the Hermès bag, and so she had to start all over again and ask the hospital switchboard to get her the international directory information operator.

It took forever to get through, and when she did, the woman who answered the phone—not Louise or Daisy, probably a housekeeper—said that Jamie wasn't home right now.

"When will he be there?" Olivia asked.

"I'm sorry, miss, I can't hear you very well," the voice in Newport said.

"When will Jamie be back?" Olivia said more loudly.

The door opened, and a nurse stuck her head around and raised a finger to her lips to hush her, and Olivia nodded, still waiting for an answer, but the woman on the phone had gone away and left her on hold, and she wanted, suddenly, to cry, which was not at all like her, but she couldn't help it.

"Hello, Olivia." Michael Arias was at the other end. "What's up?"

"I need to talk to Jamie," she said. "It's very important."

"Jamie's not here right now."

"I know, but I just want to know when he'll be back."

"Are you okay, Olivia? You don't sound quite yourself."

"I'm not," Olivia said.

"Are you sick? Has something happened? Can I do something for you, Olivia?"

Michael sounded so warm and friendly and concerned, and Olivia was about to tell him that she was in the hospital—and then, suddenly, something stopped her; something in that pleasant voice, in the extra-attentive way he was speaking to her, scared her.

"No, thank you, Michael," she said. "Just tell Jamie I called, and ask him to get back to me as soon as he can."

Except, she was perfectly aware as she put down the receiver, that he wouldn't be able to reach her, not tonight at least, because he didn't know where she was. And Olivia tried to think what exactly it was that had stopped her giving Michael the hospital's telephone number, but she couldn't think properly because all the dope in her bloodstream was weighing her down, fuzzing her brain, and she had to lie down again and close her eyes, and she was so *tired*, and she had to sleep.

She dreamed about Michael, wearing the British panama hat and sunglasses she'd seen him in at the Newport house that May afternoon all those years ago. In the dream he was smiling at her, a warm, charming smile, but his eyes were completely obscured behind the glasses, and then he walked toward her, and he took off first the hat and then the sunglasses, and his eyes were black as coal, hard as iron, and he was holding out both his arms toward her as if he were going to embrace her. And suddenly he looked so much like Jamie that she felt overwhelmed by an enormous sense of relief, and she ran straight into those welcome arms, and Jamie was holding her tightly. Except that it wasn't Jamie, it was Michael, and he was gripping her too tightly, encircling her arms and body so hard that she cried out in pain, but he kept on hugging her more and more tightly, and her left arm was agony, and he was squeezing the breath out of her, and she tried to kick him, but it only hurt her more, and she cried out again—

"Miss Segal—"

She kicked out again.

"Olivia—"

She heard the voice and opened her eyes and saw the nurse bending over her, a small flashlight in her hand.

"*Qu'est-ce qui se passe?*" the nurse asked softly.

Olivia tried to struggle up, but her plastered arm made it hard to move, so she lay back again, and forced herself to breathe normally.

"Was it a bad dream?"

"Yes."

"Can I get something for you? A warm drink, perhaps?"

"No, thank you." Olivia shook her head. "It was just a nightmare. I'm okay now."

"It's the anesthetic," the nurse said. "It gives some people bad dreams."

"Yes," Olivia said. "Was I making a noise?"

"Just a little."

"I'm sorry."

"Ne vous en faites pas, mademoiselle." The nurse patted her good arm. "Don't worry about it; just try to sleep again."

She left the room and softly closed the door. Olivia lay in the semi-darkness, eyes wide open. She tended to dream a good deal, often had wild, action-packed dreams, believed they were her subconscious encouraging her to get out and do more, but she rarely suffered nightmares.

This one was staying with her. Keeping her awake.

Michael Arias. Jamie's older cousin. Michael Arias, head of the family, as his father Juan Luis, too, had once been.

Olivia had seldom seen Michael, just at the occasional family gathering over the years when she and Annie had happened to be included. He was a man, she thought suddenly, of many faces: proud, wealthy, third-generation American businessman; Newport-style good husband with just that gentle, amusing hint of elegant, old-world British-style spy; protective, Spanish-style older relative with a whiff of Mafia-style don. All of those faces so unlike Jamie's, considering they shared almost the same blood and upbringing. There was no dark side to Jamie— there were shades, of course—but not even a soupçon of sinister; nor was there, Olivia had to admit, to Peter Arias, much as she loathed him for what he'd done to his younger brother. Peter was a swine and she felt contempt for him, but she could not imagine ever being afraid of him.

She thought again about that last letter from Carlos Arias to her father. *There are matters to be dealt with and addressed.* Had those matters included speaking to his nephew, Juan Luis's son, whose meeting with Paul Osterman back in 1964, when Michael had been just twenty-one, Carlos might only then have learned about? The meeting after which Osterman had been warned off in no uncertain terms?

Olivia sat up, careful of her arm. There was that chill again, that stinging, previously unfamiliar sensation that she'd been experiencing more and more often since the burglaries. Fear. It cleared away the last remnants of the nightmare, swept away the wish, if not the need, to sleep.

During the years in which Georg Brauner had been ransacking Emanuel Rothenburg's collection, Michael Arias had not yet been born. It made no sense to try to harness Michael to crimes committed by his father. But Carlos had written about loyalty and respect in a Spanish family. He had also written, shortly before his death, that had he had even the smallest inkling of what Juan Luis had done, all the family loyalty in the world would not have kept him silent. Perhaps Michael's sense of loyalty to his late father had been stronger than Carlos's family pride—or maybe it had been just his horror of what might come to pass if the truth came out.

For if the world had discovered what Juan Luis had done, not only would the Arias name have been tarnished forever, but their remarkable—and, by the mid-seventies, almost priceless—art collection would have had to have been broken up, perhaps surrendered completely. Pride and a fortune lost, all for the sake of honor and inherited shame.

If Olivia was right, then Michael Arias had found a legitimate way to keep Paul Osterman at bay back in 1964. But faced, twelve years later, with his Uncle Carlos's shock, moral outrage, guilt, and determination to make whatever restitution possible, Michael might have felt compelled to find a more permanent way to silence him. Together with her father. The only other person who knew the truth.

He couldn't. Olivia felt a terrible, deep shudder pass through her. *He could not, surely, have done that to his own uncle.*

Let alone to five more innocent people.

She thought about Emily, her mother, about the loss to all those sick children. She thought about Grace and Franklin Aldrich, about all that their deaths had done to Annie. She thought about Jamie, and what, if she was right, this would do to him.

"No," she said aloud, softly, into the dark.

It was too monstrous to contemplate.

Yet, of course, she did contemplate it, and it sharpened her own, now intensely personal fear with a finely hewn, technicolor clarity. For whether it had been done for the sake of a dead father's honor or for personal greed and pride, what had been priceless enough to kill for nineteen years ago was certainly worth killing for again now. And a man who could bring about the death of the uncle who had, Jamie had often told Olivia, become almost a surrogate father to his nephew, would scarcely blink at the prospect of having an outsider murdered.

The steady, throbbing ache in her left arm grew more intense. Olivia thought of ringing for a nurse and asking for a tablet for the pain, but she knew that would send her back off to sleep and she wasn't ready for that, not yet, not until she had worked it all out. She was planning, after all, to break this to Jamie as soon as she could get hold of him, tell him that his uncle had been a blackmailer, a thief, and a murderer, and that his own cousin had somehow engineered the helicopter crash that had killed Carlos and the others.

I have to get it clear in my own mind, she told herself, gritting her teeth against the pain, *because if I'm wrong, I could lose Jamie forever.*

She went over it again and again. She'd first found Carlos's note to Arthur back in 1976 while clearing out her parents' house, but she had mentioned it to no one at that time except Annie, who'd talked her into putting it away and forgetting about it. Which she had done, until she'd moved from Strasbourg to Brussels and shown the note to Jamie—and asked him to mention it to Michael, which he had. She tried to remember what Jamie had told her Michael had said about it. She couldn't remember exactly—something about Michael having agreed that the note sounded strange and asking if Olivia had found any more, similar, correspondence, and she'd said, of course, that she hadn't.

And then, after her trip to America in April, she'd come home to find the break-in. And after that the note had vanished. And the other burglaries had followed: at her office, at Jamie's apartment, at the Arthur Segal Foundation, and at Annie's house.

And Olivia had talked to Jamie about her growing suspicions, and she'd encouraged him to speak to Michael again about them, and Michael had told Jamie he'd had Carlos's personal files checked. And she remembered rather clearly what Michael had said about a week after that: that Olivia was either fanciful or that the robbery at her apartment had freaked her out and that she was working herself up over nothing.

But since then, there'd been nothing, no contact, even indirectly, with Michael Arias, and Olivia had ceased mentioning the note to Jamie. May, June, and more than half of July had gone by. Her relationship with Bernard had ended, and she'd gotten on with living in the present. Until she'd had the message from Jerry Rosenkrantz at the foundation about the safe-deposit box.

She had told no one that she was going to London, not even Jamie. So how could they have known? Unless Michael was having her watched, was maybe even bugging her apartment. Which was, of course, absurd.

Or not absurd at all, not for a man she thought might be responsible for killing six people.

The night nurse came back then, said that the doctor had written her up for pain relief if she needed it, and Olivia was ready to give in at last because she'd got it pretty much all worked out—she wished she hadn't, but she had, and now, more than anything on earth, she wanted to blot it all out, at least for a few hours.

There was nothing else to be done this long night. She could hardly try Jamie again, not after midnight, Rhode Island time. And the pain, in her arm and all over her poor, bruised body, was really bad now, was making her feel nauseous again.

The nurse gave her a pill. Olivia swallowed it. The pain began, slowly, blissfully, to recede.

She slept.

They released her the next morning, and Olivia was so eager to be dressed and out of the hospital that she lied about having someone at home to help her. But the moment she got outside fear kicked in again, made her glance over her shoulder as she climbed into the cab the hospital had called for her because her own car was still at the Gare du Midi, and even if it hadn't been, she could not have safely driven it home. Arriving at the apartment, she was almost too scared to open the front door, and she found herself wishing that Bernard were there, living with her, or better yet, that she'd agreed to go and live with him in his big, beautiful, safe mansion. But then she saw that everything in the apartment was just as she had left it, and there were no bogeymen hiding behind doors, and she grew angry with herself for even contemplating using Bernard just because she was afraid.

She fed Cleo and consoled her—poor little cat who seemed disturbed by having been left for so long without food, fresh water, or love—and then she made herself a pot of coffee. Everything took twice as long without her left arm—it would probably drive her crazy, she realized, before she got used to it, if she did get used to it before it was time for the plaster to be cut off. But the coffee tasted wonderful, and it was so good to be back in her own place, surrounded by her own things, able to lean back against her own sofa.

At one o'clock, unable to wait any longer, she reached for the telephone, then remembered there was a chance that her calls were being tapped. Which hardly mattered, since she was going to call Jamie inside Michael's own house.

She dialed the number.

"Arias residence." It was the housekeeper again.

"This is Olivia Segal calling again." She tried to sound normal, as if she made a habit of calling at seven in the morning. "I'd like to speak to James Arias, please."

"Just a moment, please, Miss Segal," the woman said.

A minute ticked by.

"Good morning, Olivia. This is Michael again."

She took a quick breath. "Hello, Michael. Sorry to call so early. Is Jamie up yet?"

"Not early enough, as it happens," Michael said amiably. "He's gone horseback riding with Louise—she enjoys this time of day."

"When do you expect them back?"

"I'm not sure exactly." Michael paused. "Are you sure there's nothing I can do for you, Olivia?"

"No, thank you, Michael."

"Are you at home? So I can ask Jamie to call you back."

"Yes," Olivia said. "Thank you."

"You're quite welcome."

She tried to gather her scattered wits together. At times like this—when had there ever *been* a time like this?—it was surely sensible to do practical, useful things. She called a local taxi firm to organize the return of her own car from Midi, took two of the painkillers the hospital pharmacy had dispensed to her, and emerged from the apartment, shortly after two o'clock, to do some one-armed grocery shopping.

She walked slowly and not at all comfortably up to rue Ernest Allard and turned into rue Watteeu, and she was doing well enough, was steadier now, back on home turf, more like herself again. She bought fresh bread, cat food, more coffee, eggs, milk, a bottle of wine, and the midday edition of *Le Soir*, and began to head home.

She knew, about halfway back, that someone was following her. A man, dark-haired, stocky, wearing a black leather jacket. She had noticed him fleetingly for the first time as she had paused to glance in the window of a shop specializing in antique mirrors and had seen him stop a little way up the street. Then again, a few minutes later when she set down her bags for a moment, trying to come to grips with being without her left hand, it had happened again. Olivia could not, dared not look at him more closely, could not see his face, except that when she turned the final corner back into rue Charles Hanssens, her heart beating too rapidly, she saw that he was wearing dark glasses and that he was clean-shaven.

She walked faster along the street to her house, glanced back, saw that he had stopped at the corner of Ernest Allard, and even as she was putting her key into the lock on her front door—and her hand was shaking, dammit—she felt—no, she *knew*—that he was watching her, and worse, much worse, was making no pretense of not watching her.

Safely inside, she closed and double locked the door, checked all the windows and the garden doors, and then rang the gendarmerie.

They sent two officers, one a woman, within ten minutes.

"Where is the man?" the male officer asked.

"He was practically right outside," Olivia said. "On the corner of rue Ernest Allard."

"You say he was following you?" the woman said.

"Definitely."

They went back out, returning five minutes later.

"No one there now," the policeman told her.

They checked around the apartment, went out into the garden, looked over the walls, found not a sign of the man. Aware that Olivia had been hit by a car just the previous evening, they helped her make a fresh pot of coffee and sat with her for a while.

"He was there," Olivia said, calmer again now, more assertive, "and there's no question that he was following me."

"It happens, regrettably," the man said. "Some men get a kick out of intimidating women."

"This was more than that," Olivia said. "I tried to tell your colleagues that last night."

"We know," the policewoman said.

Olivia looked up at her sharply. "Did they tell you they thought I was crazy?"

"Of course not," the woman said swiftly. "They said you were very upset—who wouldn't be after a hit-and-run?"

"But they still think it was someone panicking after an accident."

"They're following up all possibilities," the man told her. "We always do, mademoiselle."

"How?" Olivia asked. "When there were no witnesses."

"It makes it hard," the woman said frankly.

"So no one's doing anything at all." Olivia was blunt and angry.

"You must be very frightened," the man said.

"Yes, I am—and if you knew me even a little, you'd know that that's not a normal state of mind for me." Olivia put down her coffee cup because she could feel her right hand starting to tremble again. "What nobody seems to want to understand—and I guess I shouldn't blame you all for that, because it's such an incredible story—but I do, I'm sorry, but I *do* blame you, because this is real, and it's happening now, and it's happening to *me*—"

She stopped, knew with a thud of sick resignation, just as she had last night, that it was pointless going on. Without evidence, no one was going to believe her. And all that evidence, every last trace of it, had vanished along with the Hermès bag.

"Do you have someone who could stay here with you?" the policeman asked.

"No." Again Olivia considered contacting Bernard, realized she could not bring herself to do that. "Not really."

"Maybe," the policewoman suggested gently, "you could go somewhere else—a hotel, perhaps. Just till you're feeling stronger."

"I can't do that either." She looked at their perplexed faces and accepted that none of this was their fault. "I'm expecting a call from the United States, from a friend. It's very important."

The two officers looked at each other, appeared, without words, to reach an agreement.

"We'll try to arrange a patrol," the policeman said.

"Try?" Olivia couldn't help looking skeptical.

"We'll manage it," he said more positively. "You have cause, after all, mademoiselle, to be afraid after your experience at Midi."

"The man was there," Olivia said again.

"We believe you," the woman said.

The gendarmes made another circuit of the block, returned once more, checked around the apartment, made sure all the locks were secure, and assured Olivia that arrangements had been made for a car to patrol rue Charles Hanssens once each hour. If anything further happened, they told her, she should not hesitate to contact the local station. They would see to it, they said, that she was safe, and in the meantime they suggested that she have a rest, take care of herself.

Olivia thanked them both, locked the front door behind them, picked up Cleo with her good right arm, and went back into the sitting room. They were well meaning enough; she doubted they'd lied to her. A car on routine patrol would doubtless take a short detour once an hour to take a cursory look at her house. But she knew that, like their colleagues the previous night at the hospital, these two officers did not believe that anyone was out to kill her.

She knew, too, that if the man in the black leather jacket wanted to get to her, there would be ample time between patrol circuits for him to do so.

The rest of Wednesday afternoon passed slowly. Olivia tried, alternately, to read, to watch television, to do some work, and to sleep. Nothing lasted for long. Now and again she stood up and went to the window in the living room, looking out into the street. Twice she saw a police car, saw it slow right down outside her house and felt, briefly, comforted.

She thought, from time to time, about what she was going to do. It was so hard today, with the pain from her arm and bruises still blooming like black roses over her rib cage and legs, with the shock and fear still too fresh, still distorting her logic, to know what was right. But one thing was becoming clear enough. With Osterman's papers stolen and Jamie stuck unknowingly in the heart of what she was now almost entirely certain was the enemy camp, there was only one person left who might be able to help.

Nothing in either Carlos's or Arthur's letters had indicated that they might have taken Franklin Aldrich into their confidence, yet Annie's home had been broken into, and Annie's father had been one of Arthur's lawyers, and Richard Tyson, Franklin's partner, had told Olivia that all Franklin's old papers had been shipped after his death to the archives in their New York office.

"If Mr. Aldrich's daughter needs access," Tyson had said to her stuffily, "that could, of course, be arranged."

And Annie was there now, on the spot, in New York.

Except that if—and it was a big *if*—Arthur had passed copies of Anton Rothenburg's notebook and Paul Osterman's documents and correspondence with Carlos Arias to Franklin Aldrich, and if Annie was able to locate the proof, then if Michael Arias found that out, Annie, too, might be in danger.

It was seeing the man again that made up her mind.

Olivia wandered over to the window at ten to five, and he was there, standing directly across the road, and she gasped and dropped instinctively down to the floor, her right hand over her mouth. And when she had recovered sufficiently, when she felt able to breathe again and to risk taking another look, he was gone, and she knew there was no point calling the police because he'd vanished again and there was no evidence that he'd been there. And she thought of getting her camera, of keeping it at her side ready to shoot if he came back, and then at least she'd have *something* to show them, but she had no film in the camera or anywhere in the apartment, and she certainly couldn't go out to buy some. And she was afraid again now—truly, intensely scared—she wished, really wished, for the first time since the burglary that she'd compromised her desire for light and atmosphere and appearance and had had bars fitted over all her windows—and even little Cleo seemed to be getting antsy, skittering around all the time yet staying close, following her around like a dog.

And there really was nothing left to be done but to call Annie.

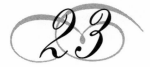

he sat, with Cleo on her lap, in the center of the sitting room floor, on the
faded Kashan silk prayer rug she'd found with Bernard at an auction
back in January, and used her tiny black Ericsson cellular phone to call
the St. Regis Hotel. It was eight minutes past five, Brussels time, just
past eleven in the morning in New York. Edward was almost certainly
out and about by this time, and there was every likelihood that Annie
would be with him.

"Mr. and Mrs. Edward Thomas, please," she told the hotel operator, and held her breath.

It rang three times.

"Hello?"

"Annie, thank God you're there."

"Livvy? How lovely. I'm just getting ready to meet Edward for
lunch." Annie paused. "Livvy, what's the matter?"

On Olivia's lap, Cleo kneaded her claws, hurting her. Olivia shut
her eyes for a moment, then opened them again.

"A great deal, Annie." She waited another instant. "I wish I didn't
have to tell you any of it. But I can't seem to find Jamie, and there is no
one else I can trust, and I can't go on alone."

"It's all right," Annie said, alarmed. "You don't have to."

And Olivia told her.

It was hard for Annie to absorb the enormity of Olivia's story, and had
it been anyone else but Olivia Segal telling it to her, she thought she

might not have believed a word of it. But Olivia was one of the most honest people in Annie's world, and Olivia was not given to flights of fancy. And Olivia was not easily frightened—in fact, Annie could not remember Olivia *ever* being frightened.

She had told Annie everything, as swiftly, concisely, and calmly as she could manage, and then she had asked her to do two things. First, to get hold of Jamie in Newport and to make sure, if she could manage it, that no one else overheard their conversation. Second, to try and get access, as quickly and discreetly as possible, to her late father's private files.

Annie had put down the telephone and had gone on, mechanically, getting ready to go out. She considered, briefly, finding Edward and telling him everything, but then she decided against it, for she realized that Edward would not let her take any risks, and getting hold of her father's files was something he could not do for her, so she would simply leave a message for him canceling lunch, telling him that something had come up and she'd see him later.

Still numb, still functioning on a strange, calming kind of autopilot, she telephoned the Arias house in Newport, was told that Jamie was out, and put down the phone before Michael or any of the others could speak to her.

Annie sat on the edge of the big hotel bed.

This could not be happening.

She forced herself to go over it again, her mind going in a wild, unwilling, nonchronological zigzag. The story about Jamie's uncle's crimes. The attempt on Olivia's life. The burglaries. And the helicopter crash that it now seemed had not, after all, been accidental.

She thought about the possible risk to herself if she got involved, made herself consider Sophie and William and Liza, not to mention Edward, and she knew that it probably was dreadfully irresponsible to think of taking a chance like this—and she wasn't the *type* to take risks ordinarily—

But then she thought about her mother and father, and how dreadfully she had missed them all these years, and if Olivia was right, then they had been murdered, for the love of God, *murdered*.

And if she could help, if her father's archives did contain the proof they needed, then she was damned if she was going to let Olivia bear the brunt of this alone, or Jamie, come to that.

Annie was trembling a little as she strode—Annie had never been a woman who strode anywhere—into the Aldrich law offices on Fifty-seventh Street, her passport in her purse in case there was no one at the office who remembered or recognized her.

"My name is Ann Aldrich Thomas," she told the receptionist, "and I need urgent access to my father's personal archives." She swept straight on before the younger woman could answer. "I'd appreciate it if you would arrange for someone to telephone Richard Tyson in London, so that he can vouch for me and make the archives available."

The receptionist opened her mouth to speak.

"When I say urgent," Annie said swiftly, "I mean urgent."

It was all there. Olivia's hunch had been accurate; Franklin had been holding copies. By four o'clock, Annie had located and skimmed through a complete set of her father's privately filed copies of Arthur Segal's correspondence with Carlos Arias, including a notarized copy of Paul Osterman's accusations against Juan Luis Arias, alias Georg Brauner, and a xeroxed copy of the pages in Anton Rothenburg's notebook. Annie was profoundly shaken, yet she knew at the same time that she had never been so dramatically galvanized by or focused upon anything.

She emerged back into the wood-paneled reception area, arms laden with papers, and found Eleanor Cohen, one of the partners, waiting for her.

"Mrs. Thomas, I'm so sorry I wasn't here when you arrived."

"That's perfectly all right." Annie smiled at the receptionist. "I was well looked after."

"Do you have everything you need?" Eleanor Cohen asked.

"Almost." Annie smiled again, apologetically. "I need to use your photocopier."

"I'll have someone take care of that for you."

"No," Annie said. "Thank you, but I'd rather do it myself."

She made two sets, returned the originals to the archive room, packaged one set to take away, and asked Eleanor Cohen to deposit the final set in the company vault.

"To be passed, with this letter, to my husband, in case—" Annie stopped.

"In case of what, Mrs. Thomas?" Eleanor Cohen asked.

"In the extremely unlikely event that I either disappear from the face of the earth or meet with an accident." She saw the concern on the attorney's face and tried to smile again. "It's just a precaution," she said. "Both those eventualities really are very unlikely."

"I should hope they are," Eleanor Cohen said.

"One more favor?" Annie asked tentatively.

"Of course."

"I have some calls to make. I have a charge card."

"That's not necessary," Eleanor Cohen told her.

"All the same," Annie said. "The calls are long-distance."

Olivia snatched up the cellular telephone. It was ten-fifteen in Brussels.

"Livvy, it's me. I have it all."

Briefly, Olivia closed her eyes. "Thank God for that. You've read it?"

"Most of it—as much as I had time to."

"So you don't think I'm crazy?"

"I never did." Annie paused. "Livvy, it's all too hideous to think about."

"Have you talked to Jamie?"

"Not yet. I've tried twice, and they say he's not there, but I think you're right—I do get the feeling someone doesn't want us to talk to him."

"Michael," Olivia said. "You think it's Michael, too."

"Unless it's Peter."

"It's not Peter's style, Annie. And he was still at school when Osterman had his meeting with Michael in sixty-four."

"And Jamie always refers to Michael as head of the family."

"It's Michael, I'm sure of it," Olivia said. "But what now?"

"I've had an idea," Annie said. "There is someone who might help us get past the others to Jamie."

"Who?"

"I don't have time to tell you any more, Livvy—I've got a plane to catch."

"Where are you going?" Olivia grew alarmed. "Annie, what are you planning? You can't do anything on your own."

"I'm not going to." Annie sounded very calm. "I'll call you later, Livvy, as soon as I know more."

"Annie, wait—"

Olivia heard the call cut out, stared at the small black phone in her hand.

"Dammit," she said. *"Dammit."*

At the Arias family compound in Newport, final preparations were under way for Michael's birthday party. Louise Arias adored throwing parties, had always entertained as often and as lavishly as possible no matter where she'd lived, even when she'd shared a small Cambridge home in her college days. But from the first moment she'd laid eyes on her husband's lovely clifftop mansion, she had vowed that no birthday, anniversary, or other cause for celebration would pass unmarked so long as she lived in that house, and it was a tribute to Louise's skills that even in Newport—even during the festive season—her invitations were received with pleasure and anticipation.

Jamie was not in the mood for a party. In the first place, he'd only recently landed the Korda Shoe Corporation account, worth at least ten million dollars a year, and he hadn't liked abandoning Maggie and David at JAA just when they were on the edge of being ready to burst their latest campaign ideas on him. In the second place, he had a lousy head cold and would infinitely sooner have been in his own home, drinking hot toddies, watching old movies, and maybe gossiping with Olivia on the phone—Olivia was the best at taking his mind off a trivial complaint like a common cold—Olivia was the best at taking his mind off most things, when he let himself think about it, which he seldom did these days. And in the third place, both he and Michael were furious with Peter for insisting on bringing Angie Rogos, his new mistress, for the whole two-day prelude to the party, which had clearly been meant for family only.

"Peter really is the prick of the universe," Daisy had said to Jamie on day one, a little drunkenly, after an interminable luncheon on the lawn during which Angie, dressed in an ankle-length but almost entirely see-through voile shift, had fawned all over her lover, heedless of his and Daisy's two young sons.

"I'm afraid he really is," Jamie agreed.

"Though it's easier for me than you, of course," Daisy had gone on. "Michael and Louise were always decent to me about Peter's infidelities, though I felt they were almost too embarrassed to bear to *look* at me after he stole Carrie from you. But now, the worse Peter's behavior gets, the more Louise seems to consider me more family than him."

"What makes you think it's harder for me?" Jamie had asked.

"Because it's easier to cope, long-term, isn't it, when you think they've left you for real love?" Daisy had paused for breath. "And because now, knowing what a dear man you are, Jamie—not even a bit like your brother—some little piece of you is bound to think you should feel sorry for Carrie—which, of course, you should not."

"I don't," Jamie had said.

"Even though you know she knows leaving you for Peter was the biggest mistake she ever made," Daisy said, and smiled ruefully. "Even bigger than Peter made leaving me."

"Carrie doesn't think that."

"Oh, yes, she does. She told me, or at least she told me she knew you were the better brother." Daisy grinned again. "Mind you, she did add that she hadn't tried cousin Michael yet."

"I'd like to see her dare," Jamie said, thinking about Louise.

"Louise wanted to invite Carrie, you know, but Michael told her it was asking for trouble."

"Thank heaven for Michael," Jamie said, and meant it.

Yet still, Michael's birthday aside, he was not in the mood for a party.

Annie had left a message for Edward at the St. Regis telling him not to worry about her, had caught the shuttle from La Guardia to Logan, and, taking the Boston rush hour into account, had jumped on a ferry across the harbor, bringing her a short cab ride from her destination.

At twenty-two minutes past six, she was rapping on the exterior glass door of the offices of Beaumont-Arias on Newbury Street, praying silently that Carrie Arias was still inside. Jamie had always said that Carrie liked to work late, claimed she got more done when the paid help—as she had called their employees, not always behind their backs—had left for the day.

She had completed eight series of raps, each series growing louder and more resonant, and was just about giving up, when Carrie's blond hair—blonder than the last time she'd seen it, Annie couldn't help noting—and her Jean Muir–clad body came stalking around the corner.

"Who the hell can't read?" Her wide blue irritated eyes grew even wider when she recognized Annie. "And what the fuck are you doing here?" She made no move to unlock the door, just stood there glowering through the glass.

"I need to talk to you," Annie said.

"Why should that be of the slightest interest to me?" Carrie asked.

"Please," Annie said. "Open the door, Carrie."

"We're closed," Carrie said. "If you want to make an appointment, call my assistant."

"Carrie, it's an emergency." Annie let the full weight of her anxiety swell that last word. "I mean it, a real emergency. Life or death."

Carrie moved an inch or so closer. "Whose life or death?"

Annie had thought about her answer to that question all the way from New York, and had decided that total, stark, if dangerous, honesty was her best and only way of tackling Carrie Arias.

"Olivia's," she said.

Carrie's eyes widened still further and she opened her mouth to laugh, then shut it again. She stepped right up against the glass. "Which option am I supposed to be backing, Annie? I have to tell you I'm considerably more inclined toward death."

Annie managed a half smile. "I guess I can't blame you for that." She paused. "Please open the door." Her smile was gone. "Please."

Carrie turned around, went over to the receptionist's desk, opened a drawer, took out a key, and held it up.

"Do I get to help?" she asked loudly so that Annie could hear her through the thick glass.

"You do," Annie replied wryly. "But maybe not in the way you might have in mind."

With deliberate slowness, Carrie opened the door.

At half past midnight on Thursday morning in Brussels, Olivia—with Cleo burrowed in beside her—was in bed, drowsy from painkillers, but too tense to sleep and unwilling to knock herself out completely with one of the pills the hospital had given her.

She had seen the police patrol car from her window several more times during the evening, and once, an officer had rung her bell to check on her, and she had felt more reassured then, had seen no further sign of the man in the black leather jacket. Perhaps, she was beginning to think, that had, after all, been coincidental; maybe he had just been a city sleaze picking on a vulnerable-looking woman—which of course she was right now with her arm in the sling—and maybe she *had* been overreacting.

And her tension now was stemming more from what Annie might be doing than from fear, and soon, soon, surely she would *have* to fall asleep from sheer, unutterable exhaustion.

"You must"—Carrie said to Annie a few minutes later in her own office, a monument to Beacon Hill–bred taste and refinement in spite of the awards and photographs displayed in a cabinet on one wall—"be crazy."

"I understand your feeling that," Annie said steadily. "But I think you may feel differently when you hear everything I have to tell you."

Carrie leaned back in her chair, her body language perfectly relaxed. She remembered their last encounter only too well, knew she would never forget, and certainly never forgive, her defeat and humiliation at the end of the Light Years fiasco. But then again, she had always known that it had been Olivia Segal's scheme, not Annie Thomas's, and now the mere knowledge that Olivia was in trouble and that Annie was here begging for her help was purest music to her ears.

"If you think," she said, "that anything you could ever tell me could possibly persuade me to lift a finger to help Olivia Segal, then you're not only crazy and incredibly brazen, but plain stupid into the bargain."

Annie sat very straight. "I gather that you and Peter are finished."

"We most decidedly are, if it's any of your business." Her voice was even more cool, clipped Bostonian than usual.

"It's not my business at all," Annie admitted. "But I imagine you'll be looking for a good settlement."

Carrie's eyes narrowed coldly. "That really is none of your business."

"I imagine"—Annie ignored what she'd said—"you'll be hoping to squeeze him dry. Lord knows he deserves it."

"Surely what you really mean is that I deserve it, Annie."

"At this precise moment," Annie said, "I'm not in the least interested in what you do or don't deserve."

"I'm surprised," Carrie said. "I mean, I'm surprised by you. I thought you were such a mouse, Annie Aldrich Thomas, Jamie's gentle, trank-gulping little friend. Even when you came to the Ritz-Carlton that day with Olivia, even when you had your say, I knew you were just hanging on to Olivia's coattails, still a mouse. What are you on these days, Annie, to make you so bold?"

Annie felt strangely calm. "Even a mouse has to stand up and be counted sometimes." She paused. "I have ammunition for you, Carrie, to use against Peter. All the ammunition you could ever dream of, and more."

"I don't think I need much more than I have," Carrie said confidently. "Given that my husband's been flaunting his mistress over half of New England and Manhattan."

"Twelve mistresses would be nothing compared with what I have for you, Carrie," Annie told her, "nor would a half dozen of their children."

For the first time, Carrie permitted herself a flicker of interest.

"Go on," she said.

At a quarter to seven, already dressed in his damned tuxedo—Louise always insisted on black tie for her major parties; if she could really have her way, Michael said that she'd have every Arias man, preferably every male guest, wearing white tie and tails—Jamie blew his cold-blocked nose, looked at his watch, and wondered if he had time to call Olivia. They hadn't spoken for several days, and there was a problem with the phone extension in his room, and he missed her, and suddenly it seemed to him that the long, long evening ahead for which he still was no more in the mood than he had been, might be made more bearable if he could just snatch a few minutes of conversation with her first.

He wandered down the handsome winged staircase, past the haunting painting by Puvis de Chavannes that Michael had once told him his late father, Juan Luis, had personally helped to hang about a year prior to his death. Louise had placed a huge bowl of lilies on the stand beneath it, and as Jamie glanced down to the grand entrance hall below he thought for an instant that, for his personal taste, the house was looking just a touch too weddinglike for a man's birthday party. But then he remembered Louise telling him at a previous celebration that she regarded all parties, no matter what their raison d'être, as the province of females. "Women," she had told Jamie, "understand how to make people feel welcome and comfortable and light-hearted far better than men, except, I suppose, gay men, and their parties—their *top* parties—are the best of all."

He went into the library to use the telephone, sat down in the cool, dark peace and quiet, finding it just what his poor banging head needed, savored it for just a moment, picked up the phone, and began to dial.

The door opened and Michael came in.

"Jamie, just the man." He looked apologetically at his cousin. "Is that urgent or can it wait?"

Jamie put down the receiver. "It's not urgent."

"Not calling the office?"

Jamie shook his head. "Olivia."

"Pretty late for her, isn't it?"

"Not really—we often speak around this time." Jamie looked up at Michael. "What can I do?"

"I need a second opinion on the champagne," Michael said. "Louise just brought me a glass for a private toast and I'm not certain if it's quite right."

"I'm not sure if I'm the man for the job this evening," Jamie said. "This damn cold's playing havoc with my taste buds."

"I'm afraid you're the only man," Michael said firmly. "Since

Peter's locked in his bedroom with Miss Rogos. Besides, champagne's an excellent cure-all."

Jamie stood up. "I guess it can't hurt."

Michael opened the door. "You're sure you don't mind leaving that call for now? I really could use your opinion."

Jamie shook his head.

"It's nothing that can't wait till tomorrow," he said.

"I don't believe it," Carrie said about a half hour later. "I really don't believe it."

"I think perhaps you should," Annie said. She indicated the package resting on the desk in front of her. "It's all there, after all. All the proof you could ask for."

She felt suddenly drained. She had given Carrie an edited version of the long, dreadful tale, had told her and shown her just enough and no more, but she had observed its ever growing impact on the other woman's now taut and paler face.

"I've shocked you," she said.

"Of course you've damn well shocked me," Carrie said sharply. "What do you take me for? I'm not soft, God knows, and I have no wish to be, but even I draw the line at murder." She shook her head. "Jesus, I can't *believe* it—Michael? Solid as a Spanish rock, pillar of the community Michael Arias, a *murderer?*"

"You do realize, don't you," Annie said slowly, "that whether or not you decide to use this to get what you want from Peter, you're very much better off knowing about this ahead of its getting out." She paused. "Which it will, Carrie, one way or another. After which being a member of the Arias family may not be quite the bonus it's been in the past."

"It's reasonably common knowledge," Carrie said, "that I'm finished with the Arias family."

"You're still married to Peter."

"Meaning what exactly?" Carrie spoke slowly, still allowing Annie's story to sink in.

"That you might be wise to distance yourself from them more completely," Annie said. "Before it's too late."

"I think that's a little melodramatic, from my standpoint," Carrie said. "After all, no one's going to believe that I knew about any of this. We don't even know for sure yet if Peter knows about it."

Annie trod as carefully as she could, fully conscious that it was only Carrie's shock that was allowing her to remain there, and that, knowing Carrie, the situation could alter at any moment. "Let's just say," she went on, "that Peter's going to have to prove his ignorance." She paused. "And we both know that a lot of wives have been found guilty by association."

Carrie was silent.

"Of course, Olivia and I could help you out," Annie went on, "by speaking for you. We could make it absolutely clear—we could even testify, if that became necessary—that you knew nothing about either the Rothenburgs or the helicopter crash until we told you."

Carrie's eyes grew chillier again. "I take it this is where my help comes in." She paused. "The implication being that if I don't help you get Olivia out of trouble, you might suggest that I did know something."

"I didn't say that," Annie said, far more calmly than she felt.

"You're getting rather good at this, Annie," Carrie said. "Blackmail becomes you."

Annie couldn't help flushing.

"So what do you want me to do?"

"Come with me to Newport and help me get to Jamie. I know he's there, at the house, but I haven't been allowed to speak to him."

"And you expect me to persuade them to let you in?"

"Yes."

"When?"

"Now."

"Now?" Carrie looked startled. "It's after half past seven."

"So we could be there by nine-thirty or ten."

"It's out of the question," Carrie said crisply. "I have two engagements this evening, and I have no intention of canceling them."

Annie looked at her, saw the familiar coldness back in her blue eyes, and knew she still had work to do if she was going to talk Carrie round.

"Someone has to warn Jamie," she said quietly. "I understand your not caring about Olivia, but I can't imagine you'd want to see Jamie in actual danger."

"I can't imagine that James is in any danger," Carrie said.

"Can't you?" Annie asked pointedly.

Carrie glanced at her antique Cartier watch, then shook her head impatiently. "There's no purpose in even considering going to Newport tonight, not with Louise giving a birthday party for Michael."

"We could join the party," Annie said.

"Even you must have heard of security, Annie," Carrie said. "These parties are scrupulously guarded. No invitation, no entrance."

"But you're still Mrs. Peter Arias." Annie paused. "You're still Caroline Beaumont Arias. Are you going to tell me you'd let some security guard stop you from walking into an Arias family party?"

"Certainly not," Carrie said.

Annie held her breath.

"I don't like being bulldozed, Annie."

"And I don't like my two best friends being in danger."

"Do you honestly believe," Carrie asked, "that Michael would go so far as to harm his own cousin?"

"I don't know," Annie answered. "I'd like to think he wouldn't."

"But if Michael had his own uncle killed . . ." Carrie's voice trailed off.

"Exactly." Annie sat in an agony of suspense.

Carrie was silent for several seconds.

"Wait outside," she said at last. "I have some calls to make."

Annie picked up her bag and the package and stood up.

"Are you going to come with me, Carrie?"

Carrie looked up at her. "I think, perhaps, this is one confrontation I would like to witness firsthand."

Annie felt weak with relief. "So you're coming?"

"Not if you don't get out and let me make my calls."

Olivia answered the telephone just after two. She was still so groggy with sleep that she thought she heard Annie telling her that she was on the way from Boston to Newport with Carrie, and that she was using Carrie's car phone, and that one way or another they'd have Jamie out of there within a few hours; and Olivia was to go back to sleep now, she was no longer in this on her own, she could get some rest, and Annie would get back to her as soon as there was any news to pass on.

"Did you say Carrie?" Olivia asked fuzzily.

"That's right," Annie answered.

Olivia put the receiver down again and lay back and half smiled into the dark on her way back down into the luxurious escape of sleep. She knew now, was comfortable in the knowledge that she was in the middle of the strangest dream. Which only went to prove how crazy dreams could be. Because the very notion of Carrie Beaumont Arias coming to Annie's and Olivia's aid was one of the wildest, craziest things that anyone's subconscious could possibly dredge up.

Annie and Carrie encountered their first obstacle at the outer entrance of the Arias compound where the gateman asked for their invitations or, failing that, their names, so that he could check them off on his list, and two armed security guards hovered in the background as if Al Capone were going to leap from the trunk of Carrie's car any second.

"You're not on my list, ma'am," the gateman said, leaning down to Carrie's window. The sound of distant music filtered through the warm summer night air.

"I didn't say I was," Carrie said.

"It's invitation only, ma'am. I'm sorry."

Carrie nodded toward the gatehouse. "Why don't you call the main house and ask permission to let us in?"

"No point, ma'am. As I said, it's strictly invitation only."

Carrie stuck her head a little farther out of the window. "What are the names of the hosts of this party?"

"Mr. and Mrs. Michael Arias, ma'am." The man managed to blend courtesy and snobbishness into his tone.

"And what did I say my name was?" Carrie's acidity was soft, gentle.

"Mrs. Peter Arias, ma'am."

"Do you know who Peter Arias is?"

"Mr. Michael Arias's cousin."

"Whose wife I am," Carrie said.

"Yes, ma'am." There was a hint of a sigh behind the words.

"So don't you think you could, after all, make an exception and let us in?"

"No, ma'am, I don't think I could." The man observed the slow, dangerous narrowing of Carrie's eyes. "But I will call the house and check with them."

"Well, thank you," Carrie said sweetly.

"You're welcome, ma'am."

In less than four minutes, the time it had taken to get Louise Arias to give the okay, they were heading up the long driveway toward the house, the music growing louder, sounding, Annie thought, like Duke Ellington—though of course it couldn't be Ellington because he was dead, and from what she'd heard about Louise's parties, she'd rather be dead than play recorded music.

"You were great back there," Annie said weakly. She was still scarcely able to believe that she'd talked Carrie into coming all that way with her, and now, watching and listening to her in fighting form and—on the face of it, at least—on her side, was almost too much to take in. "I'd never have got this far without you," she added.

"No, you wouldn't," Carrie agreed.

"I owe you already."

Carrie shrugged, driving on. "Nothing to it, not for a hard-nosed bitch like me. Though you're right. You do most certainly owe me."

"Oh, God," Annie said, her throat tightening as they slowed down again. "There's Louise."

Mrs. Michael Arias stood in the doorway in slender, immaculate, cream silk glory, her silhouette almost entirely merged with the dazzle of chandeliered brilliance in the entrance hall behind them.

"When in doubt," Carrie told Annie, "leave it to me."

She got out of the car, handed the keys to the waiting attendant, and walked up the stone steps, followed by Annie.

"Carrie, what an unexpected surprise," Louise said, and leaned forward to give her a careful air kiss on both cheeks. "And with Annie Thomas, of all people—how lovely."

"I hope you don't mind too much, Louise." Annie held out her right hand. "I was in Boston and bumped into Carrie, who said she was coming up for the party."

"Jamie didn't mention that you were in Boston," Louise said.

"He didn't know."

Michael appeared behind his wife. "Good Lord," he said. "It's true."

"Happy birthday, Michael," Carrie said. "May we come in?"

"Of course you may." Louise stepped back graciously. "Isn't this a lovely surprise, Michael."

Michael closed the door, his face impassive. There were no guests to be seen in the hall—just two waitresses hurrying past—but the sounds and scents of a large party, still distant, a heady combination of music, conversation, and laughter, of food and a score of predictable perfumes and smoke, lapped around Annie and Carrie, enveloping them.

"Everyone's having dinner, I'm afraid," Louise said.

"So what can we do for you?" Michael asked a little brusquely.

"Michael." Louise sounded reproving. "That's not very hospitable."

"We're in the middle of a party," Michael said reasonably. "For which they're hardly dressed."

"I can take care of that," Louise said, and smiled at Carrie. "If you wouldn't object too violently to borrowing something of mine."

"Not at all," Carrie said, "but I won't, thanks just the same, Louise. I've always believed Jean Muir can take me just about anywhere."

"I'm quite happy as I am, too," Annie said, not remotely happy in the daytime Escada suit she'd put on that morning—an eternity ago—to meet Edward for lunch, though her unease, of course, had little to do with her clothing. "I've only come to see Jamie."

"We've really come," Carrie said quickly, "for a family talk."

"Tonight?" For the first time, Louise looked disconcerted. "You can't be serious."

"Not tonight," Michael said firmly.

"Definitely tonight," Carrie said.

Louise lowered her voice. "I know you have good cause to feel hostile towards Peter, but surely Michael's birthday is not the right time."

"It's the perfect time," Carrie said softly. "But it has nothing to do with my hostility towards my husband." She paused. "Where is Peter, by the way? Tête-à-tête somewhere with his mistress, I suppose?"

"I'm not sure." Louise was growing flustered. "In the gardens, having dinner, I imagine."

"If you've come here with the idea of creating some kind of spectacle, Carrie," Michael said, "then we'll have to insist you leave."

"No spectacle, Michael." Annie answered instead of Carrie. "Just a small family gathering."

"You're not family," Michael said, dislike showing. "What does this have to do with you?"

"I thought you said you'd come along to see Jamie," Louise said.

"I have," Annie agreed. "Do you know where he is, Louise?"

"Jamie has a bad cold," Michael said abruptly. "I think I saw him going up to bed awhile back."

"Did you, darling?" Louise was surprised. "I'm sure I just saw him dancing."

"Perhaps, Louise, you could find him for Annie?" Carrie asked sweetly.

"I'd rather go myself, if you don't mind," Annie said.

"Then perhaps you could go rustle up Peter," Carrie suggested to Michael. "We really do need to have this little talk as quickly as possible."

"It's completely out of the question," Michael said tightly.

Louise was growing more baffled than annoyed. "We can hardly disappear from our own party to have a meeting, Carrie—surely even you must see that."

"Not really," Carrie said. "I heard you say once, Louise, that if a party's properly organized, it should be able to run perfectly all on its own." She paused to listen to the sounds coming from beyond the house. "They all seem to be getting on with things rather well without you right now."

"All right." Michael's anger became more open. "That's enough. You'll have to leave."

"I don't think so," Carrie said.

"Don't make me throw you out, Carrie."

"Michael, please," Louise protested. "Let's not have a scene."

"Don't worry, Louise," Carrie said confidently. "He won't throw us out. Unless he wants us to bring in the police."

"Oh, stop, Carrie," Louise said, upset and vehement. "This is getting out of hand. You know, I wanted to invite you tonight, but

Michael said it would just create embarrassment—I do hope you're not going to prove him right."

"I'm rather afraid I am," Carrie said. "Though not in the way you mean."

Annie, having kept silent for a time, letting Carrie, as she'd suggested, take the lead, knew it was time to speak up.

"You haven't asked after Olivia, Michael," she said.

His dark eyes hardened. "Why should I have done that?"

"Is something wrong with Olivia?" Louise asked, growing ever more confused.

"She's not very well," Annie answered. "After her accident."

"Oh, dear," Louise said. "Nothing too serious, I hope."

"Not as serious as it might have been," Annie said, and took a breath. "She was hit by a car." She looked directly at Michael. "Do you think we can have that talk now?"

"I suggest the library," Carrie said.

"And I suggest," Michael said, "for the last time, that you leave."

Louise tossed her perfect auburn hair. "Oh, for heaven's sake, darling, let's talk to them and get it over with." She looked at Carrie. "How long is this going to take? I really do have to get back to our guests."

"Why don't you get back to them right now?" Michael said. "I can take care of this meeting without you."

"No, Michael, you can't," Carrie said.

Annie reached out, unexpectedly, and touched Louise's left arm gently. The older woman was cold, and Annie, feeling suddenly quite certain of her innocence, felt intensely sorry for her. "I really do think that you should stay, Louise," she said.

"For goodness' sake, let me throw them out," Michael said to his wife. "Carrie's trouble; she's always been trouble."

"And glad of it," Carrie said coldly, "knowing what I do now."

"I'm going," Annie said abruptly, "to find Jamie."

Jamie was dancing with Daisy, the worst of his cold chased away temporarily, at least, by champagne and atmosphere. Louise had drawn her white lily theme like a lovely, pure, luxuriant chain throughout the house and gardens, so that everywhere guests wandered, from the hallways to the pool house to the bathrooms, the chaste, yet oddly seductive flowers nestled around them, never intrusive, just promoting a sense of having stepped into some nameless, exotic land where beauty and pleasure ruled and outside concerns had no place.

"I want to go swimming," Daisy said.

"Really?" Jamie looked down at her in surprise. "And risk ruining your lovely hair? That's not like you."

"I think I'm a bit drunk."

"You've been drunk quite a lot the last few days, Daisy Arias."

"It must be the company."

"Thank you," Jamie said.

"Not you, Jamie. Certainly not you."

"I thought you enjoyed being around the family," he said affectionately. Daisy sometimes tended toward prissiness, yet Jamie found, as time went by, that he liked Peter's first wife more and more.

"I do, usually," Daisy said, clinging to him a little more tightly, as if she might fall down otherwise. "But I haven't this time, not as much, and it really isn't because of Peter and Angie."

"What then?"

"Michael's been in such a grouchy mood."

"Has he?" Jamie hadn't noticed.

"You've not been yourself either," Daisy said, "but that's probably just your cold."

"I'm sorry," Jamie said.

"Not your fault," Daisy told him politely.

The music stopped.

"Hello, Jamie."

Jamie let go of Daisy and turned around.

"Annie!" A smile of pleasure and surprise lit up his face, then vanished when he saw the expression in her eyes. "Annie, what's happened?"

For the first time since she and Carrie had arrived in Newport, Annie felt herself go weak at the knees.

"Oh, Jamie," she said. "Thank God I've found you."

The sound of breaking glass woke Olivia just after four-fifteen. Instantly, icily awake, without a hint of grogginess now, she turned on the bedside light.

The cat was wide awake, too, standing by the door, her tortoise-shell fur standing on end, her tail erect, and the green of her eyes almost completely swallowed up by huge, black, fully dilated pupils.

"It's okay, Cleo," Olivia whispered.

She heard another sound.

Olivia reached for the phone, dialed 100 for the police, heard nothing. Quickly, tucking the receiver between her ear and her chin, she pressed her finger on the cut-off button and released it again. There was no tone.

"Oh, God," she said, then remembered the cellular phone. It was there, where she'd left it after Annie's call, on the other night table. Swift as she could, hampered by her arm, she snatched it up. The battery was drained and the spare, she knew, was in her study.

"Oh, God," she said again.

And the light went out.

Peter Arias was half drunk. Jamie, knowing only that Olivia was in some kind of trouble, was distraught and confused. Louise was having a hard time keeping her outrage, dismay, and embarrassment under control. Michael was tight-lipped and patently furious. They were all sitting in the library on dark leather chairs, and they were waiting.

"Well," Carrie said, closing the door. "Since the gang's all here, Annie, you may as well begin."

"What the fuck," Peter asked, "has she got to do with us?"

"If by 'us,' " Carrie answered, "you mean you and me, nothing at all."

"Annie?" Jamie was pale. "What is going on?"

Annie stood up. If anyone had asked her how she felt at that moment, she could only have answered that she felt entirely outside herself, like an observer. If Olivia had been there with her, she knew she would have been glad to melt into the background, to let Olivia take over. But Livvy wasn't there—Livvy was in Brussels with her arm broken and lucky to be alive. Because of one of these people.

"I'll keep it short," she began, "which is not easy, when you're telling people about more than fifty years of evil."

Michael got to his feet. "What is this nonsense?"

"Sit down, Michael," Carrie said from her chair near the door.

"Don't tell me what to do in my own home."

"Please, Michael," Annie said, "sit down."

Louise reached out for her husband's hand to draw him back down. "It's all right, dear. The sooner we let her have her say, the sooner we can get back to the party."

"I'm not sure," Annie said gently, "that you'll be feeling much like a party when I've finished."

Peter swiveled around in his chair, trying to get comfortable. "I must say, your friends have a weird sense of timing," he said to Jamie. "This one's the junkie, isn't she?"

"Ex-junkie," Carrie said, uncharacteristically fair.

"Shall I get on with it?" Annie asked them all.

"No," Michael said flatly.

"Oh, for pity's sake, please do," Louise said desperately, and drew her husband down beside her again.

Annie looked down at Jamie, into his soft, dark eyes. "I'm so sorry to have to tell you this, in this awful, cold way. To be honest, I didn't think I had it in me." She paused. "Carrie says she's always thought I was a mouse, and I tend to agree with her." She paused again. "But I suppose that discovering that your parents have been murdered to cover up a war crime tends to toughen up even the most timid mouse."

"What," Jamie asked, "are you talking about, Annie?"

"What *is* she talking about?" Peter asked.

"I think she's hallucinating," Michael said.

"What are you *talking* about, Annie, dear?" Louise asked.

"She's talking about your husband," Carrie answered for Annie. "She's telling you all that Michael arranged the deaths of six people nineteen years ago—including his own Uncle Carlos—"

"Dear God." Michael shook his head and stared at Annie as if she were entirely mad.

"Don't be such a fucking idiot, Carrie," Peter said loudly.

Louise's hazel eyes were huge with horror. "I never heard anything so *disgusting* in my entire life! Such *lies!*"

Michael patted her arm. "Don't worry, sweetheart. The woman's obviously deranged."

"I'm afraid not, Louise," Annie said quietly.

Jamie was ashen-faced. "Annie, I don't know what's going on—I don't know what's wrong with you—"

"There's nothing much wrong with Annie," Carrie said. "Though it does pain me a little to admit that, as you can imagine, James." She looked at Annie. "Go on. No point stopping now."

"No," Annie said. "I know there isn't."

She told it briefly and starkly, told her stricken, appalled audience what she was now more certain than ever Michael already knew. That Juan Luis Arias had been a thieving, opportunistic, blackmailing murderer. And that when Arthur Segal had told Carlos Arias what his brother had done, and when Carlos had gone to Michael, to his trusted, beloved nephew, to tell him what he had learned and what he planned to do about it, Michael, acting either in defense of his father's honor, or simply because he was unwilling to lose everything because of his uncle's crisis of conscience, had arranged the helicopter crash.

"And no one else would ever have been any the wiser," Annie told them, nearing the end of her story, "if Olivia hadn't happened on a note that Carlos had sent to her father." She looked straight at Michael, now sitting rigid with anger. "It was only after Jamie asked you if you knew what the note meant that her apartment was broken into and the note was stolen."

At last Michael moved. He stood up and stared down at her, and his eyes were black with anger.

"And that," he said, "is just about enough, Mrs. Thomas." His hands, down by his sides, were tightly clenched. "I've listened quietly and patiently to your ramblings about Nazis and Jews and paintings. I've sat still while you accused me of murdering my own uncle—my own *uncle* and five other people, for the love of God—"

"Michael—" Louise was standing, too, reaching for her husband's left hand. "Don't upset yourself. You were right; the woman's obviously deranged. She's probably not even responsible for what—"

"She's a goddamned drug addict, for fuck's sake," Peter said.

Annie stood her ground, went on as if no one else had spoken. "And then Olivia found out about the other break-ins, and she began to realize that someone was trying to make sure that there were no more notes or proof—"

"So now I'm a burglar, too, am I?" Michael asked dryly.

"Not personally, of course not." Annie felt her legs beginning to buckle, knew that she was almost finished, and she hadn't really figured beyond this; she didn't know, did not have the faintest notion what was going to happen next. "Just as you didn't personally run Olivia down at the Gare du Midi in Brussels yesterday, or steal her bag—"

"For God's sake," Louise burst out, still clutching Michael's hand for dear life. "Have you no shame, Annie? Is there to be no *end* to this lunacy?"

"The bag," Annie went on, "that contained all the evidence of everything I've just told you."

"Which has gone, I take it," Michael said. "How inconvenient for you."

"Not really," Annie said. "Not anymore. Not once I found that my own father had copies of everything." She paused. "I have one set here with me, Michael." She bent down to pick up the package she'd brought from the New York office. "Proof. Absolute proof." She paused again. "And there are paintings, Olivia tells me, all over this house, that once belonged to Emanuel Rothenburg."

"The Gauguin, for one," Carrie said softly, with gentle malice. "The one in your drawing room, Louise."

Louise sat down again. Everyone in the room went completely silent. From outside, the sounds of music and partying continued.

"It is true," Carrie said. "Hard as it is to swallow, it really does seem to be quite true."

"Michael," Louise said faintly, "tell them they're wrong."

"Of course they're wrong." Michael's voice was stiff.

"No," Carrie said. "We're not. Are we, Michael?"

Annie had that odd feeling again, as if she were watching everyone in the room from a distance. Jamie, lost in his nightmare, engulfed by disbelief, struggling to comprehend the total annihilation of all his foundations, not knowing whether to be more aghast by what had happened to Olivia or what had gone on so many years ago. Louise, her face, her whole immaculate cream silk body seeming to crumple, as she sat slumped in her chair, staring at her husband as if he were a stranger. Peter, his face on the edge of green, plainly as appalled as the rest of them, wishing he were more drunk than he was.

Michael was still standing. Annie made herself look at him again and fancied for a moment that she saw it all behind those black eyes, the fury consuming him, his mind racing, calculating, planning what to do to her.

"I don't think there's anything you can do now, Michael," she said softly. "The truth's going to come out, whichever way you turn."

"Unless, of course," Carrie said, "you're planning to kill everyone who knows."

"But even that wouldn't be enough," Annie said, holding firmly to the package of her father's papers, "because this is not the only set of copies, and I have, of course, made arrangements for the information to be passed on if anything should happen to me."

She sat down at last, finished, and simply, suddenly, quite unable to go on. She stared down at the package of papers on her lap and felt her mouth quivering. She found that she could not, any longer, look at anyone else in the room. She could not, more than anything, bear to see Jamie's face.

Michael looked down, for a moment, at his wife, but Louise was just gazing now, unseeing, into the distance, and so he turned to Peter, but Peter only shook his head. He looked past Annie, toward the door, where Carrie still sat like a sentry, perfectly composed in her Jean Muir dress.

"Thinking of leaving, Michael?" she said.

Peter's eyes were suddenly quizzical. "How in hell," he asked Carrie, "did you get in on this act?"

"Annie figured I might help"—his estranged wife's smile was cool and unruffled—"because I might want to use this against you. Which, of course, I might."

"Christ." Peter shook his head again. "Oh, Christ."

Louise began to weep, and Jamie, automatically, pulled out a crisp white handkerchief and passed it over to her.

The door opened.

"Am I family enough," Daisy Arias inquired scathingly, "to be allowed to join this little private party?"

"Only," Carrie answered, "if you've brought a stiff drink with you."

Olivia, fear-chilled in her sleeveless nightdress, knew that she had to leave her bedroom. She couldn't just wait there like some pathetic sacrificial lamb for him to come to get her. She had to at least *try* to get either to her study for the telephone battery or to the kitchen for a knife or—best of all—to the front door for freedom, whichever was easiest, whichever was *possible*.

It had been a good half hour since she'd heard the breaking glass, and maybe, just maybe, it had come from somewhere outside, maybe from a neighboring house or a car.

But the lights had gone out. And the telephone was dead.

She opened the door slowly, stood very still on the threshold, and listened. Nothing. Uncertain whether nothing was better than something—for at least if she could hear him, she might know where the son of a bitch was—

Unless nothing meant that he'd come for something rather than her, and that he'd already gone. But she didn't really believe that. Her broken, plaster-weighted, painful arm told her otherwise. The man in the black leather jacket had tried to kill her once and had failed. He had, presumably, been ordered to come back and finish the job.

Something brushed her ankle and Olivia gasped, couldn't help gasping, even when she realized it was only Cleo, moving on past her. Cleo, her little feline advance guard, all stealth and claws and speed when she needed it.

Olivia listened for another long minute and went after her.

Halfway along the corridor, with her first choice to make—*study to right, kitchen to left, front door straight ahead*—she stopped.

She could hear something.

Her eyes, wide and terrified, stared into the darkness, her ears strained to identify the sound.

Breathing? Not breathing.

It was hissing. It was Cleo, only Olivia had never heard a sound like it coming from her cat, part hiss, part growl.

She felt him coming too late, felt the movement of air from the left— *he's been waiting in the kitchen*—and then he was on her, one strong leather arm around her throat, one glove over her mouth, stopping her from screaming.

She heard the cat again, heard a yowling, felt the man kicking, heard a small thud, and Olivia wanted to kill him then, felt all the rage she'd been suppressing for the past thirty-six hours or so against Juan Luis and Michael Arias, and summoning all her strength she twisted around and kicked her attacker, Cleo's attacker, as hard as she could.

"*Pute!*"

He punched her, twice, once in the face, once on her left shoulder, and Olivia saw light then, dazzling, whirling light, but all the pain was in her broken arm. Jesus, it hurt, she'd never, never, *never* felt such pain before in her entire life.

"Please," she gasped, sobbing. "*Please.*"

"Shut up," he said in English.

"Please don't kill me," she said.

He did not kill her. He gripped her hard with one arm, gripped her bad side so that she shrieked with the pain—"Shut *up!*" he said again—and turned on a flashlight with his other hand, and then he dragged her along the corridor to the wood-paneled hall. And Olivia thought he must be going to take her out into the street, that he was going to kidnap her, and hope kindled inside her for a moment because maybe, just *maybe*, the police patrol car might come along at the right moment—it was only a chance, but it was better than nothing—

But then he stopped, right in the middle of the hall. He bent down, dragging Olivia down as he went, and the pain shot through her again—

"God!" she cried out.

"*Ferme ta gueule!*"

He set down the flashlight and took a key from his pocket, and through her tears of pain, Olivia saw that he was unlocking the door to the cellar that she had never seen, the door that had never been opened in all the time she'd lived there. And it wasn't as good as the front door would have been, but maybe if he was just going to lock her into the cellar she stood a chance, because it had to be only a matter of time before Annie and Jamie found out she was in trouble, and—

"*Viens.*"

He went ahead of her, sideways, keeping his grip on her, went down the steps, shining the flashlight as he went so that he didn't fall. Olivia struggled to keep her footing, stumbled once, yelped again as he dragged at her poor arm, and then they were down in the cellar.

It smelled, of damp and disuse and something else, rats, perhaps, but then Olivia remembered the mouse that Cleo had caught a couple of months back, and she'd once heard that mice and rats never lived together, and she thought she could handle mice if she had to, could handle anything so long as he gave her some time.

"*Voilà,*" he said.

He raised the flashlight and shone it straight ahead.

Olivia looked. There was a safe in the middle of the floor. A big, open, walk-in safe with a heavy, solid steel door that reminded her of the vault door at the Britannia Safe Deposit in London. She remembered that the real estate broker had told her that the owner of the house was an Antwerp diamond merchant; this, presumably, was where he had kept his jewels on the premises.

She looked again, saw that there was something inside the safe. She tried to focus, and recognized the pair of Georgian silver candlesticks she had bought with Bernard after the robbery—and there, too, was the lovely Victorian silver biscuit box he'd bought her as a gift.

"*Un p'tit accident,*" the man said. "While you were putting them away."

She stared at him and suddenly understood.

"No," she said, shaking her head violently. "I never had a key—no one will believe it."

"Maybe they will, maybe they won't," he said. "*Allez.*"

He pushed her hard from behind, and then, when she struggled to stand firm, he seized her by her plaster cast and hauled her, screaming with agony, into the safe.

"Best to try and sleep," he said.

And closed the door.

24

At midnight, they were all still in the library, with the exception of Louise—who had dragged herself sufficiently together to return to their guests and try to wind down the party without too much fuss.

"I shall tell everyone," Louise had said to the room in general before leaving, "that Michael has a bad migraine." She had not looked at her husband. "Please will someone lock the door behind me so that no one else can wander in." She had glanced down at Peter, half sitting, half lying in his leather armchair, his eyes glazed over with drink, fatigue, and shock. "If Miss Rogos asks, what would you like me to tell her?"

"To go home," Peter had answered. "That would be best, don't you think, Louise?"

"I wouldn't like to say what I think about anything anymore, Peter," Louise had said.

The library was one of the smallest rooms in the Arias mansion, but it was still large enough for the six people who remained to have split into three camps. In one, Jamie and Annie sat on either side of the mahogany desk as Annie tried, for the third time in ten minutes, to telephone Olivia. In the second, Peter sat over by the shelves housing Carlos Arias's old collection of Spanish literature, one ex-wife on either side of him: Daisy—briefly but succinctly filled in by Carrie—sat bolt upright with a glass of champagne in her hand, her fascinated, horrified eyes roaming around the room; Carrie, bored for the moment but with no intention of leaving, leafed idly through a leather-bound edition of Ramón José Sender and waited for things to heat up again.

Michael's camp was a solitary affair. He was still strangely immaculate, superficially, at least, untouched by all that had gone on, a handsome middle-aged man in a tuxedo. He had confessed to nothing, was for the moment displaying no emotion at all, yet already he seemed isolated by the crimes of which he had been accused. He might still, Daisy thought, watching him, be boiling with rage inside, or maybe he was being consumed by the hellfires of guilt, or maybe he was just calculating like mad how to get out of the god-awful mess he seemed to have gotten himself into. But if he was doing any of those things, they did not show.

"There's still no answer," Annie, her eyes afraid, said to Jamie at ten past midnight.

"Maybe she's really sleeping," Jamie said.

Annie shook her head vehemently. "She was pretty much asleep when I spoke to her last time, but she still managed to answer the phone."

"Perhaps she's taken a pill," Carrie suggested from across the room. "They can knock you out—you should know that, Annie."

"Olivia hates sleeping pills," Annie said, ignoring the jibe.

"Did you try her mobile?" Jamie asked.

"No answer. Just that damned voice that takes messages when the phone's out of range or whatever."

"Did you leave a message?" Daisy asked.

"I left two messages," Annie said tersely.

"Sorry," Daisy said. "Stupid question."

"No, I'm sorry," Annie said. "It isn't your fault."

"You're really worried about her, aren't you?" Jamie asked.

"Aren't you?" Annie said.

"Yes," Jamie said. "Of course I am."

Annie stood up. "Something must be wrong. It's six o'clock in the morning in Belgium, and Olivia wasn't in any condition to get up and go anywhere, and she was incredibly anxious to hear from you or me." Her fear, now that she had accepted it, given voice to it, grew rapidly, gathered force. "Something's really wrong, Jamie. I know it is."

"Okay," he said, his own alarm growing with hers. "Okay, let's call the Brussels police."

"Just a minute." Carrie put down the Sender novel. "I have a question for Michael."

Michael did not acknowledge her.

"Is the person who tried to kill Olivia still after her?"

Michael did not move.

Jamie stood up. "Michael?"

Slowly, Michael looked up at his cousin, and for the first time there was a flicker of uncertainty in his eyes.

"Michael?" Jamie's voice was disbelieving. "Is Carrie right?"

"How should I know?" Michael said quietly.

With a roar Jamie was on him, dragging him out of his chair, and he realized that though he'd experienced rage, he had never in his whole life known what it felt like to want to kill another human being, but he felt it now, he wanted to kill Michael—he wanted nothing more. His right fist smashed into his stomach, his left into his face, and he heard Michael groaning with pain, but pain just wasn't *enough*, so Jamie, maddened, out of control, went for his throat, fastened both his hands around his neck and started to squeeze—

"Jamie, *stop* it!" Annie was trying to pull him off, but he wasn't listening, wasn't coherent, wasn't really Jamie. "Somebody stop him before he *kills* him!"

"Peter!" Daisy shrieked, still holding on to her champagne for dear life. "Peter, do something, for God's sake!"

"I should let him carry on, if I were you," Carrie said calmly.

"Jamie, *no!*" Annie tried to get between the two men. "Jamie, think of Olivia—what about *Olivia?*"

He stopped instantly, just stopped dead and let go and Michael fell back onto the floor, gasping for air, slumped against the bookshelves behind him. No one helped him. No one went near him. Annie put her arms around Jamie, held him, felt him shaking violently.

Peter stood up.

"What can you do, Michael?" His voice was very hard. "What are you going to do to stop this?"

"Nothing," Michael said hoarsely, and for the first time since Louise had left the room, he looked really afraid. "How can I do anything to stop something I know nothing about?"

"Of course you know something," Peter said.

"Even if I did," Michael said, "I probably couldn't do anything."

"Why not?" Peter asked. "Why *not*?"

"Because if any of this were true," Michael answered, picking his words carefully, "I imagine that a man would have been paid to do a job. In which case, there might be no way of contacting him."

Jamie pulled away from Annie. "What do you mean, no way?" The worst of the physical rage was spent now, but the hate was still there simmering in his dark eyes. "There must be a way."

Michael still sat on the floor with his back to the bookshelves. His black tie hung loose, the top two buttons of his shirt were undone, and there was blood on his lower lip and around his left nostril.

He shook his head slowly, looking straight up at his cousin.

"I doubt it," he said.

The crisp, hard quality of Carrie's voice was almost a welcome breath of sanity in the wild atmosphere in the room.

"I must say, Annie," she said, "that if you don't need a Valium or three after this little show, then I really do have to hand it to you."

Annie made a small sound, half laughter, half despair.

And Jamie turned back to the desk and picked up the telephone.

It was a little after seven o'clock in Brussels. Four or five feet above Olivia's head, above the roof of the safe, above the cellar, the man in the black leather jacket had completed his work awhile back. He had closed but not locked the cellar door (since it was intended that the woman's death should be regarded as accidental), pocketing the key, and then he had flipped the lever at the main fuse box back to ON. He had reconnected the telephone, had fixed the pane of glass he'd smashed to gain entry, and he had made her bed and generally tidied up the place to look normal. And all the while, Cleo, still in pain from where he had kicked her, crouched in a corner of the entrance hall, behind the coat stand, and quivered with fear and loathing until he had gone.

The safe, Olivia had long since figured out, was made the way refrigerators had been in the past, had the kind of door that, even unlocked, was impossible to open from the inside once closed. Inside it was pitch black. The air was still cool enough but musty, and although the fingertips of her right hand had located two tiny holes on the back wall—too tiny and dust-caked to allow any significant air through—Olivia had long since concluded that if no one came in time she would die of suffocation. There was, she thought, some mathematical formula for calculating how long a person could survive on a limited supply of oxygen, but she didn't know what the formula was, which was probably just as well. She knew there was no point in screaming for help because there was no one to hear, and screaming would, almost certainly, use up more oxygen than just sitting still and waiting. But Olivia had never been much good at sitting and waiting for anything in life. Olivia liked—she *needed*—to get out and do things for herself, to make things happen.

The way she had gone to London and opened the box. And made this happen.

She wondered how Annie was doing, wondered if Jamie had by now learned the truth about Michael and Juan Luis. She thought that they had, in all probability, been trying to reach her, and she thought it was not unduly optimistic to believe that they would, in time, become concerned about her and send someone to check on her. And she tried, very hard, not to dwell on the likelihood that even if someone did come, and even if they came into the apartment, they were not terribly likely to think of opening an old, never used door to a cellar that did not even belong to her property.

Olivia sat down in the black, cold, claustrophobic safe and allowed a huge all-enveloping wave of panic to engulf her. And then, several minutes later, after the last of it had ebbed away, she tried valiantly to persuade herself that the worst of the fear was over now, that she could go on now, could survive without losing her mind; because the idea of that—of growing so demented with terror that she got hysterical and went crazy—seemed almost worse than dying. But if she was honest with herself—and stupid, *stupid* Olivia Segal was always so fucking honest with herself and everyone else, wasn't she?—she knew that the fear was anything *but* over.

And she had no way of knowing how much time she had left.

★   ★   ★

An inspector with the Police de Bruxelles told Jamie that they had been patrolling rue Charles Hanssens all through the night, and no problems had been reported.

"I can send a car to check the place again," the inspector said. "If there is any indication of a problem—"

"But there may not *be* any indication," Jamie yelled, trying but failing to keep his temper for Olivia's sake. "For Christ's sake, I've told you that someone is trying to kill her—I've told you that there's every likelihood that they may try again—for all we know they already have!"

There was a soft knocking at the door as he slammed the phone down, and Daisy got up to open it. Louise came in looking pale and drawn.

"The party's finally over," she said. "There's no one left. It's not easy throwing people out and staying tactful." She paused. "They all seemed to have a good time."

"So no one missed the birthday boy," Carrie commented. "I told you, Louise, it's a tribute to the way you organize your parties."

Louise looked over at Michael, saw the smear of blood still on his face and on his shirt, but did not remark on it.

"Any more developments here?" she asked no one in particular.

"What's happening here"—Peter got to his feet again, walked over to where Michael was now sitting in a chair, and kicked him hard on the sole of his left Bennis and Edwards shoe—"is that this skunk is going to wake up our fucking company pilot and tell him to get his ass over to Newport State Airport and get our plane ready to fly these people to Boston in time for the first damned connection to Brussels."

"Why?" Louise asked.

"Because your husband says that if there is a hit man after Olivia, there's probably no way of stopping him."

"Then of course they must go." Louise was exhausted but superficially calm now and in command. "But Peter, why not raise the pilot yourself?" She looked down at Michael briefly, with something approaching disdain. "After all," she added, "you are in charge now, surely."

★   ★   ★

Olivia had lost all track of time. She had, for a while, sat in a kind of cramped half-lotus position trying to do some basic yoga relaxation in an attempt to stave off the terror, but then it had struck her that she was breathing too deeply, was probably using up too much precious air, and she was neither skilled enough nor calm enough to drill herself into taking shallow breaths. And the thought that she had been wasting oxygen had pushed her into new panic, had sent her adrenaline pumping crazily. She had given in to that for a few minutes, had let herself pound on the steel walls and roof of her prison, had wept and railed and yelled for someone to help her, for anyone to come. And then she had settled down again, numbed and dulled by the exertion and the pointlessness of it all, and for quite a good long time she stayed that way, and it was easier, far easier. And maybe it might be better to do what the man had told her to. Just go to sleep, give in, and go easy.

She slept then—maybe for minutes, maybe hours—but she woke up with the sudden realization that she had been missing something, had been sitting there just waiting to be rescued or to die when she could, instead, have been doing something to help herself.

The candlesticks. She fumbled around, found one of them, and clambered awkwardly to her feet.

The two tiny holes on the back wall. She'd had a tool all along and she hadn't thought to use it. *For crying out loud, Olivia, what's wrong with you?*

She felt over the candlestick searching for sharp edges, but it had an ornate foliage decoration, and it was all too rounded, too smooth, and the only remotely useful part was at the candleholder end. *So use that then, damn you, woman.*

There was no contest. The silver was too soft, the steel wall too rigid and thick, and Olivia found that she was weeping again as she fought and failed to enlarge those two little holes, and of course it was useless, because it was a *safe*, for fuck's sake, a reinforced box built to withstand the custom-made tools of professional thieves, and all she was doing was wasting more air, and all that would happen was that she would die sooner.

★   ★   ★

The Brussels police reported that since the officers who'd rung Olivia's doorbell just after eight A.M. had received no reply, they were assuming that Olivia had taken their earlier advice and left the apartment, perhaps for a hotel.

"Bernard Martens," Annie said shortly before she and Jamie were due to take off from Newport State Airport in the Arias jet. "Bernard will want to help."

They located him at his home, and Annie was right; they didn't need to tell him too much, little more than that they believed Olivia might be in danger, because although Bernard had kept communications with her to a minimum since his return from the Far East, he still cared for Olivia and always would.

"I'll go straight away," he had told Jamie.

"Tell the police," Jamie had said. "Maybe you can persuade them to help you break in."

"That won't be necessary," Bernard said. "I still have her key on my ring, so I can let myself in, if need be."

"That's great, Bernard." The relief was immense. "Thank you."

"Don't thank me." Bernard was already reaching for his jacket. "Call me when you reach Boston, if you can—I'll hope to have good news."

"She's not there," he told them when they called from Logan at five-thirty local time. "I've been inside, and I've looked everywhere, and the police are perfectly right—there's no sign of any problem. As a matter of fact," Bernard added, "I have never seen the apartment looking so immaculate."

"Maybe the police are right," Annie said to Jamie after he'd hung up. "Maybe she has gone to a hotel."

"Maybe," Jamie said.

It was not until they were airborne en route to Paris that he sat up with a violent jolt of fresh alarm.

"Annie."

Annie, who had been dozing fitfully, opened her eyes. "What?"

"Can you remember ever—I mean *ever*—seeing any home of Olivia's looking immaculate? That's the word Bernard used."

Annie sat up straighter. "No. You're right. Livvy likes chaos—or at least controlled chaos."

"And even if she did feel like tidying up to take her mind off things—"

"She couldn't have done that much because of her arm," Annie finished for him.

"Which means"—Jamie swallowed hard, feeling sick at the thought—"that if the place really is as immaculate as Martens said it was—"

"Then someone else must have cleaned it up."

It was hardly a conclusion they could ask the Air France pilot to radio through to the Brussels police.

Olivia, dozing uncomfortably on the floor of the safe, thought she had heard a noise, faintly, from somewhere above her head. She had sat up quickly, feeling dizzy, had listened hard, then heard it again.

Footsteps, maybe?

She had climbed to her feet and shouted for help, but she was so weak now, and, though her voice had echoed inside the safe, there was no real power left in it. Yet she had gone on calling, over and over again, pausing to listen some more, hearing nothing and trying again. She had gone on calling through the tiny, inadequate holes, and then she had remembered the candlesticks, had picked one up and banged it on the steel roof, but the sound had almost deafened her, had made her cringe with the reverberations, and the movements had sent new pain shooting through her broken arm. Yet still she had gone on screaming, using up her ebbing reserves of strength and oxygen.

But Bernard Martens, checking meticulously over every inch of the apartment, had heard nothing at all, and he had not given a thought to the cellar, because he, like Olivia, knew that it had never been used, knew that the door had always been locked and that there had not even been a key.

And it was not until after he was long gone that Cleo, still too shocked to risk confronting any man, emerged from her hiding place behind the coat stand in the hall and padded slowly and cautiously, her tail swishing from side to side, to the cellar door.

Where she lay down, curled neatly in the most comfortable, comforting position she could find, to wait for her mistress to come upstairs again.

While down below, in the dark, Olivia slept, waiting to die.

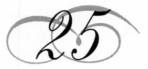

It was almost eight in the evening when their connecting flight from Paris finally touched down at Zaventem Airport. Jamie and Annie had long since stopped talking about what might have happened to Olivia. Their imaginations, already so horribly inflamed by all they had learned over the past twenty-four hours, were running too painfully wild and they were both, by now, superstitiously afraid that voicing their worst fears might somehow make them more real than bottling them up.

"Shouldn't we call the police again?" Annie asked at passport control, breathless from running, as Jamie seethed beside her in the queue. "Or what about Bernard Martens?"

"No more delays," Jamie said through gritted teeth. "Let's just *go*."

With no luggage to claim and no holdups by customs officials, they ran for the exit. Annie had never seen Jamie like this before, pushing luggage trolleys out of his way, almost sending strangers flying, cutting through the line of passengers waiting for taxis, and giving the driver of the first car in the line a wad of dollar bills to get them to Olivia's street fast, whatever the traffic. And the wildness in his eyes and the increasingly desperate set of his jaw sent shivers through Annie, because she realized it meant that Jamie had a powerful sense that time was running out, and that terrified her almost more than anything else.

It was almost dark when they got to rue Charles Hanssens.

"How will we get in?" Annie asked, standing on the cobbled

pavement outside Olivia's house as the taxi drew away and disappeared into rue des Minimes. "I knew we should have called Bernard."

"I'll smash a window." Jamie was already taking off his jacket and winding it around his right hand to protect it.

"You really think Bernard missed something, don't you?" Annie stared wide-eyed around the empty street as Jamie marched straight up to the sitting room window and punched through the glass. "You really think she's in there."

"I don't know." Jamie tried to reach the catch.

"Let me—my arm's thinner."

"It's okay," he said, his voice strained with the effort of stretching. "I've got it." It was a sash window, it pushed up easily enough, and in another moment he was inside and letting Annie in at the front door.

"Get the lights," Jamie said, and headed for the sitting room.

"Bernard was right." Annie was right behind him. "It is immaculate."

Everything was in its place, every cushion plumped, every newspaper neatly folded, not a coffee cup in sight.

"Olivia didn't do this," Jamie said. "Not in a thousand years."

Annie stopped in her tracks. "Cleo. Did Bernard say anything to you about the cat?"

"No."

Jamie was out of the room and on his way to the bedroom, but Annie found she could not bring herself to follow him there. In all her waking nightmares on the plane, the bedroom was where she had pictured Olivia. She knew it was impossible—she knew Livvy couldn't be there because Bernard had looked, and yet Annie still had gone on imagining her there, hurt and frightened or worse, much worse.

"Cleo!" she called tersely.

"No sign," Jamie said, coming back from the bedroom.

Annie breathed again, called the cat again.

"Maybe Olivia took her," Jamie said.

"So you think maybe she has gone somewhere, after all?" Annie asked hopefully.

"No." Jamie shook his head in confusion. "Yes. I wish to God I knew."

"I'll check the kitchen," Annie said.

That, too, was uncharacteristically tidy, but the little cat was in the corner, cowering under the table, black-eyed with fear.

"Cleo's in here," Annie called to Jamie.

The cat hissed at her.

"Sweetie, what's wrong?" Annie crouched down, and the tortoise-shell arched her back and hissed again, her tail erect and warning.

Jamie came in behind her.

"Be careful," Annie said softly, still crouching. "Something's upset her. She's always been such a friendly little thing."

Slowly, gently, she held out her hand. Very tentatively, Cleo sniffed at it and jumped a little, but Annie just stayed quite still and waited patiently, making soothing, comforting sounds, and after a few moments, the cat stood up and came out from under the table.

"That's a good puss," Jamie said softly.

Cleo rubbed her head against Annie's hand.

"Maybe she's just hungry," Annie said.

"She can eat when we've found Olivia," Jamie said.

The cat walked past Annie, gave Jamie a wider, more suspicious, berth, and skirted out of the kitchen into the hall, stopping beside the cellar door.

She meowed.

"Okay, sweetie," Annie said, looking down at her. "I know you're starved, but Jamie's right, you'll have to wait."

Cleo meowed again and crouched low.

"What do we do now?" Jamie asked, emerging from the kitchen.

"Call Bernard—see if he's heard anything." Annie paused. "And check in case Livvy's been back and turned on her answering machine."

Jamie headed back to the sitting room.

Cleo extended her right paw and scratched at the cellar door.

Annie looked at the door.

"There's no access to the basement, is there?" she called out to Jamie.

"No," he called back. "Olivia said the door was always locked."

Cleo stood up, hunched low, and started scraping with both paws.

"Jamie," Annie said, still quietly but with urgency. "Come out here."

He came back out into the hall and looked down at the cat. All the tension was back in him.

"Try the handle," he said.

It turned in Annie's hand. She pulled, but nothing happened.

"It's locked," she said.

Jamie licked his dry lips. "Try pushing," he said.

She pushed hard. The door opened with a groan. Cleo jumped, hissed, and ran for the kitchen. Annie's heart began to race.

"Oh, God," she said softly.

Jamie stepped past her, looking for a light switch. He found one, just inside the door, and flicked it. Nothing.

"We need a flashlight," Annie said.

"Kitchen," Jamie said.

They opened cupboards, banging the doors. Cleo raced out, back to the cover of the coat stand in the hall, just as Annie opened the last one. "Got it," she said, and tossed a flashlight at Jamie.

They ran back out into the hall and for one more instant they looked into each other's eyes, sharing their thoughts and fears, and then Jamie switched on the beam and started down the steps.

"Olivia!"

"Jamie, be careful," Annie cautioned, right behind him.

"Olivia?" he called again. He reached the bottom, turned to help Annie down, then shone the beam slowly around from left to right and then back again. It was a large cellar, with a lot of empty racks—probably once used for wine—along all its walls. There were four—no, five—wooden crates piled up in front of one of the racks, but otherwise, apart from an ancient safe to the left of center, the cellar had been cleared entirely. It was empty, and there was nowhere to look.

"There's nothing here." Annie's voice echoed Jamie's feelings: half relief, half disappointment.

Jamie walked around for a few moments, shining the flashlight up to the ceiling, then, once again, into each corner.

"Nothing," he said flatly.

"I really thought—" Annie stopped.

"I know. Me, too."

Jamie turned around. "We'd better get back upstairs, call Bernard, check a few hotels."

"Maybe Livvy's been in touch with the police."

"Let's hope."

Annie started up the steps first, then stopped.

"What?" Jamie asked.

"I thought I heard Cleo."

"Dumb cat," Jamie said. "For a moment back there, I really thought she knew something."

The sound came from behind them. Jamie, on the third step up, turned around and shone the flashlight back down into the cellar.

"There she is," Annie said, pointing. "She must have come down with us."

Cleo was beside the old safe, crouched low again, tail swishing, nose sniffing at the dusty black steel.

"Oh, God," Annie said. "You don't—" Terror closed her throat, made it impossible to speak.

Jamie said nothing, went back down slowly, walked over to the safe. He registered dimly that his heart seemed to have stopped; his thoughts were coming at him vaguely, as if they hardly belonged to him, were going on without him.

They both stared at the safe. There was no combination, just a lock and no key, and they both knew, looking at it, that there was no way on earth even a far stronger man than Jamie could get it open without help.

"Try the door, Jamie," Annie said, her voice hoarse with fear.

He did not, could not seem to move.

"Jamie, try it."

He shook his head. If Olivia was in there—

"*Try* it," Annie said again.

Jamie, ice cold with dread, put out his right hand and gripped the handle. It turned and clicked. Cleo gave one of her little startled jumps and backed off. *Hail Mary, full of grace,* his mind prayed silently, unexpectedly.

"Open it, Jamie." Annie's voice was suddenly hard.

He pulled the door open.

Olivia lay curled up on the floor, her face cushioned by her right arm and hidden from view by the fractured left arm, still in its grimy sling.

She wore a flimsy, sleeveless nightdress, and her legs and feet were bare, and she was not moving.

She did not, from where Jamie and Annie stood, seem to be breathing.

Neither of them said a word.

Jamie passed Annie the flashlight and stooped to get inside. Numbly, tenderly, he put his arms around Olivia, and she was so cold, so lifeless, and he knew, suddenly, as he lifted her out of the safe, what people meant when they talked about hearts breaking.

Annie shone the light on Olivia's face and touched the side of her neck.

"Put her down," she said tersely.

Jamie cradled Olivia closer, bent his head so that his face touched her hair. Somewhere inside him anguish was waiting to be let out, but there was too much rage ahead of it, building and building—

"Put her down, Jamie," Annie said more sharply. "Quickly."

He looked up at her, startled.

"Jamie, for God's sake, do as I say."

He laid Olivia gently down, and Annie pushed him firmly away, and Jamie had seen so many new sides to Annie in the past day and night, and she was being so strong again, so self-possessed, so *competent*, and he saw that she was feeling for Olivia's pulse.

"She's alive," Annie said, hope blazing. "We need help, Jamie. Call an ambulance." She looked up at him, saw that he was in shock, and hardened her voice still more. "Jamie, *move*. Call an ambulance and tell them suffocation and hypothermia and maybe more."

He raced up the steps.

"And bring down a blanket!" Annie called after him.

She was vaguely aware of the cat over by the wall, too nervous to approach, but Annie was no longer thinking about Cleo or Jamie or about anything except Olivia. She knew what she was doing, she only needed to *remember*, because she'd learned about first aid and CPR when Sophie and William had been little, and she just had to keep calm and remember what she was supposed to do, and then it would come back—

She saw a flutter then, saw that Olivia was definitely breathing and there was no need for CPR, and Annie gave a quick, loud, involuntary sob of relief, and then quickly, deftly she got her into the recovery position. And there was nothing more to do now than stroke Livvy's hair and speak to her softly and gently, and try to keep her warm, and wait for the ambulance to come.

It really was mostly hypothermia, they said at Saint-Jean Hospital, trying to answer Jamie's still wild-eyed questions gently and calm-ingly—and exhaustion, and, of course, shock, but the young lady seemed to be a most resilient person. And no, Jamie could not see her again just yet—he and Madame Thomas had spent enough time with her already—but it might be possible a little later, so long as he promised not to stay too long.

When they finally let him into the room again, Olivia was lying back, her eyes closed, her plastered left arm in a fresh, clean sling propped on a pillow.

Very quietly, anxious not to wake her, Jamie sat down on a chair.

"Don't sit so far away," she said, her eyes still shut. "Come sit on the bed—just mind the arm."

"I thought you were asleep." He sat down carefully at her good side.

Olivia opened her eyes. "Where's Annie?"

"She's talking to the police again."

"Have they caught the man?"

"I don't think so. Not yet. But they will."

"The doctors said there's a guard outside."

Jamie nodded. "There is. There will be until it's over."

Olivia looked into his face. "And how are you doing?"

"Better, now that I know you're okay."

"What about the rest of it?"

"Michael, you mean?"

"And your uncle." She paused. "It must have been a terrible shock."

"You could say that," Jamie said softly, his eyes very dark. "I'm so sorry, Olivia. So desperately sorry."

She was startled. "What do you have to be sorry for?"

"They're my family. Michael killed your parents and Annie's."

Olivia tried to sit up then but found she could hardly manage it.

"Jamie, stop that. You're not responsible for any of it. Your father died, too."

"Yes."

"Then stop it, do you hear me? No guilt. No collective family shame."

Jamie gave a small, bleak smile. "Easier said than done."

Olivia reached for his hand. "I love you, Jamie," she said.

"I know. I love you, too." He paused. "Bernard's here, you know."

"Is he? Poor Bernard."

"He feels terrible," Jamie said. "Because he didn't think to try the cellar door."

"No reason he should have," Olivia said. "I hope you told him."

"I think he needs to hear it from you."

Olivia nodded. "Later, maybe."

The door opened, and Annie came in, treading carefully.

"You're allowed to breathe," Olivia said warmly.

Annie embraced her, mindful of the arm, then stood back to look at her. "You look okay—I can't believe it."

"You look like hell," Olivia said, and squeezed Annie's hand. "Come to think of it," she added, looking at Jamie, "you both do."

Annie sat on a chair. "We're not supposed to stay long."

"What did the police say?" Olivia asked.

"Not much. I told them the whole story. It took a while."

"What are they doing?" Jamie was grim faced again. "Have they contacted the Rhode Island police yet?"

"Not yet," Annie said. "They say it's too early."

"Too early for what?" Olivia asked.

Annie looked uncomfortable. "I think we should leave this till morning. You have to sleep, Livvy, and we could both use some rest, too."

"What's going on, Annie?" Olivia asked.

"You may as well tell us," Jamie said. "You know she's not going to rest till you do."

Annie waited another moment. "They say they don't have enough proof to take action against Michael."

"Not enough *proof*?" Fresh anger and disbelief revived Jamie. "How much more do they need?"

"All the papers we have accuse Juan Luis of war crimes, but there isn't any solid evidence of what Michael's done." Annie paused. "Not until they get the man in the leather jacket."

"But Michael as good as admitted that he'd set it up," Jamie said.

"As good as may not be enough." Annie paused. "Especially if the rest of the family decide not to back us up."

"There wasn't any doubt in that room, Annie," Jamie said tautly. "We all knew. Even Louise believed it."

"I know," Annie said softly. "But Michael didn't actually confess."

"And even if he had"—Olivia spoke up—"the others might decide to rally round Michael."

Neither Annie nor Jamie spoke.

"They all have a lot to lose, Jamie," Olivia said, feeling his anguish.

"Look," Annie said. "Let's not get too upset too soon. The police haven't said they don't believe us—just that they can't ask the Rhode Island police to arrest Michael without something positive to go on." She paused. "The helicopter crashed nineteen years ago. The investigation decided it was mechanical failure."

"We'll get the case reopened," Olivia said.

"It won't be easy," Annie pointed out.

"None of this has been easy," Olivia said.

"It might get easier," Jamie said, "if they catch the man."

"Or if Michael confesses," Olivia said.

THE PACT

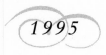

1995

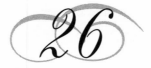

*O*ne week passed. Olivia was released from the hospital and went home to rue Charles Hanssens with Jamie, while Annie agreed to fly back to England, where Edward, shocked almost beyond words, wanted her safe and sound with him and the children.

A second week went by. The man in the black leather jacket had not been caught by the Brussels police, and with no other force involved, either in Europe or in the United States, no one thought there was a realistic likelihood of his capture unless he tried again—which Olivia, Jamie, and Annie were now all pretty much agreed he would not. The hit, they reasoned, must by now have been called off, and with so many more people now in possession of the facts—not to mention the file on Juan Luis Arias—there was simply no more purpose to be served by killing Olivia.

Jamie, still in Brussels, made numerous calls to Peter and Louise, but whether he called them in Newport, Boston, or New York, and whether he called Arias Shipping or their respective homes, neither was ever available to speak to him. The same applied to Daisy, and though Carrie was quick to return his call when Jamie tried her, she was equally swift to point out that her version of what they all knew had gone on in the library that night would mean fuck-all if the others had all decided to lie their heads off.

"They've closed ranks," Olivia told Annie on the phone on August 10, with Jamie on the bedroom extension. "I knew they would."

"I don't see how they can." Annie was appalled all over again.

"Simple," Olivia said. "Michael will have told them how he did it all for the whole family. For their future, for their children. For the Arias name. He'll have reminded them how much they enjoy their wealth—how much they'd hate losing their standing in the community—how awful it would be for them all if he went to prison."

"What about Peter?" Jamie said bitterly. "Michael killed *our* father, for God's sake."

"Peter has his children to consider," Annie said quietly.

"And Peter has no backbone," Olivia pointed out. "That's no surprise."

"I can't bear it," Jamie said. "It's intolerable."

"I know," Olivia said.

It was not the only thing that both Olivia and Jamie found intolerable. Left alone together, with so much residual tension still humming inside them and with the rawness of their trauma-heightened emotions still vivid in their minds, both Olivia and Jamie had become abruptly, almost unbearably, aware of the other, silent agitation between them: the sexual energy that had been quieted but never wholly laid to rest. Love was not the issue now. There had never been any doubting the intensity of their feelings for each other. They loved each other, as they loved Annie, more, they supposed, than they had ever been able to love any outsider. Love, pure and simple, had never been the problem. But the memories of that one night in Boston had never ceased to simmer in the back of both their minds, and somehow, the hell they had been through in the past two weeks had turned the heat back on high.

Olivia's body was still sore and her arm in its cast, and Jamie was still drained and shocked, still yearning for disbelief. And yet suddenly—after having coped more than adequately with spending platonic, affectionate but sexless time together for over six years—neither she nor Jamie seemed capable of being in the same room as each other for more than a few minutes without feeling weak with lust.

It blew up, finally, at breakfast one morning.

"I think I might go back to bed," Olivia said as Jamie filled the electric kettle with water and switched it on.

"Why?" Jamie looked at her sharply.

She shrugged. "I just feel like it."

"Is the arm hurting?"

"Not much." She smiled at him. "I'm fine, Jamie. I just feel like indulging myself."

He nodded. "Good idea. You head on back, and I'll bring you a tray."

"I can manage." She wandered over to the cupboard where her two big pine trays were kept.

"No, you can't," Jamie said.

"Sure I can."

"How are you going to carry a tray?"

"Easy." She took out the tray and put it on the table. "I take one thing at a time—first the tray, then the coffee, then the toast."

"I'll bring it all to you. Go back to bed, Olivia."

She looked at him. He was wearing gray shorts and a gray Calvin Klein T-shirt and his forearms and face were a little more tanned than his legs, and his feet were bare—such nice, neat, strong feet—and his dark hair was rumpled. Olivia felt desire kick her again, more violently even than it had the previous evening and afternoon and morning, and she knew that she'd never longed for any man as she longed for Jamie now, at this instant—that even the hunger she remembered during that long-ago afternoon and evening with him had been a weak and trifling hunger compared to this.

"For God's sake," she said suddenly, fiercely.

"What?" He looked startled.

"What's *wrong* with us?"

Jamie granted himself permission to look at her. She was wearing a man-size white shirt with one sleeve hanging useless, and her hair was still wet from the shower, and the beauty of her high cheekbones and slender neck was even more pronounced than usual because she'd lost weight since the hit-and-run, and there was an area just over her left collarbone that seemed to be crying out to be kissed.

"What's stopping us now, Jamie?" Olivia's voice was husky with yearning. "Carrie's a hundred years ago—*everything* that stopped us is a hundred years ago—"

"I know."

She walked over to him. And without the slightest hesitation, looking straight into his eyes, she laid her right hand on his erection. He thought he would explode, but not even a groan left his lips. She took her hand away.

"Why are we still fighting this, Jamie?" Her green, slanting eyes blinked. "I can hardly breathe for wanting you, and you have a big enough hard-on to take on Sharon Stone, and yet you still just stand there and look at me."

"I don't want Sharon Stone," Jamie said.

"But you do want me."

"I've never stopped wanting you."

Her eyes softened, seemed to melt. "Then for God's sake, kiss me."

The kettle boiled and turned itself off.

"No," Jamie said softly.

"Why not?" Olivia stared at him. "Why the fuck *not*, Jamie?"

For one long moment, Jamie closed his eyes. And then he opened them again, turned away, and switched the kettle back on.

"Go back to bed, Olivia."

"No, I won't go back to bed." Her cheeks were hot, as if she had a fever. "Not until I know what is *wrong* with you." Her voice was tight, strangling in her throat. "You just said you've never stopped wanting me, and you know how much I want you—and we both know we love each other just about every way there *is* to love someone."

"If you won't go to bed," Jamie said, still softly, "then at least sit down at the table, and I'll pour us both a cup of coffee and I'll tell you what's wrong."

"Okay." She nodded her head, fighting a sudden urge to cry.

"Sit."

Olivia felt a warm, furry body against her legs. She swallowed hard. "Cleo needs breakfast."

"I'll feed Cleo."

"Thank you."

"You're welcome."

Olivia drew back one of the chairs and sat down. "Shit, Jamie."

Jamie smiled wryly. "I agree." He spooned cat food into Cleo's bowl in the corner, poured fresh water into her second bowl, then got their coffee and sat down opposite Olivia.

"I'm not going to kiss you," he tried to explain, "because I couldn't stop. I wouldn't want to stop."

"I wouldn't want you to."

His dark eyes were filled with pain. "I can't take another one-night stand with you, Olivia."

"It's morning," she said.

"I mean it."

"I know," she said unsmilingly. "I couldn't take it either. I think it would just about kill me." She paused. "I don't understand how you can even think that could happen, Jamie. When we both love each other, when we both know that and accept it."

"Unfinished business," Jamie said.

"What kind?" Olivia took her first sip of coffee.

"You know what kind."

She put down her cup. "So are you going to let Michael destroy us, too?" The tightness that had been in her throat was in her chest now. "Hasn't he done enough to us already?"

"It isn't just Michael," Jamie said. "It's me. And you, too."

"I don't have a problem."

"You're post-traumatic."

"No, I'm not."

"Sure you are."

"Even if I am," Olivia said, "I know how I feel about you. In every way."

"Maybe you do, maybe you don't," Jamie said. "Either way, what harm can it do to wait a little longer?"

She drank some more coffee. "Is that what you're proposing? That we wait?"

"Yes."

"How long?"

"I'm not sure."

Cleo jumped up onto Olivia's lap and began to knead her claws against her bare thighs.

"Doesn't that hurt?" Jamie asked.

"Yes."

"Want me to take her?"

"No, thank you. It takes my mind off wanting you."

Jamie reached over and picked Cleo up. Unfazed, the cat continued where she'd left off, content enough with his soft gray shorts.

"I guess I'm post-traumatic, too," he said, "in a way."

"You're still feeling guilty for being an Arias," Olivia said flatly. They'd had a few conversations in the past week about Jamie's guilt and shame, and she had tried repeatedly to put him straight, but she knew she had not succeeded.

"There's still so much to be resolved," Jamie said. "I know you feel it, too."

"Of course I feel it." She shook her head slowly. "I just don't connect any of that with our feelings for each other."

"I'm not denying our feelings," Jamie said. "I know what we have. I think I always did, deep down—"

"Not so deep," Olivia said.

"No," he admitted.

"But now, surely, it's out in the open—at least between us—"

Jamie laid his right hand on the table, as if he were reaching for her, then changed his mind and took it away again.

"I want it to be perfect, Olivia."

"It will be."

He shook his head. "Not yet." He grimaced as Cleo dug her claws into his left leg. "I want to be able to come to you when I can face myself in the mirror in the mornings without remembering what my family has done."

"Michael is your cousin, not your brother. You barely remember Juan Luis—and your father didn't do anything, except try to help."

"That doesn't help me now," Jamie said.

She looked at him accusingly. "This is crap, Jamie."

"Maybe."

The tears came back, stinging, hot behind her eyes, but the thought of crying now, in front of him, made her angry. "I mean, this is *really* crap. We should be getting each other through this, not turning each other away."

"We are getting each other through it," Jamie said.

"I'd get through it better with your arms around me."

"I wouldn't."

"Then you'd better go home," Olivia said abruptly.

Jamie flinched. "I don't want to leave you."

"Are you going to change your mind?"

"No. I can't."

"Then I mean it." Olivia stood up, and Cleo, her good mood disturbed, jumped off Jamie's lap. "You'd better go back to Boston, because I don't think I can stand having you around."

"That isn't what I want," Jamie said softly.

"Right now," Olivia answered, "I don't think I care what you want."

Her mood was gentler by the time he left the next day, August 14, though right until the last moment before check-in Jamie pleaded to stay to take care of her, and she remained adamant that she would not be alone with him until he was ready to act on his feelings for her.

"I love you," he said, for the dozenth time that day, before he went through to passport control.

"I know you do," Olivia said. "Our love isn't in question."

"Maybe now I'm going back, I'll be able to get through to Michael or the others."

"I doubt you'll even get close."

"They'll have to talk to me sooner or later," Jamie said.

"Maybe."

Olivia knew that she had not the slightest intention of accepting the Ariases' new and outrageous status quo, but when Jamie, who was still hoping against hope that decency would ultimately prevail, called from Boston to ask for more time, she saw no good reason not to agree.

"After all," Olivia said to Annie later on the phone, "what's another four weeks after nineteen years?"

"Does Jamie really believe Michael may still confess?" Annie asked.

"No, not really. I think his hopes are hingeing on Peter developing some kind of a conscience. Or maybe Louise."

"What do you think, Livvy?"

"I think there's not a hope in hell. Not unless they're pushed."

"I think you're right," Annie agreed. "But you're still willing to wait?"

"I think it's as good an idea as any other," Olivia said. "Let them think we've given up."

"Lull them into a false sense of security, you mean," Annie said.

"It can't hurt," Olivia said.

"And then what?"

"Then we'll see."

Annie's antennae went up. "Whatever we do decide, ultimately," she said firmly, "promise me we'll act together."

"Of course," Olivia said.

"Promise me, Livvy," Annie persisted. "No more solo stunts."

"Definitely not."

"Promise me."

Olivia smiled into the phone.

"I promise," she said.

The month passed, and apart from the cast being removed from Olivia's arm, nothing altered.

"We can't wait any longer," Olivia told Jamie on the telephone.

"I know," he said.

"Annie wants us to come to her place to talk over our plans."

"Do we have any plans?" Jamie asked.

"I have a kind of plan," Olivia said.

"I thought you might," Jamie said.

"Is that all right with you?" Olivia asked.

"Is what all right with me?"

"Putting your life on hold again."

"It's what you're doing, isn't it?"

"It's different for me," Olivia said. "You have JAA to consider—all I have to do is find a stand-in, which isn't too hard in Brussels—and Bernard's already agreed to take Cleo for as long as it takes."

"You're talking about arrangements, not life," Jamie said. "All our lives are on hold, as you put it, until this is over: yours, mine, and Annie's."

"See you in Stone Bridge, then," Olivia said.

"When?"

"I can leave tomorrow."

"I'll need two days," Jamie said.

They were both acutely, painfully aware that the other subject closest to their hearts had not even been mentioned.

They started out with a gentle, English country weekend with Edward and the children. The hot summer was holding, and much of Stone Bridge life seemed to be happening outdoors, with Banbury Farm House being used more for cooling-off purposes than anything else. They picnicked and barbecued and swam and cycled and went horse riding, and Annie gave everyone reflexology sessions—though in Olivia's case it was impossible because Olivia was ticklish and shrieked with laughter every time Annie touched her feet—and the slaughter of the Rothenburgs, the murder of their parents, and the attempts on Olivia's own life seemed, just for those few happy days, a million years away.

And then, on the evening of Sunday, September 17, Edward returned to London. And it was time to talk.

"I have a kind of plan," Olivia said. "It's not much, but it's better than trying—and probably failing—to get the crash investigation reopened—"

"And even if we do get them to look at it all again," Annie said, "it'll take forever."

"So what is this plan?" Jamie asked.

They were sitting around the table in Annie's kitchen, and it reminded Olivia and Annie of another time, back in the winter of early 1990, when they had sat, without Jamie, plotting their revenge against Carrie. Then, Olivia remembered, Leo and Boots, the two cats, had slept beside the stove for heat, and Bella, the retriever, too, had snoozed in the toasty warmth, but this September evening, the kitchen seemed the coolest, least heatwave-draining place to be.

"First," Olivia began, "we need to be sure that we all want the same end result."

"Which is?" Jamie asked.

She looked at him very directly. "I want to see Michael pay for what he's done. I don't care how, exactly—I'm not baying for blood, and the thought of a trial makes me sick to my stomach—"

"Me, too," Annie said softly.

"But I just can't bear the thought of him getting off scot-free," Olivia went on. "I mean, he's gone unpunished for nineteen years, for Christ's sake, but at least none of us knew the truth." She paused. "But we know now."

No one spoke.

"Okay." Olivia gave a small smile. "Here's my plan, for what it's worth, which may not be a damn." She paused. "I want us to sit on them—all of them, except Michael. I want us to be wherever they are, all the time. I want us to fly to Boston and hire investigators to do the legwork, so that we can just move in at all the right moments. I want them to see us wherever they go. I want to bug them, to haunt them, to goad them. I want us to drive them nuts." Her face was very serious now. "I want them to know that we haven't gone away. That we're never going to go away. That they can't just bury what you told them on Michael's birthday and forget it ever happened."

"Why not Michael?" Jamie asked. "You said all of them except Michael."

"Because sitting on Michael would be a waste of time and effort," Olivia answered. "Because Michael has no conscience—he might even have enough nerve to sic a lawyer, or even the police, on us. But Louise and Peter and Daisy are different—you both told me how shocked they were that night in the library."

"They managed to forget quickly enough," Jamie said, bitter again.

"They haven't forgotten," Annie said. "They're just weak and unprincipled and afraid—"

"And greedy," Jamie added.

"And probably very confused," Olivia said, surprisingly gently. "I've had a lot of time to think about it from their side, Jamie, and I think I can almost understand the temptation to try to forget it."

"I can't," Jamie said.

"I said *almost*—and of course you can't understand," Olivia said. "You're so different from them—you're as different from Peter as Carlos was from Juan Luis. Peter is unprincipled, and he's a bastard, but I think he's more of a fool than actively wicked. There may just be hope for Peter."

Annie was warming to the plan. "Thinking back to that night, and the way she reacted, I don't think it would take too much to sway Louise."

"Or Daisy," Jamie added. "Daisy's fundamentally decent."

"Provoke them all enough, make them all uneasy enough—*panic* them enough," Olivia said, "and who knows, they may just turn on Michael."

Less than six days later, on Saturday, September 23, when Peter emerged from Angie Rogos's apartment on Park Avenue where he'd spent the night, Olivia, waiting outside on the sidewalk, looked right through him. And when, two and a half hours later, Daisy Arias stepped blithely out of B. Loren where she'd just had her nails wrapped, Annie was standing out on Newbury Street doing the same thing. And when, an hour or so after that, Louise came away from her homeless charity luncheon at the Ritz-Carlton, she saw Jamie leaning against a lamppost directly opposite where her chauffeur was waiting with her gray Bentley.

Each of them looked disturbed.

"It's Peter's birthday on Monday," Jamie told Olivia at the end of the first day, "and Carrie says she knows they're all going to be in New York having dinner at Le Bernardin."

"You told Carrie about our plan?" Olivia was startled.

"She called me about some Beaumont-Arias business," Jamie explained, "and I made a snap decision. She's on our side in this, Olivia—I think she proved that back in Newport—and she thinks it would really freak them all out if the three of us got a table close by."

"She's right," Olivia admitted.

"But don't you have to book weeks in advance to get reservations at Le Bernardin?" Annie said.

"I'll get us a table," Olivia said, "even if I have to buy the place."

They all agreed, late on Monday night in the suite they were sharing at the Plaza, that the collective discomfort of the Ariases had indeed been wondrous to behold. Which was not, they decided, all that surprising when they considered that during the course of that same day—many hours before Annie, Olivia, and Jamie had been shown to the next table at Le Bernardin—Louise had been startled and openly upset to see Olivia at La Guardia getting off the same Boston–New York shuttle she'd just flown in on; Peter had looked jolted when he'd spied Annie buying the *Times* in the lobby of the Arias Shipping building on Third Avenue; and Daisy, pink-faced with embarrassment and unease, had spotted Jamie watching her paying for three brassieres and matching panties in Bloomingdale's lingerie department.

"It's working," Olivia said. "I really think it's working."

"What's really getting to them all," Jamie said, "is that we haven't made a single attempt to speak to any of them."

"Did you see Michael's face when we sat down tonight?" Annie said with satisfaction.

"Talk about *wrath*," Olivia said.

"I thought he looked a little sick," Jamie disagreed.

"I was talking about Louise," Olivia said, with pleasure. "Daisy's just mortified by the whole thing and Peter's obviously feeling like hell. But I still think it's Louise who holds the most power when it comes to Michael—and Louise is most definitely getting mad."

"With us or with Michael?" Annie asked.

"With us, obviously, but she has to be starting to ask herself if staying with Michael is quite the decision she thought it was."

"How did you think Michael looked?" Jamie asked Olivia.

"I don't know." The pleasure went out of her eyes. "I don't think I can judge anything too well when it comes to Michael. He's too sly—he has too many faces."

It seemed to go on and on, the three of them darting back and forth between Boston, Newport, and Manhattan, constantly alerted to their subjects' whereabouts by the electronic pagers issued by the investigation agency.

"How much longer?" Annie, losing confidence, asked Olivia over breakfast on the terrace at the Stanhope on Friday morning. "How much longer before we give this up and take the long-haul approach?"

"Not much longer," Olivia said, refilling her coffee cup and starting on her scrambled eggs.

"You still think there's hope?" Jamie, too, was growing pessimistic and increasingly depressed about his family. "Nothing's happening."

"We don't know that for sure," Olivia said. "A lot may be happening behind closed doors." She looked at them. "Am I the only one eating here?"

"I'm not really hungry." Annie pushed her plate to one side.

"They may be fighting," Jamie said. "Louise and Peter probably are giving Michael a hard time, and Daisy's probably on the phone every day wanting to know what they're going to do. But I'll bet you Michael's probably telling them right back that all they have to do is hold on and we'll go away."

"Which we will," Annie said, "sooner or later."

"I won't," Olivia said quietly.

"You'll have to, ultimately," Jamie said.

"No," Olivia said. "I won't give up."

"What do you mean?" Annie asked.

"What I say." Olivia bit off a piece of bagel and cream cheese. "Don't look like that, Annie—I'm not going to do anything crazy— I'm not going to buy a gun or buy my own hit man, tempting as the thought is—"

"Not just to you," Jamie said.

"I don't see the joke," Annie said. "And what do you mean when you say you won't give up or go away?"

"I don't know," Olivia answered frankly.

"You don't have some other plan, then?"

Olivia smiled. "No, Annie, I don't. Just this one."

"But don't you think we may have to change our tactics soon?" Jamie asked. "If we don't achieve anything this way." He paused. "I mean, maybe it's time to stop trying to psych them out from a distance—maybe we need to start attacking close up."

"Maybe," Olivia said. "Except that once we actively harass them, we'll be giving Michael grounds to take out an injunction against us."

Annie sighed. "So we keep on as we are."

"I guess," Jamie said, "for the time being."

"So we're all agreed?" Olivia asked.

"I guess," Jamie said again.

Olivia glanced at him again, surreptitiously, anxiously. "Are you okay?" she asked him quietly.

"Just about." Jamie looked into her eyes, then swiftly looked away again. "How about you?"

"Hanging in," Olivia said.

Annie looked from one to the other and longed, abruptly, to kick them both. But she said nothing at all.

That Saturday night, while Annie stayed at the Plaza so that she could dog Peter's movements over the weekend and while Jamie stayed home so he could go on giving Daisy the jitters, Olivia chose to overnight at the Inn at Castle Hill in Newport. Ostensibly, she was there to spend a restful morning and early afternoon and still be on hand for when Louise and Michael left the house to return to New York as they often did on Sunday evening. But her real intention—which she had shared neither with Jamie nor Annie—was to attend the eleven o'clock Sunday morning mass at Saint Mary's Roman Catholic Church, because she remembered Daisy telling her—an hour or so before she'd fallen off Cliff Walk all those years ago—that when Louise and Michael weekended in Rhode Island, they generally made a point of going to the midmorning mass at the old Catholic church where Jacqueline Bouvier had married John F. Kennedy.

Olivia sensed, even before she left the Inn, that if this too vague, too imprecise plan of hers was ultimately to succeed, this encounter might be the most telling, perhaps the most crucial of all. She gathered from Jamie that even more than her husband, Louise Arias was a devout Catholic, and Olivia was not particularly proud of using religion to her own ends. But on the other hand—given that she was dealing with a man who had, in all probability, been receiving absolution for all of the nineteen years since he had killed Arthur and Emily, Grace and Franklin, Carlos Arias, and the pilot of their helicopter—she found that she was not particularly ashamed either.

She watched their arrival, watched the chauffeur open the rear doors of Michael's limousine, watched Louise straighten her black skirt with one gloved hand, watched Michael place a supportive hand beneath his wife's elbow, and knew the instant when they both simultaneously saw her, observed the look of true desperation on Louise's face and the flash of hot rage on Michael's, and relished it all.

Olivia stood perfectly still, waiting, her eyes cool and remote, and she realized, as the Ariases recovered and turned their backs and walked slowly and decorously up the steps into the church, that they believed they would be safe from her once they were inside.

Oh, no, she thought, *you don't get off that easily.*

She waited five minutes more, and then, just before the service was due to begin, she took a Hermès head scarf from her shoulder bag, unfolded it, and tied it, fittingly Jackie Kennedy–style, over her dark hair, and then she, too, walked into Saint Mary's.

It was cool and peaceful and three-quarters filled. Ahead of her, men, women, and children were dipping their fingers into holy water, were making the sign of the cross and then genuflecting before taking their seats, and Olivia felt out of place, felt almost tempted to go through the motions, but she refrained, looking around instead for Michael and Louise. And they were pretty much where she had expected them to be—almost at the front, in the second pew over to the right of the altar—and pretty much as she had pictured them, on their knees beneath one of the stained-glass windows, the picture of piety.

Olivia looked for a seat—the right seat—and it was there, and it was even more perfect than she'd hoped for, right behind Michael in the third pew. Slowly, smoothly, she made her way down the center aisle and slid into the seat just as both Ariases rose from their knees.

"Good morning," she said.

They turned. Louise's face was white, her lips tightly compressed. Michael's was unreadable, except for the hate in his dark, almost black eyes.

I wish you dead, those eyes said.

Olivia smiled.

"What time's confession?" she asked.

Louise looked as if she had been slapped.

The mass began.

Olivia went out ahead of them when it was over, and her stomach was churning a little, but she felt, on the whole, quite calm. She waited on Memorial Boulevard, close, but not too close, to where the limousine was waiting, several cars away from the church; watched them emerge, exchanging swift, tight-lipped greetings and smiles with acquaintances and friends, watched them walk toward her slowly, arms linked—not, Olivia felt, for closeness—more, she thought, because Louise required the support.

"Have you no shame?" Michael asked softly, menacingly, when they were about a foot away.

"Hello, Michael," Olivia said. "Hello, Louise. No time for confession this morning?" She almost felt the other woman's tremor but felt no compassion. "Maybe you can come back later, or doesn't it work like that?"

"I'm surprised at you," Michael said. "I was sure you'd have learned your lesson by now."

"Which lesson is that?" Olivia looked at Louise. "Does he mean having my arm broken, do you think? Or being locked in a safe to suffocate?"

"Michael, I want to go," Louise said, still holding on to his arm.

"What if Peter's children had been with us?" Michael asked Olivia.

"Michael—" Louise was whiter than ever.

"What *about* the children, Louise?" Again, Olivia ignored Michael. "What will they think when Michael's put on trial for murder? When the whole truth comes out?"

"Please," Louise said. *"Please."*

"Please what, Louise?" Olivia asked quietly. "Please leave you alone so that you can protect your murderer husband?" She looked around, saw that there were still a number of people standing around, and it was a lovely morning, and no one seemed in any rush to go home. "Shall I say it more loudly, Louise?"

"Do that," Michael said violently, "and you'll regret it."

"Will I? I don't think so."

"Get in the car, Louise." Michael removed his arm from his wife's.

"I will start saying it more loudly soon, Louise," Olivia said. "We all will. Jamie, and Annie and her family, and I—and there are just too many of us for Michael to silence now."

"Louise, get in the car," Michael said again.

Louise started moving towards the car, but Olivia moved with her. "Surely you must realize, Louise," she kept on at her, "that it can only be a matter of time before all this shit hits—"

Still sidling along the sidewalk, Louise began to cry, and Michael put out his right hand and pushed Olivia hard—

"Go on, Michael." She almost fell, recovered, kept on moving with Louise. "I dare you, I *dare* you—and you, too, Louise—I warn you, for your own sake and for your children's sake, do something about this man soon, before it's too late for you all—"

"Michael!" Louise tried to grab at his sleeve. "*Do* something!"

"Get away from my wife," Michael spat at Olivia.

"Dump him, Louise." Olivia was getting breathless now, but she wasn't through yet. She knew this was it, this was her one big chance, sensed that she had all but penetrated this poor woman's remaining defenses, that she was almost there. "Distance yourself before he destroys you all. Do it whichever way you like—I don't care, I really don't care how you do it, but stop protecting him before it's too late."

They were almost at the limo, and the chauffeur had the back curbside door open, and Olivia saw from his face that he'd heard what she'd been saying.

"See him, Louise—he's heard us, and he's wondering what's going on, and he won't be alone—"

Louise scrambled and half fell into the back of the limousine.

"Think of your reputation, Louise. Don't let him drag you down. You didn't know my father, did you? But you knew Carlos—of course you knew Carlos—he was a good Catholic, like you—"

"You go to *hell*," Michael said.

He pushed her again as he passed her to get into the car after his wife, and Olivia felt the weight of his body against her shoulder, and again she staggered a little and almost fell, and again she felt the force of his loathing, his unspoken wish for her death.

But bending down, looking into the dim car, past his livid, furious, bitter face, and seeing Louise Arias's eyes for the last time—staring, weeping, horrified eyes—Olivia felt nothing but triumph.

It was Monday evening, back at Jamie's apartment, before Carrie telephoned to give them the news.

That Louise and Michael had stayed over in Newport on Sunday night, and that Louise had woken up later than usual that morning, and that when she had realized that her husband had not yet come back from the early swim he took most mornings in an inlet near the house, she had raised the alarm.

Michael's body had been found late that afternoon. It was clear that death had been by drowning. There were, according to the Newport police, no suspicious circumstances, and when questioned about her husband's state of mind, Louise said that Michael had been in an excellent mood following a peaceful weekend—so peaceful that they had made their decision to stay at the house for one more night.

"Seems we did it," Annie said very quietly.

"I guess so," Jamie said.

"Are you okay?" she asked him.

"I don't really know," he answered.

They both looked over at Olivia. She was standing in the glass-enclosed alcove in Jamie's sitting room, staring out over Boston Harbor. She had hardly spoken since the call.

"Livvy?" Annie said. "Are you all right?"

She didn't answer.

Jamie stood up, went over to her, laid a hand on her right shoulder.

"What are you thinking?"

Olivia didn't turn around, didn't trust herself to look at him.

"That I killed a man," she said.

"No." Jamie's voice was clear and firm. "No, you didn't."

"As good as."

She had told them about Saint Mary's, had told them what she had said and done, and neither of them had blamed her for going as far as she had, for both Jamie and Annie had shared the same sense of relief because that part of this awful time was over now.

"None of us thought Michael would kill himself," Annie said from the middle of the room.

"You couldn't have known what was going to happen," Jamie said.

"Couldn't I?"

At last, Olivia turned around.

"I don't think either of you understands." Her eyes seemed darker with the intensity of her self-examination. "It isn't the knowledge that I pushed Louise to the point where she must have told Michael he had little choice. It isn't even the fact that I as good as dragged him into the ocean for that last swim—"

"Livvy, don't," Annie said, distressed.

"It's the fact"—Olivia wasn't finished yet—"that I can't pretend to feel a scrap of remorse for it. Oh, sure, I feel bad for Louise and for the family—that's easy enough to do. But the fact is—the cold, hard truth—is that I'm glad, really *glad*, that Michael Arias is dead."

"And do you think I'm not?" Jamie asked gently.

"Do you think we don't both feel that way about it?" Annie moved closer.

Olivia shook her head. "It isn't the same."

"Why not?" Annie asked.

"Because you didn't do it," Olivia said, simply. "I did."

The coroner's verdict was death by misadventure. At the funeral, one week after the inquest, Jamie, back in England with Olivia and Annie, was the only member of the Arias family who did not attend. The eulogies, Carrie reported to them afterward, were glowingly panegyric.

The man in the black leather jacket was never found.

EPILOGUE

DUKESFIELD FELL: JULY 4, 1996

27

"Do you think," *Olivia asked the others, nearly ten months later, as they* stood on the familiar, windswept, rugged hillside, "we've done the right things since then, made the right decisions?"

"Don't you?" asked Annie.

"I asked you first," Olivia said.

Annie waited a moment. "Yes," she said. "Under the circumstances, yes, I do."

"Jamie?" Olivia asked.

"You know what I think."

"I'd like to hear it again. Here, in this place."

Jamie nodded. "Then no, I don't think anything we've done has been exactly right. None of it's been fitting, or proper. Justice has not been served." He paused, felt the cool summer wind ruffle his hair. "But I think we did the best we could."

"Livvy?" Annie looked at her. "What about you?"

Olivia's green eyes were very distant, her wide mouth a hard, straight line. "I hate it all so much," she said. "I still hate it so much that it hurts me, physically, to think about it. To think that Juan Luis got away with it, and then Michael—"

"Michael didn't exactly get away with it," Annie said.

"Oh yes, he did," Olivia said. "That's exactly what he did. And I hate it. And I hate, almost more than that, that Jamie still feels responsible for what those two men did—even if you say you don't, Jamie, I see it in your eyes. And I hate it." She shook her head. "And yet—"

"And yet?" Jamie nudged her gently.

"And yet I know we did do the best we could." Olivia looked down at the ground, at the place where their parents had died. "And that it has to be enough."

They had done what they could. They had, for the sake of Peter's children, gone along with Louise's pleas for silence, and in exchange, Louise had agreed that part of Juan Luis's collection should be auctioned for the most fitting of the charities sponsored by the Arthur Segal Foundation, and the remainder donated, in Emanuel Rothenburg's name, to museums in New York, Berlin, Paris, Tel Aviv, and Zurich.

They had done what they could, yet in the months that had followed Michael Arias's death, as the three friends had come to see—if not to fully accept—that it was too late for true justice to be done, Jamie had suffered more than the others, living as he had to with the knowledge of his family's crimes. Olivia and Annie reminded him, over and over again, how much they loved him, told him that it was insane for him to feel even the remotest shred of guilt, yet still he could not seem to shed the shame. He felt, he tried to explain to them, as if he needed to give up everything he owned, to scrub away every trace of the blood money that had helped make him the man he was.

"For heaven's sake," Olivia told him impatiently on the phone one day before Thanksgiving, "you're not a goddamned monk—stop whipping yourself and get on with your life."

"That's almost exactly what Carrie told me last week," Jamie said.

"You're in touch quite a lot these days," Olivia said, jealousy rising as it always did now, had, against her better nature, ever since Carrie had redeemed herself by coming to their aid.

"We have lunch," Jamie said, "every now and again. It's easier now that her divorce from Peter's been finalized."

"Anyway," Olivia said grudgingly, "Carrie's right. You should listen to her and stop giving yourself such a hard time."

"Maybe," Jamie said, but they both knew he didn't really believe it.

★   ★   ★

"Isn't it time," Annie said when she called Olivia a few days later, "you shook him out of this?"

"How can I? We've both tried often enough."

"You know how."

"What do you mean?"

"Be honest with him," Annie said. "About your feelings for him." She paused. "Don't you think it's time you both opened up about the fact that you're in love with each other?"

Olivia was startled. "How did you know?"

"Don't be absurd, Livvy," Annie answered. "I've known for years."

Olivia thought about it for a few moments. "It won't work, you know, Annie. Even if he does still feel the way I do, Jamie doesn't think he deserves anything good to happen to him anymore."

"You'll find a way," Annie said positively.

Olivia had found it by courtesy of Paul Osterman. She had been trying, for a few months, to trace his family in Philadelphia, and early that December she learned that his wife had died some years back but that his son now lived in Florida with his own family. She wrote to Simon Osterman at the end of the month and received, in response, the warmest of letters, inviting her to bring Jamie and Annie to his home in Fort Lauderdale.

They all went together in March—Annie accompanied by Edward and their children—but Jamie, Annie, and Olivia went alone to their first meeting with Osterman, and they talked, at great length, about the burden that his father had carried to his grave, and they talked, too, about culpability and restitution and guilt. And Simon Osterman advised Jamie to focus his mind on the goodness of his father rather than on the evil of his other relatives, for it was transparently clear to him that Jamie was his father's son; and by the time they were ready to go home, Jamie had begun to feel a little easier in his mind, had begun to look toward the future.

"So what about you two?" Osterman's wife, a warm, easygoing woman, had asked Jamie and Olivia in their back garden on their last evening. "Any plans to get married?"

"Not yet," Olivia answered, and the look that Jamie threw at her was so filled with surprise and confusion and, underscoring it all, with purest love, that she had to suppress her own sudden urge to crow with delight.

And Jamie had reached for her hand.

"But soon," he had said.

They made love that night, at long last, in Jamie's room at their hotel, and it was not the way it had been all those years before in Boston, nor was it as either of them had pictured it during those hot, frustrating days and nights they'd spent denying themselves in Brussels. There was passion, and there was desire, and, ultimately, there was the most glorious staving of the hunger they had both experienced for so long, but it was less wild, less driven than they had anticipated, and there was a peacefulness about it, a sweetness and rightness that spoke volumes about what they could expect in the years to come.

They had been married less than two months later, in May, after Olivia had given up her apartment in Brussels and moved, with Cleo, into Jamie's place in Boston, and they were making plans to move JAA to New York, where Olivia knew there would never be a shortage of clients for the Segal Translation Agency.

And on the Fourth of July they all went together, as they had ten years earlier, and almost ten years before that, up to Dukesfield Fell, where the helicopter had plunged back to earth and scattered their parents' remains over the hillside, and they held each other in the chill but sweet-smelling summer wind, and remembered.

"I find myself wishing sometimes," Olivia said, "that I'd never found Carlos's note and that I'd never opened my father's box."

"But if you hadn't," Annie said, "we would never have known any of it."

"But are we better off for knowing?" Olivia asked. "Is anyone?"

"I think so," Jamie said. "I think Anton Rothenburg would think so."

"I'd like to believe that," Olivia said.

·A NOTE ON THE TYPE·

The typeface used in this book is a version of Bembo, issued by Monotype in 1929 and based on the first "old style" roman typeface, which was designed for the publication, by the great Venetian printer Aldus Manutius (1450–1515), of Pietro Bembo's *De Ætna* (1495). Among the first to use octavo format, making his books cheaper and more portable, Aldus might have grown rich printing as he did a thousand volumes per month—an extraordinary number for the time—had his books not been mercilessly pirated. The counterfeits did, however, spread the new typefaces throughout Europe, and they were widely imitated. The so-called Aldine romans were actually designed by the man who cut the type for Aldus, Francesco Griffo (d. 1519). Griffo fought with Manutius over credit for the designs and was later hanged after killing his brother-in-law with an iron bar.